ADULT ATTACHMENT

Adult
Attachment

THEORY, RESEARCH, AND CLINICAL IMPLICATIONS

Edited by
W. STEVEN RHOLES
JEFFRY A. SIMPSON

THE GUILFORD PRESS
New York   London

© 2004 The Guilford Press
A Division of Guilford Publications, Inc.
72 Spring Street, New York, NY 10012
www.guilford.com

Printed in the United States of America

This book is printed on acid-free paper.

Last digit is print number: 9 8 7 6 5 4 3 2 1

Library of Congress Cataloging-in-Publication Data

Adult attachment: theory, research, and clinical implications / edited by W.
Steven Rholes, Jeffry A. Simpson.
   p. cm.
  Includes bibliographical references and index.
  ISBN 1-59385-047-6 (hardcover)
  1. Attachment behavior. I. Rholes, W. Steven (William Steven) II. Simpson,
Jeffry A.
  BF575.A86A38 2004
  155.9′2—dc22

                               2004007721

To Ramona, for her support and inspiration
And to Eric and Ted, for making their old man happy
–W. S. R.

To my family–Cindy, Chris, and Natalie–for their love
and support over the years
–J. A. S.

About the Editors

W. Steven Rholes, PhD, is Professor and Head of the Department of Psychology at Texas A&M University. He has conducted research programs in social cognition, children's social development, and adult attachment since receiving a degree in psychology from Princeton University in 1978. In 1992, along with his colleague Jeffry Simpson, Dr. Rholes published one of the first studies to confirm predictions about avoidant attachment style, using behavioral observations as evidence. For the past decade, the impact of attachment styles on emotional support sought and provided by couples has been the central focus of his research program. Dr. Rholes has also served in two administrative positions, department chair and associate dean, during this period.

Jeffry A. Simpson, PhD, is Professor of Psychology at Texas A&M University. He received his doctorate in psychology from the University of Minnesota in 1986. His research focuses on interpersonal relationships, evolution and social behavior, and social influence. Dr. Simpson also serves as Associate Editor for the *Journal of Personality and Social Psychology*.

Contributors

Austin W. Albino, MA, Department of Psychology, University of Missouri, Columbia, Missouri

Lisa Feldman Barrett, PhD, Department of Psychology, Boston College, Boston, Massachusetts

Claudia Chloe Brumbaugh, BA, Department of Psychology, University of Illinois at Chicago, Chicago, Illinois

Mary Campa, MA, Family Life Development Center, Cornell University, Ithaca, New York

Jude Cassidy, PhD, Department of Psychology, University of Maryland, College Park, Maryland

Rebecca J. Cobb, PhD, Department of Psychology, University of California, Los Angeles, California

Nancy L. Collins, PhD, Department of Psychology, University of California at Santa Barbara, Santa Barbara, California

M. Lynne Cooper, PhD, Department of Psychology, University of Missouri, Columbia, Missouri

Joanne Davila, PhD, Department of Psychology, State University of New York at Stony Brook, Stony Brook, New York

Lisa M. Diamond, PhD, Department of Psychology, University of Utah, Salt Lake City, Utah

Brooke C. Feeney, PhD, Department of Psychology, Carnegie Mellon University, Pittsburgh, Pennsylvania

Judith A. Feeney, PhD, School of Psychology, University of Queensland, Queensland, Australia

Maire B. Ford, MA, Department of Psychology, University of California at Santa Barbara, Santa Barbara, California

R. Chris Fraley, PhD, Department of Psychology, University of Illinois at Chicago, Chicago, Illinois

Dara Greenwood, MS, Department of Psychology, University of Massachusetts, Amherst, Massachusetts

AnaMarie C. Guichard, MA, Department of Psychology, University of California at Santa Barbara, Santa Barbara, California

Nurit Gur-Yaish, MA, Department of Human Development, Cornell University, Ithaca, New York

Cindy Hazan, PhD, Department of Human Development, Cornell University, Ithaca, New York

Angela M. Hicks, MA, Department of Psychology, University of Utah, Salt Lake City, Utah

Susan M. Johnson, EdD, Department of Psychology, University of Ottawa, and private practice, Ottawa, Ontario, Canada

Roger Kobak, PhD, Department of Psychology, University of Delaware, Newark, Delaware

Mario Mikulincer, PhD, Department of Psychology, Bar-Ilan University, Ramat-Gan, Israel

Holly K. Orcutt, PhD, Department of Psychology, Northern Illinois University, DeKalb, Illinois

Paula R. Pietromonaco, PhD, Department of Psychology, University of Massachusetts, Amherst, Massachusetts

W. Steven Rholes, PhD, Department of Psychology, Texas A&M University, College Station, Texas

Phillip R. Shaver, PhD, Department of Psychology, University of California at Davis, Davis, California

Jeffry A. Simpson, PhD, Department of Psychology, Texas A&M University College Station, Texas

Natalie Williams, MA, Department of Psychology, University of Missouri, Columbia, Missouri

Yair Ziv, PhD, Department of Psychology, University of Maryland, College Park, Maryland

Contents

xi

PART III
Intrapersonal Aspects of Attachment
Cognitive Organization, Structure, and Information Processing

PART IV
Interpersonal Aspects of Attachment
Intimacy, Conflict, Caregiving, and Satisfaction

PART V
Clinical and Applied Issues
Therapy, Psychopathology, and Well-Being

PART I

INTRODUCTION

New Directions and Emerging Issues
in Adult Attachment

CHAPTER 1

Attachment Theory

Basic Concepts and Contemporary Questions

W. STEVEN RHOLES
JEFFRY A. SIMPSON

Attachment theory is among the most sweeping, comprehensive theories in psychology today. It offers a biosocial, lifespan account of how close relationships form, are maintained, and dissolve and how relationships influence, sometimes permanently, the persons involved in them (Bowlby, 1979). The theory addresses these issues from a variety of perspectives, including physiological, emotional, cognitive, and behavioral. The theory articulates constructs and processes that are relevant to understanding elements of social development, interpersonal behavior, relationship functioning, psychosocial adjustment, and clinical disorders. The chapters in this volume address many of these multifaceted issues.

This introductory chapter comprises two sections. In the first, we review some of the basic concepts that anchor attachment theory. This section is targeted to readers who might be new to the attachment field. It focuses in large part on the seminal theoretical and empirical attachment work involving young children, but it also reviews some of the major principles of attachment processes in adults. Readers who are familiar with attachment theory and research may want to skip to the second section, which highlights some of the critical questions and emerging issues that are addressed in the chapters of this volume.

BASIC ATTACHMENT CONCEPTS

Before we begin, some comments on nomenclature are in order. Throughout this volume, "attachment behavior" refers to efforts to achieve physi-

3

cal or psychological contact with attachment figures. "Attachment bonds" refer to the emotional ties that exist between individuals and their attachment figures. The terms "attachment styles" and "attachment orientations" are used interchangeably throughout the chapters. Briefly, they refer to stable, global individual differences in (1) tendencies to seek and experience comfort and emotional support from persons with whom one has an attachment bond and (2) presumptions about the responsiveness of attachment figures to bids for comfort and support.

Self-report adult attachment measures can be scored to create four attachment categories: secure, anxious, dismissive–avoidant, and fearful–avoidant. Two continuous dimensions—commonly labeled "avoidance" and "anxiety" (or "ambivalence")—define a two-dimensional space that underlies these categories (Brennan, Clark, & Shaver, 1998). "Avoidance" is defined in large part by discomfort with psychological intimacy and the desire to maintain psychological independence, even in close relationships such as marriage. "Anxiety," or ambivalence, refers to a strong need for care and attention from attachment figures coupled with a deep, pervasive uncertainty about the capacity or willingness of attachment figures to respond to such needs. The "secure" attachment style category involves the combination of low avoidance and low anxiety, the "anxious" style consists of high anxiety and low avoidance, the "dismissive" style reflects high avoidance and low anxiety, and the "fearful" style involves high scores on both dimensions. Many contemporary adult attachment studies focus on the two attachment style dimensions rather than on the four categories.

The most widely used interview measure of adult attachment, the Adult Attachment Interview (AAI; Main & Goldwyn, 1994), assesses how memories of childhood experiences with attachment figures are organized mentally. The AAI places individuals into one of three primary categories: dismissive, secure (free/autonomous), or preoccupied. The "dismissive" AAI category is similar conceptually to the dismissive–avoidant group in the self-report measures and the underlying attachment dimension of avoidance. It is marked by efforts to keep the need for comfort and support from attachment figures deactivated through repression of memories of vulnerability and of rejection by attachment figures in childhood and through denial of the importance of attachment relationships. The "preoccupied" AAI category is most analogous conceptually to the self-report "anxious" category and the underlying anxiety dimension. It is defined by an inability to come to terms with adverse experiences with attachment figures in childhood and adolescence, which leads to a sometimes lifelong enmeshment, and often deep-seated anger, with parents and other attachment figures. The "secure" AAI group is most closely related conceptually to the secure self-report group and to low scores on both the avoidant and anxious dimensions. Secure people are marked by a sense of personal autonomy and the ability to examine past and present attachment issues objectively, free from both repression and enmeshed, unresolved feelings and thoughts. Although most secure people have relatively benign experiences with attachment figures in childhood and adolescence, some have found ways to free themselves from the effects of rejection, neglect, and even physical abuse.

Attachment theory was initially formulated by John Bowlby (1969, 1973, 1979, 1980) and subsequently extended in important directions by Mary Ainsworth (Ainsworth, Blehar, Waters, & Wall, 1978). The theory begins with the premise that human beings, similar to many other primate species, have an innate orientation to social life. Specifically, attachment theory claims that human beings have an evolved, biologically based predisposition to direct "attachment behaviors" (e.g., searching for, promoting physical contact with, looking at, following, visually tracking) toward persons who serve as their primary caregivers. The attachment behavioral system is a loosely organized set of behaviors whose primary feature in common is that they serve the goal of increasing physical and psychological proximity to a primary caregiver. This system presumably evolved because it increased physical proximity between vulnerable infants and children and their stronger, wiser caregivers. The attachment system is one of three biologically based systems that Bowlby discussed. The other two are the caregiving and exploratory systems, which have received much less study than the attachment system.

According to attachment theory, primary caregivers become increasingly differentiated from other people in the minds of infants during their first year of life. Infants are believed to form attachment bonds with their primary caregivers in all but the most extreme of conditions (e.g., when infants are socially isolated for long periods of time, or when they have multiple short-term caretakers). To have no attachment bond means that all caregivers or social partners are equivalent. No individual has been singled out as special. By the end of the first year, attachment figures typically are the center of most infants' social worlds. The process of forming emotional bonds with attachment figures is proposed in attachment theory to be fundamentally universal, even though it may vary in detail across cultures. Nevertheless, one central premise of attachment theory is that natural selection favored infants who became attached to their caregivers because doing so most likely afforded greater protection from danger and predation in ancestral environments.

Not all attachment bonds are the same. According to attachment theory, different patterns of attachment should emerge in response to the way caregivers react to their infants' attachment behaviors (Ainsworth et al., 1978). Infants tend to develop "secure" attachments to caregivers who serve as good, receptive targets for their attachment behaviors. Caregivers who foster greater security tend to read their infants' cues of distress more accurately and find effective ways to comfort them. When their infants are not distressed, the caregivers remain physically and emotionally "available" to their infants without being disruptive or intrusive. Caregivers who promote security accept the difficulties and stress of child care, including the limitations that attentive infant care imposes on their lives. Infants who form secure patterns of attachment with their attachment figures differ from insecure infants in numerous ways. For example, they readily seek comfort from their attachment figures when they are distressed, and they are calmed more quickly and completely by their attachment figures (Ainsworth et al., 1978).

According to Ainsworth and colleagues (1978), there are two principal types of insecure attachment: anxious–ambivalent and avoidant. Ainsworth's typology is assessed by the Strange Situation test, which involves a series of distressing separations and reunions between mothers and their 12- to 18-month-old children. Children classified as having secure relationships directly seek comfort from their mothers, are calmed easily, and then resume other activities (e.g., playing, exploring the room). Children classified as having anxious–ambivalent relationships display decidedly mixed reactions to their mothers (i.e., approach–avoidance behaviors), remain agitated, and fail to resume normal activities. And children classified as avoidant disregard or ignore their mothers, show signs of emotional disengagement and withdrawal, and engage in behaviors that keep them distracted from the distress they are feeling. The Strange Situation measures characteristics of the *relationship* between infants and their primary caregivers rather than the characteristics of the infants themselves. Thus it is technically incorrect to refer to infants (or children) as being secure, avoidant, or anxious–ambivalent.

As individuals grow and mature, they develop an orientation toward attachment figures in general as a function of their unique history with attachment figures. Some attachment histories, whether good or ill, are simple and uncomplicated; individuals have only a few attachment figures, and the behavior of their attachment figures is relatively consistent from infancy through adolescence. Some attachment histories, however, are more complex. Individuals with these histories, for example, may have received very different patterns of caregiving from their mothers and from their fathers, producing a different attachment pattern with each parent. Alternatively, the behavior of their primary attachment figure(s) might have varied dramatically across time, leading them to experience major changes, from attachment security to insecurity and perhaps back again. Individuals may have been separated long term from attachment figures, or attachment figures may have been lost through permanent separations, death, or divorce. In response to losses, new potential attachment figures may enter into an individual's life. From these varied histories and through processes of combination that are still not fully understood, a generalized attachment orientation—an attachment style—develops.

Individual difference measures of general attachment styles have not been developed for children. Procedures for assessing attachment in children assess relationship-specific attachment patterns. Nonetheless, children who manifest different attachment patterns to attachment figures even in infancy behave differently at later points in development with their attachment figures and others. For example, elementary-school children who have been classified as secure, avoidant, or anxious–ambivalent with their mothers in the Strange Situation at age 1 respond differently to, and form different kinds of relationships with, their schoolmates in early childhood (see Thompson, 1999). Though it remains unclear precisely when general "attachment styles" can be said to have developed, they can be assessed and used to predict social behavior in theoretically meaningful ways starting in the early teenage years (see Crowell, Fraley, & Shaver, 1999; Feeney, 1999).

The psychological structures that underlie different attachment styles are known as "working models" (Collins & Read, 1994; Collins, Guichard, Ford, & Feeney, Chapter 7, this volume). These structures provide rough-and-ready blueprints for what should be expected and what is likely to occur in different kinds of interactions with attachment figures. Working models have both conscious and unconscious components and, therefore, they are believed to influence both consciously controlled and automatic, unconscious mental processes. Working models orchestrate behavior, cognition, and affect in close relationships, providing guidance about how to behave, what should be expected or anticipated, and how to interpret the meaning of ambiguous interpersonal events. Working models also control attention to and memory for information associated with attachment-relevant events, and they regulate affect—especially negative affect—when attachment-relevant stressors are encountered. According to Bowlby (1980), working models should be fairly accurate reflections of the experiences that individuals have had with attachment figures.

Working models are termed "working" because they remain open to correction and revision. They are never immutably "fixed" by one's attachment history. Similar to scientific theories, working models allow people to formulate expectations, develop hypotheses, and explain relationship outcomes. As with scientific theories, working models tend to be conservative in that new experiences are assimilated into existing models more readily than models are accommodated to fit new experiences. Working models, therefore, are situated at the juncture of existing premises (many of which have served well to explain interpersonal events and guide behavior) and new information (some of which may challenge, contradict, or refute existing premises). New information can come from new relationships, from new insights (e.g., reinterpreting the meaning of past attachment relationships), or from major life events that expose individuals to radically new situations or experiences. Thus working models operate at the intersection of past experiences, new experiences, and revised conceptualizations of the past.

Finally, among the core propositions and hypotheses of attachment theory, the five listed below are perhaps the most central.

1. *Although the basic impetus for the formation of attachment relationships is provided by biological factors, the bonds that children form with their caregivers are shaped by interpersonal experience.* This proposal has withstood challenges from those who have proposed that attachment patterns in young children are merely by-products of differences in temperament (see Vaughn & Bost, 1999).

2. *Experiences in earlier relationships create internal working models and attachment styles that systematically affect attachment relationships.* Thus, at any given point in adulthood, experiences in childhood, adolescence, and earlier adulthood partially determine the nature of one's attachment relationships through their impact on working models and attachment styles. This so-called "prototype" hypothesis has received considerable support in the adult attachment literature, although the mechanisms by which it operates need further clarification (see Feeney, 1999). This proposition does not assert that attachment styles fully determine attachment relationships; they are also influenced by the experiences with the attachment figure in question. Thus it is possible for a person with an insecure attachment orientation to have a secure attachment relationship. Working models and attachment styles are most directly pertinent to behavior in close relationships, but they may become integrated into basic values or personality and thus affect behavior in other contexts.

3. *The attachment orientations of adult caregivers influence the attachment bond their children have with them.* This hypothesis is derived from the propositions that attachments are the product of social experience and that adult attachment orientations influence behavior, including behavior with infants and children, in close relationships. This "intergenerational transmission" hypothesis has received clear support, especially in the work of Main and her colleagues (see Hesse, 1999).

4. *Working models and attachment orientations are relatively stable over time, but they are not impervious to change.* When change occurs, it is expected to be the result of new experiences with attachment figures or reconceptualizations of past experiences with attachment figures. Evidence reported in this volume supports this view (see Davila & Cobb, Chapter 5, and Fraley & Brumbaugh, Chapter 4, this volume).

5. *Some forms of psychological maladjustment and clinical disorders are attributable in part to the effects of insecure working models and attachment styles.*

Adult attachment orientations correlate with a variety of clinical and subclinical disturbances (see Dozier, Stovall, & Albus, 1999). The processes through which they create or exacerbate different psychological problems, however, requires further clarification.

CONTEMPORARY QUESTIONS

This volume is organized into four major sections. The first (Part II) deals with change in attachment orientations across the lifespan and theoretical issues associated with the measurement of attachment orientations. The second (Part III) addresses intrapersonal aspects of attachment, in particular the working models construct and physiological aspects of attachment orientations. The chapters in Part IV explore interpersonal behaviors, specifically caregiving and responses by couples to stress and conflict. Part V addresses the relations of attachment styles to vulnerability to clinical and subclinical disturbances and the processes of therapeutic change.

Hidden under the seemingly mundane cover of a measurement issue lies one of the most hotly debated controversies in the adult attachment field today. In the mid–1980s, two measures of adult attachment orientations were created. Mary Main and her colleagues (Main, Kaplan, & Cassidy, 1985) developed the AAI, which assesses generalized adult attachment orientations based on recollections of experiences with attachment figures in childhood. At about the same time, Hazan and Shaver (1987) introduced the first self-report measure of adult attachment. The purpose of their instrument was to assess the adult versions of the emotional and behavioral features identified by Ainsworth in children with secure, avoidant, and anxious–ambivalent attachments to their primary caregivers. Theoretical and empirical questions about how these measures relate to one another have been of concern for nearly two decades (see Shaver, Belsky, & Brennan, 2000).

Attachment theory states clearly that internal working models have both conscious and unconscious components. An important question, therefore, is whether attachment styles identified by self-report contain unconscious elements. Shaver and Mikulincer (Chapter 2) address this issue and the larger controversy between adherents of the AAI and self-report measures. They establish that attachment styles identified by self-report means are associated with automatic and uncontrolled, or unconscious, processes. In doing so, they provide additional evidence for the construct validity of self-report measures.

In addition to being a theory of individual differences, attachment theory also provides an explanation of how attachment bonds develop between individuals. This topic has received relatively little attention. Individual differences in attachment style have been studied far more often. Hazan, Gur-Yaish, and Campa (Chapter 3) attempt to correct this imbalance. They describe the development of attachment bonds from physiological, emotional, cognitive, and behavioral perspectives. They present a compelling case that, by focusing almost exclusively on individual differences in attachment orientation, the field has ignored vital aspects of attachment theory.

The work reported by Fraley and Brumbaugh and by Davila and Cobb (Chapters 4 and 5) takes up the challenges of longitudinal research. Their chapters are concerned with how, why, and when lasting changes in attachment orientations occur. Early in the history of attachment research, attachment theory was often misunderstood to say that attachment orientations form early in life and remain largely unchanged into adulthood. This misconception may have had its roots in Bowlby's original theoretical ties to neo-Freudian psychology. Regardless of its origin, many early criticisms of attachment theory arose from the failure to understand that systematic changes in attachment orientations can and should occur under conditions that successfully challenge the assumptions on which working models are based.

Marshaling compelling support for this premise has proven challenging because of the complexity of longitudinal research and the difficulty of measuring change. Fraley and Brumbaugh, in Chapter 4, provide a valuable service by translating Bowlby's ideas about stability and change into testable, mathematical terms. Their work helps clarify the nature of the hypotheses that can be derived from Bowlby's writings. In Chapter 5, Davila and Cobb describe the processes that generate change in attachment orientations. They also suggest that understanding how change unfolds naturally will have important implications for clinical interventions that focus on revising the mental structures that encourage maladaptive behavior in relationships.

Perhaps the most important intrapersonal construct in attachment theory is the working model. In his 1980 book, Bowlby outlined the structure and function of these models based on the evidence then available in psychiatry and psychology. Within the past decade, significant advances have been made toward understanding how working models affect relationship processes and outcomes. Integrating many of these advances, Collins, Guichard, Ford, and Feeney (Chapter 7) describe the components of working models, explain their organization in memory, and articulate the processes through which they guide behavior, affect, and cognition. Mikulincer and Shaver (Chapter 6) deal with similar issues. They present a model that describes how security-enhancing interactions with attachment figures might produce self-concepts that incorporate a strong sense of autonomy and the capacity to engage in healthy self-calming and self-regulation. Diamond and Hicks (Chapter 8) discuss intrapersonal elements of attachment from a physiological, rather than a cognitive, perspective. Their chapter suggests that attachment processes may at least partially account for the biological conditions that contribute to psychological disorders and physical health.

Attachment theory's most important interpersonal proposition is the prototype hypothesis. Without it, the theory would be relevant to relationships but not to the persons involved in them, making the theory far less comprehensive. Consistent support for this hypothesis has been central to the proliferation of attachment research. Chapter 9, by Pietromonaco, Greenwood, and Feldman Barrett; Chapter 11, by Judith Feeney; and Chapter 10, by Brooke Feeney and Nancy Collins extend this hypothesis in new directions. Pietromonaco and colleagues focus on the ways in which relationship conflicts can pose both threats to and opportunities for relationships. They also discuss the consequences of these perceptions for conflict resolution and long-term relationship functioning. Judy Feeney's chapter addresses associations between attachment styles, stress, and relationship functioning. She reviews the ways in which individuals with different attachment styles perceive stressful events and then cope with them. Brooke Feeney and Nancy Collins explore caregiving in adult attachment relationships. They present a new model that describes pathways between the caregiving, attachment, and exploratory systems that can guide future research on this neglected topic. The topics covered in these chapters—conflict, stress, and caregiving—are critical to the long-term happiness and stability of intimate relationships.

Several chapters in the final section of this volume address how attachment orientations are associated with health and well-being. The first generation of research on adult attachment and mental health asked whether attachment orientations correlate with the clinical and subclinical disorders discussed by Bowlby. This initial work demonstrated that persons with insecure attachment orientations are more vulnerable to a variety of psychological problems. The chapters in this volume are representative of the second generation of research. They go beyond documenting associations to investigating the processes that render insecurely attached persons more susceptible to problems. Many of these chapters also clarify the way in which concepts in attachment theory can be used to treat attachment-related disorders.

Drawing on empirical research guided by attachment theory and clinical case studies, Johnson (Chapter 12) describes a new and very important model of couple therapy. Kobak, Cassidy, and Ziv (Chapter 13) introduce the concept of "attachment trauma," which they relate to posttraumatic stress disorder (PTSD). They discuss important parallels between this disorder and their new construct. Simpson and Rholes (Chapter 14) present a process model that outlines how anxious–ambivalent people might perceive and interact with their partners in ways that exacerbate depressive symptoms, particularly during periods of stress. Cooper, Albino, Orcutt, and Williams (Chapter 15) report the results of a major longitudinal project that examines adjustment and risk taking in African American and European American adolescents. Their chapter shows that different attachment styles are uniquely related to certain types of problematic behavior.

CONCLUSION: EMERGING THEMES

The research reported in this book is the continuation of approximately three decades of effort to study attachment in humans. In its first stage, attachment research focused almost exclusively on infants and addressed issues related to the measurement, origins, and consequences of infants' attachments to their primary caregivers. Its second stage began with the extension of the theory to adults. This stage has been marked in large part by research on the consequences of individual differences in attachment style for interpersonal relationships and mental health.

What kinds of studies will the next stage of attachment research include? Based on the chapters in this book, we believe that new research will include more longitudinal studies that address how attachment styles change and how relationships between adults become attachment relationships; that is, how attachment bonds develop. In the next stage of research, we anticipate more empirical and theoretical work on the caregiving and exploratory systems and the interactions between them and the attachment system. To date, most research on clinical issues has asked whether insecure attachment orientations are associated with increased vulnerability to disturbance. The processes that link attachment orientations to emotional and mental disturbance have been largely ignored. Process research will, we believe, become an important theme in clinically oriented investigations. Finally, although research on the impact of working models on information processing and on automatic, uncontrolled thought processes is not new, it is still in its infancy in attachment research and will continue to be an important topic.

In conclusion, the chapters contained in this volume accomplish several important goals. As a group, they clarify and expand some well-established theoretical constructs; they introduce new theoretical constructs; they address issues of attachment stability and change across time; they explicate how attachment styles may guide and regulate behavior in adult relationships; and they propose several new process models that link adult attachment styles to psychological and health-related disorders. By approaching these issues from different perspectives—evolutionary, biological, physiological, cognitive, emotional, behavioral, and interpersonal—these chapters showcase some of the most important new directions and emerging issues in adult attachment today. We hope you will enjoy the intellectual adventure.

ACKNOWLEDGMENT

W. Steven Rholes and Jeffry A. Simpson contributed equally to this chapter. The writing of this chapter was supported by National Institutes of Health Grant No. MH49599–05.

REFERENCES

Ainsworth, M. D. S., Blehar, M. C., Waters, E., & Wall, S. (1978). *Patterns of attachment: A psychological study of the Strange Situation.* Hillsdale, NJ: Erlbaum.

Bowlby, J. (1969). *Attachment and loss: Vol. 1. Attachment.* New York: Basic Books.

Bowlby, J. (1973). *Attachment and loss: Vol. 2. Separation: Anxiety and anger.* New York: Basic Books.

Bowlby, J. (1979). *The making and breaking of affectional bonds.* New York: Methuen.

Bowlby, J. (1980). *Attachment and loss: Vol. 3. Loss: Sadness and depression.* New York: Basic Books.

Brennan, K. A., Clark, C. L., & Shaver, P. R. (1998). Self-report measurement of adult attachment: An integrative overview. In J. A. Simpson & W. S. Rholes (Eds.), *Attachment theory and close relationships* (pp. 46–76). New York: Guilford Press.

Collins, N. L., & Read, S. J. (1994). Cognitive representations of attachment: The structure and function of working models. In K. Bartholomew & D. Perlman (Eds.), *Advances in personal relationships: Vol. 5. Attachment processes in adulthood* (pp. 53–90). London: Kingsley.

Crowell, J. A., Fraley, R. C., & Shaver, P. R. (1999). Measurement of individual differences in adolescent and adult attachment. In J. Cassidy & P. R. Shaver (Eds.), *Handbook of attachment: Theory, research, and clinical applications* (pp. 434–465). New York: Guilford Press.

Dozier, M., Stovall, K. C., & Albus, K. E. (1999). Attachment and psychopathology in adulthood. In J. Cassidy & P. R. Shaver (Eds.), *Handbook of attachment: Theory, research, and clinical applications* (pp. 497–519). New York: Guilford Press.

Feeney, J. A. (1999). Adult romantic attachment and couple relationships. In J. Cassidy & P. R. Shaver (Eds.), *Handbook of attachment: Theory, research, and clinical applications* (pp. 355–377). New York: Guilford Press.

Hazan, C., & Shaver, P. R. (1987). Romantic love conceptualized as an attachment process. *Journal of Personality and Social Psychology, 52,* 511–524.

Hesse, E. (1999). The Adult Attachment Interview: Historical and current perspectives. In J. Cassidy & P. R. Shaver (Eds.), *Handbook of attachment: Theory, research, and clinical applications* (pp. 395–433). New York: Guilford Press.

Main, M., & Goldwyn, R. (1994). *Adult attachment scoring and classification systems* (2nd ed.). Unpublished manuscript, University of California–Berkeley.

Main, M., Kaplan, N., & Cassidy, J. (1985). Security in infancy, childhood, and adulthood: A move to the level of representation. *Monographs of the Society for Research in Child Development, 50*(1 & 2, Serial No. 209), 66–104.

Shaver, P. R., Belsky, J., & Brennan, K. A. (2000). The Adult Attachment Interview and self-reports of romantic attachment: Associations across domains and methods. *Personal Relationships, 7,* 25–43.

Thompson, R. A. (1999). Early attachment and later development. In J. Cassidy & P. R. Shaver (Eds.), *Handbook of attachment: Theory, research, and clinical applications* (pp. 265–286). New York: Guilford Press.

Vaughn, B. E., & Bost, K. K. (1999). Attachment and temperament: Redundant, independent, or interacting influences on interpersonal adaptation and personality development? In J. Cassidy & P. R. Shaver (Eds.), *Handbook of attachment: Theory, research, and clinical applications* (pp. 198–225). New York: Guilford Press.

PART II

ATTACHMENT PROCESSES ACROSS THE LIFESPAN

Continuity, Discontinuity, Change,
and Measurement Issues

CHAPTER 2

What Do Self-Report
Attachment Measures Assess?

PHILLIP R. SHAVER
MARIO MIKULINCER

The measurement of adult attachment patterns got off to a rousing start in the 1980s. George, Kaplan, and Main (1985) created the Adult Attachment Interview (AAI) to assess "current state of mind with respect to attachment," and Main and her colleagues (e.g., Main, Kaplan, & Cassidy, 1985) demonstrated that a parent's AAI classification (secure/autonomous, preoccupied, dismissing, or unresolved) predicted the quality of attachment shown by a child to that particular parent. (See Hesse, 1999, for a comprehensive description and history of the AAI.) Hazan and Shaver (1987), working independently, proposed a theory of romantic attachment and created a simple self-classification question, responses to which were systematically related to mental models of self and partner, beliefs about romantic love, and memories of childhood relationships with parents. Armsden and Greenberg (1987) developed a multi-item, multiscale self-report Inventory of Parent and Peer Attachment (IPPA), which could be used to assess security, or perceived quality, of adolescents' relationships with their parents and peers. West, Sheldon, and Reiffer (1987) created a multi-item, multiscale measure for clinically analyzing an adult's relationship with a particular attachment figure. Bartholomew and Horowitz (1991) created interview measures of both parent and peer attachment histories. And Pottharst and Kessler (cited in Pottharst, 1990) created an Attachment History Questionnaire (AHQ) to assess adults' memories of attachment-related experiences in childhood—for example, separations from parents, loss of parents, and quality of relationships with parents and other attachment figures.

Out of these initial efforts, two somewhat independent lines of research emerged (see descriptions and summaries in Bartholomew &

Shaver, 1998; Crowell, Fraley, & Shaver, 1999; Shaver & Mikulincer, 2002). In one of the lines, based primarily on the AAI, developmental and clinical psychologists repeatedly showed that AAI classifications of parents can predict the Strange Situation (infant attachment) classifications of their children. Some insights have been gained about the nature of this cross-generational transmission process (e.g., George & Solomon, 1999; van IJzendoorn, 1995), although the details are still somewhat sketchy. Researchers in this tradition have also shown that certain kinds of psychopathology are related systematically to AAI classifications (e.g., Lyons-Ruth & Jacobvitz, 1999). When this approach to assessment is extended to the romantic/marital domain (Crowell et al., 2002; Crowell, Treboux, & Waters, 2002; Simpson, Rholes, Orina, & Grich, 2002; Waters, Crowell, Elliot, Corcoran, & Treboux, 2002), connections between the AAI and behavior in couple relationships emerge.

In the second line of adult attachment research (reviewed by Mikulincer & Shaver, 2003), personality, social, and some clinical psychologists have used either Hazan and Shaver's (1987) very brief self-report measure of what came to be called "adult attachment style" (secure, anxious, or avoidant) or some extension or refinement of that measure (e.g., Bartholomew & Horowitz, 1991; Collins & Read, 1990; Feeney, Noller, & Hanrahan, 1994; Simpson, 1990). Some measures are based on a four-category typology of attachment styles (secure, preoccupied, fearful, and dismissing) instead of the three assessed by Hazan and Shaver, and some yield scores on two, three, or five dimensions.

In 1998, Brennan, Clark, and Shaver conducted a factor analysis of all existing English-language dimensional measures of attachment style created up to that point and discovered, in line with the two-dimensional model proposed by Bartholomew and Horowitz (1991), that all of the measures could be reduced to two orthogonal dimensions, attachment anxiety (fear of separation and abandonment) and attachment avoidance (e.g., discomfort with intimacy and dependency). The resulting Experiences in Close Relationships scale (ECR) has been used in many studies since 1998 and has been found to be highly reliable and to have high construct and predictive validity (Shaver & Mikulincer, 2002).

The two lines of attachment research have remained separate because of the different research questions motivating investigators—intergenerational transmission of attachment patterns versus social-cognitive dynamics affecting feelings and behavior in close, especially romantic/ marital, relationships—and the belief that the AAI and self-report attachment measures are unrelated. This belief is based on the substantial differences between the AAI and self-report attachment measures in targeted relationships (parent–child vs. adult–adult relationships), method (intensively coded interview transcripts vs. brief self-reports), and analytic focus (structural properties of coherence, believability, and vagueness of a person's narrative of attachment experiences vs. content of a person's perceptions, feelings, and self-observed behavior).

The belief that two very different domains are being measured is also based on recent findings indicating that self-reports of attachment anxiety and avoidance are not significantly associated with AAI classifications (Crowell, Treboux, & Waters, 1999; Simpson et al., 2002; Waters et al., 2002). However, other studies have found significant associations between self-report and interview measures of attachment patterns (Bartholomew & Horowitz, 1991; Bartholomew & Shaver, 1998; Griffin & Bartholomew, 1994; Shaver, Belsky, & Brennan, 2000). For example, Shaver and colleagues (2000) found that self-report attachment scores could be predicted from AAI coding scales with multiple *R*'s of .48 and .52.

Another barrier to integration of the two lines of attachment research is AAI researchers' supposition that self-report measures cannot plumb the psychodynamic depths probed by the AAI. As Jacobvitz, Curran, and Moller (2002) wrote in a recent article, "the AAI classification coding system assesses *adults' unconscious processes for regulating emotion*. . . . Unlike the AAI, the self-report measures of attachment tap adults' *conscious appraisals* of themselves in romantic relationships" (p. 208, emphasis in original). Such researchers have tended to infer that because self-report measures involve conscious, deliberate answers to explicit questions, they are probably limited to indexing conscious mental processes. On this assumption, it is easy to reach the conclusion that self-report measures are unlikely to relate to the psychodynamic processes of interest to Bowlby (1969/1982) and other clinicians, especially those with a psychoanalytic orientation.

In order to challenge this view of what is tapped by self-report measures of attachment style and to demonstrate what can be accomplished when these measures are used in research, we (Shaver & Mikulincer, 2002) published a target article in which we showed that self-report measures, when used in conjunction with other kinds of measures, such as behavioral observations and implicit priming techniques, can reveal a great deal about implicit, unconscious processes. As we said in that article:

> [Our review of recent studies] indicates that considerable progress has been made in testing central hypotheses derived from attachment theory and in exploring unconscious, psychodynamic processes related to affect-regulation and attachment-system activation. The combination of self-report assessment of attachment style and experimental manipulation of other theoretically pertinent variables allows researchers to test causal hypotheses. (p. 133)

In the target article, we also showed that findings derived from self-report measures of attachment style can be coherently integrated within a theoretical model of the activation and dynamics of the attachment behavioral system in adulthood (Shaver & Mikulincer, 2002). This model (see Figure 2.1) includes three components. The first component involves the monitoring and appraisal of threatening events, which can lead to activation of the attachment system. The second component involves the monitoring and appraisal of attachment-figure availability and is responsible for individual differences in the sense of attachment security. The third component involves monitoring and appraisal of the viability of proximity seeking as a way of dealing with attachment insecurity. This component is responsible for individual variations in the use of hyperactivating or deactivating strategies of affect regulation. The model also includes excitatory and inhibitory "neural circuits" (shown as arrows on the left-hand side of the diagram) that result from the recurrent use of hyperactivating or deactivating strategies, which in turn affect the monitoring of threats and of attachment figures' availability or unavailability.

According to this model, individual variations in self-reports of attachment anxiety and avoidance reflect the underlying action of hyperactivating and deactivating strategies. On the one hand, self-reports of attachment anxiety reflect the appraisal of proximity seeking as a viable option, which leads to increased efforts to attain closeness and support by insistently expressing vulnerability, need, and anxiety. The main goal of these efforts is to get an attachment figure, who is viewed as insufficiently concerned and available, to pay attention and provide protection. The basic means for attaining this goal is to maintain the attachment system in an activated state until an attachment figure is perceived to be available and responsive. These strategies involve physical and psychological proximity seeking, heightened vigilance regarding actual and potential threats, and intense monitoring of attachment-figure availability or unavailability, because these cues are highly relevant to security attainment. On the other hand, self-reports of attachment avoidance reflect the appraisal of proximity seeking as a nonviable option, which leads to defensive independence and self-reliance, denial of attachment needs, and suppression or deactivation of attachment strivings. This deactivation effort includes the downplaying of actual or potential threats and refusal to monitor the availability or unavailability of attachment figures, because thinking about threats or attachment figures might reactivate the attachment system.

Although some of the 11 commentaries on our article (Shaver & Mikulincer, 2002) were supportive, others were skeptical or critical. Some authors familiar with the AAI tradition (Belsky, 2002; Bernier & Dozier, 2002; Jacobvitz et al., 2002; Waters et al., 2002) continued to suspect that their approach is superior in (1) tapping unconscious processes, (2) delineating the information-processing strategies of dismissing and preoccupied adults, (3) evoking rich narrative accounts of attachment relationships that directly reflect interviewees' internal working models, (4)

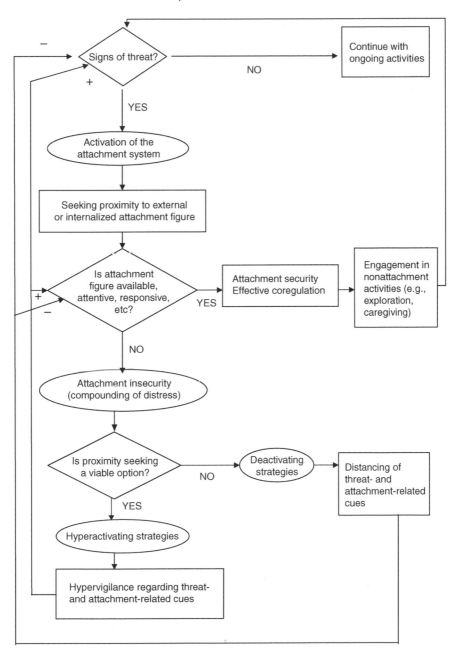

FIGURE 2.1. Shaver and Mikulincer's (2002) integrative model of the activation and dynamics of the attachment system in adulthood.

relating attachment working models to social behavior, and (5) discovering how adult attachment patterns emerge from a person's attachment history. These critics also claimed (6) that self-report measures of attachment style suffer from a lack of discriminant validity, as they tend to be correlated with self-report measures of other psychological constructs such as depression and trait anxiety.

The purpose of this chapter is to continue this important dialogue by examining the research literature in the self-report tradition to see if the AAI researchers' criticisms stand up to the evidence. In each of the following sections, we address one of the six kinds of criticism advanced by AAI researchers and review empirical evidence related to that criticism.

IMPLICIT, UNCONSCIOUS CORRELATES OF SELF-REPORTS OF ATTACHMENT STYLE

A number of authors have questioned the validity of self-report measures of attachment style for assessing implicit, unconscious aspects of attachment-system functioning (e.g., Crowell & Treboux, 1995; Hesse, 1999; Jacobvitz et al., 2002). In their view, self-report measures tap only a person's conscious appraisals of feelings and behaviors in close relationships, which can be inaccurate reflections of the underlying dynamics of the attachment system. We agree that it is possible that some people defensively report that they do not worry about rejection and separation when actually they do worry about these issues, and some may have no conscious access to such worries, even though they exist. Because of such problems, critics claim that self-report measures of attachment style cannot be considered valid measures of a person's "true" working models of self and others or of attachment-related strategies of affect regulation (which Cassidy & Kobak, 1988, called hyperactivating and deactivating strategies). Many of the critics prefer to use the AAI, which they believe is a reliable and valid measure of unconscious processes revealed when a person discusses attachment-related experiences recalled from childhood, such as separations from attachment figures (Hesse, 1999).

Although, like every self-report measure, attachment-style scales can be somewhat biased by social desirability concerns and other motivational and cognitive tendencies, there are several reasons for continuing to use them to index implicit aspects of attachment-system functioning, as Crowell and colleagues (1999) have explained. First, most adults have sufficient experience in close relationships to provide valuable information about their relational cognitions, emotions, and behavior. Their characteristic feelings and behaviors may be useful reflections of unconscious processes, even though these processes cannot be perceived directly. Second, conscious and unconscious processes typically operate in the same direction to achieve a goal, and unconscious motives are often manifested in conscious appraisals (Chartrand & Bargh, 2002). Third, even in the case of people who defensively deny attachment needs or claim they do not suffer from attachment insecurities, "it is possible to use attachment theory to derive the kinds of conscious beliefs that defensive people may hold about themselves" (Crowell et al., 1999, p. 453). In this way, one can predict from self-reports how a person is likely to behave under particular conditions even if the people providing those reports are not able to make the same predictions. This kind of prediction is commonly made in studies based on other kinds of self-report scales, such as measures of narcissism (see Morf & Rhodewalt, 2001, for a review). It is not unique to the attachment domain.

Beyond these conceptual considerations, research using self-report measures of attachment style has already revealed many theoretically predictable and coherent associations between attachment style and indices of implicit, unconscious processes. If the proof of the pudding is in the eating, as the adage says, or the proof of the measure is in the theoretically significant findings it generates, then the value of self-report measures of attachment style has been solidly demonstrated.

One line of research has focused on the cognitive accessibility of attachment-related representations at a particular moment—that is, their readiness to be used in information processing. According to Wegner and Smart (1997), a concept or thought can be activated and can influence mental processes before the person undergoing that activation recognizes it in his or her stream of consciousness. Therefore, the extent to which a concept or thought influences performance in cognitive tasks can serve as a measure of cognitive activation. In our case, it can provide a valid indication of implicit correlates of self-reports of attachment style.

Many attachment studies that examine implicit mental processes related to self-reported attachment style rely on the lexical decision task (Meyer & Schvaneveldt, 1971). In this task, participants view a string of letters and try to determine as quickly as possible whether it forms a word. Reaction times (RTs) serve as a measure of the accessibility of thoughts related to the target words—the quicker the RT, the higher the inferred accessibility. Using this method, six studies have clearly shown that self-reports of attachment style are related in theoretically coherent ways to implicit, unconscious attachment-related thoughts (Baldwin, Fehr, Keedian, Seidel, & Thomson, 1993; Baldwin & Meunier, 1999; Mikulincer, 1998a, 1998b; Mikulincer, Birnbaum, Woddis, & Nachmias, 2000; Mikulincer, Gillath, & Shaver, 2002). In these studies, people with a self-reported secure attachment style have exhibited relatively short lexical decision latencies (indicating heightened accessibility) for words connoting positive, relationship-enhancing responses from a partner (e.g., care, acceptance), proximity-related words (e.g., love, closeness), and names of security-enhancing attachment figures. People with a self-reported anxious attachment style, like those classified "preoccupied" on the AAI, evince heightened accessibility of concepts connoting negative responses on the part of a relationship partner (e.g., hurt, rejection) and other attachment-related worries.

Lexical decision studies have also revealed avoidant individuals' negative models of others and defensive suppression of attachment-related worries. Specifically, people with a self-reported avoidant attachment style easily access words connoting negative partner responses but are slow to access worries about separation and abandonment. They also exhibit slow RTs to attachment-related worries, even after being subliminally primed with the word "death," which for other people is a potent activator of attachment-related fears. However, these same avoidant individuals are quick to access attachment-related worries when a "cognitive load" is added to the lexical decision task (i.e., when study participants must perform an additional cognitively demanding task, which appropriates mental resources from the defensive exclusion processes normally used by avoidant people). These findings indicate that a person's self-report of avoidant attachment is a useful predictor of unconscious suppression of worries related to separation and abandonment. In other words, although the self-report measures depend on conscious self-observations, they point to individual differences in unconscious mental processes, as well.

In a second kind of study, Dolev (2001) used the well-known Stroop color-naming task (Stroop, 1938) to examine implicit, automatic manifestations of attachment styles identified with self-report measures. In this task, participants look at a word and are asked to identify as quickly as possible the color in which it is printed. Research consistently indicates that activation of a specific thought increases attention to thought-congruent stimuli and mental representations (such as words), thus leading to slower color-naming RTs for thought-relevant words in the Stroop task (e.g., Mathews & MacLeod, 1985). That is, interference with color-naming responses in the Stroop task is a valid indicator of cognitive accessibility. Dolev found that self-reports of attachment anxiety were associated with slower color-naming RTs (heightened accessibility) for words connoting worries about separation and abandonment. She also found that self-reports of attachment avoidance, which were not associated with the accessibility of attachment-related worries, became related to heightened accessibility of these worries when a "cognitive load" was added to the color-naming task.

Once again, therefore, self-reports of attachment anxiety validly predicted automatic preoccupation with attachment-related worries, whereas self-reports of attachment avoidance validly predicted defensive suppression of these worries. This suppression could be overcome by adding a cognitive load that interfered with defensive suppression. These effects are so closely related to the theoretical conception of anxiety and avoidance in attachment theory that they would be difficult to explain, as a whole, by any other theory.

Recently, Zayas, Shoda, and Ayduk (2002) used the Implicit Association Task (IAT; Greenwald, McGhee, & Schwartz, 1998)—a categorization task designed to measure the strength of automatic associations between a target concept (e.g., romantic partner) and an attribute (e.g., positive or negative traits). In this task, a strong automatic association between a target concept and an attribute implies that activation of the target concept automatically and effortlessly also activates the attribute (indicated by faster RTs to the attribute in the presence of the target concept than in the presence of a different concept). Zayas and colleagues found that self-reports of attachment avoidance, which are hypothesized to reflect negative models of others, are related to stronger automatic associations between, on the one hand, two target concepts—current romantic partner and mother—and, on the other hand, negative personal attributes. That is, self-reports of attachment avoidance accurately reflect the extent to which a significant other automatically activates representations of that person's negative attributes. It is especially interesting that this activation occurred for both romantic partner and mother, both of whom are likely to be attachment figures for most adults.

In another line of research, investigators have assessed physiological correlates of self-reports of attachment style. In particular, they have used measures of physiological arousal (e.g., heart rate, blood pressure, and skin conductance) to discover how attachment style is related to activation of the autonomic nervous system (ANS). Findings indicate that self-reports of attachment style are not just conscious fabrications. For example, Carpenter and Kirkpatrick (1996) and Feeney and Kirkpatrick (1996) found that women with self-reported anxious or avoidant attachment styles reacted with higher heart rate and blood pressure to the presence of a romantic partner in a stressful situation than did securely attached women. Moreover, Mikulincer (1998a) found that people with anxious or avoidant styles had higher heart rates following negative partner behaviors than securely attached people. These findings indicate that self-reports of what we theoretically view as insecure attachment, including avoidant attachment (which, as explained earlier, we view as defensive), are reasonable indicators of a person's discomfort in a current close relationship. The findings also confirm Bowlby's (1988) hypothesis that insecurely attached people are often distressed rather than soothed by close relationship partners.

Fraley and Shaver (1997) measured galvanic skin response (GSR), or skin conductance (caused by increased perspiration), while people sought to suppress thoughts about their romantic partner leaving them for someone else. These researchers found that self-reports of attachment style predicted underlying activation of attachment-related strategies of affect regulation. Specifically, self-reports of attachment avoidance were associated with less frequent thoughts of loss following the suppression task and lower skin conductance during the task. This study used a fairly direct measure of avoidant individuals' defensive exclusion of distress-eliciting material (a deactivating strategy) and also an indirect measure of affect regulation (decreased autonomic arousal). In contrast to attachment avoidance, attachment anxiety was associated with more frequent thoughts of loss following the suppression task and higher skin conductance during the task. This finding is compatible with the theoretical notion that anxious individuals hyperactivate attachment-related processes and then have a difficult time calming themselves down after separation-related concerns have become salient (Shaver & Mikulincer, 2002).

Another promising strategy for examining the unconscious correlates of self-reports of attachment style was used in a recent study by Gal (2002), in which 72 Israeli undergraduates completed an attachment-style scale and the well-known Rorschach (1942) Inkblot Test. The Rorschach is one of the most frequently used projective instruments for assessing a person's implicit cognitive representations, unconscious motives, and underlying mental organization (Exner, 1993).

In Gal's (2002) study, Rorschach protocols were analyzed using Exner's (1993) comprehensive scoring system, the reliability of which has been extensively documented, and the results fit well with attachment theory. First, self-reports of attachment anxiety, which are assumed to reflect hyperactivation of negative emotions, rumination on distress-related thoughts, and negative models of the self (Shaver & Mikulincer, 2002), were indeed found to be associated with Exner scores indicating distress and emotional outbursts, a tendency to react with strong emotions to person–environment transactions, lack of ability to regulate and control emotional experience, and distorted perception of the self as helpless, weak, disgusting, and unlikable. Second, self-reports of attachment avoidance, which are thought to reflect deactivation of negative emotions and defensive maintenance of self-esteem (Shaver & Mikulincer, 2002), were found to be associated with Exner scores reflecting inhibition of emotional expression, a tendency to hide behind a façade, and maintenance of a grandiose, inflated self-representation. Once again, therefore, a measure designed to tap unconscious processes, one used frequently in clinical settings, produced results that were highly compatible with both attachment theory and the validity of self-report measures of attachment style.

Although not yet definitive, the studies reviewed in this section strongly suggest that self-reports of attachment style are coherently associated with measures tapping implicit and automatic mental processes. Thus we reject the criticism that self-report measures of attachment style reflect mainly response biases or conscious attitudes and fail to correlate with implicit, unconscious aspects of attachment-system functioning.

DISMISSING AND PREOCCUPIED
INFORMATION-PROCESSING STRATEGIES

Another criticism of self-report measures of attachment style is that they do not tap the same information-processing strategies assessed by the AAI (e.g., Bernier & Dozier, 2002; Crowell & Treboux, 1995; Hesse, 1999; Jacobvitz et al., 2002). Specifically, self-report scales are viewed as ineffective instruments for assessing what Main and colleagues (1985) called "dismissing" and "preoccupied" states of mind with respect to attachment. This critique is based on the weak to moderate correlations between, on the one hand, AAI scales characterizing dismissing states of mind (parental idealization, lack of recall of attachment experiences, derogation of attachment experiences) and preoccupied states of mind (anger and passivity) and, on the other hand, self-reports of attachment style (e.g., Shaver et al., 2000). Bernier and Dozier (2002, p. 173) concluded, for example, that "the AAI and self-reports of adult attachment tap related but distinct manifestations of the attachment system."

We agree that self-reports of attachment style are not identical to the AAI. As stated before, these instruments differ in their methodology (coded interview vs. self-report questionnaire) and in the foci of the mental representations they assess (child–parent relationships vs. romantic relationships between adults). This does not mean, however, that attachment-style scales fail to relate to the information-processing strategies assessed by the AAI. In fact, although there are only modest to moderate correlations between AAI coding scales and self-report measures of attachment, recent studies that have assessed the strategies characteristic of dismissing and preoccupied attachment using techniques other than the AAI have turned up theoretically coherent associations with self-report scales. These studies, reviewed in the following paragraphs, corroborate our claim that attachment-style scales differ from the AAI in content and method but not in the core attachment-related processes they index.

One important AAI coding scale that identifies the dismissing state of mind is called "idealization of the primary attachment figure" (Main et al., 1985). According to Hesse (1999), "this scale assesses the discrepancy between the overall view of the parent taken from the subject's speech at the abstract or semantic level, and the reader's [i.e., coder's] inferences regarding the probable behavior of the parent" (p. 403). That is, parental idealization is operationalized as the discrepancy between the positivity of the traits a participant uses to describe his or her childhood relationships with mother or father and the positivity of remembered childhood experiences recounted during the interview and evaluated later by coders who have no additional knowledge about the participant's actual history.

In a recent study, we operationalized parental idealization in terms of Hesse's (1999) guidelines and examined its association with self-reports of attachment avoidance. Specifically, 60 Israeli undergraduate students completed a brief 10-item attachment-style scale (Mikulincer, Florian, & Tolmacz, 1990) during class time and were individually interviewed 2 weeks later by another researcher. In this interview, they were asked to generate five adjectives or traits that describe "your relationship with your mother during childhood." After participants wrote the five adjectives, the experimenter asked them to retrieve a "memory or experience that led you to choose each one of the traits." The experimenter then read the five adjectives and, for each one, asked participants to write a story exemplifying the way the targeted adjective applied to the childhood relationship with mother.

Participants' adjectives and narratives were subjected to content analysis. First, two psychology graduate students, who were blind to participants' attachment scores and narratives, read all of the generated adjectives and rated the hedonic tone of each one on a 7-point scale ranging from 1 (*highly negative*) to 7 (*highly positive*). Because the correlation between the two judge's ratings was high ($r = .75$), the ratings were averaged to form a single score. We then computed a total score for each participant by averaging the ratings of the five adjectives he or she generated (Cronbach's alpha = .71). The higher the score, the higher the positivity of the traits a participant generated to describe his or her relationship with mother. Second, two other psychology graduate students, blind to participants' attachment scores and the adjectives they generated, read all of the narratives and rated the hedonic tone of each narrative on a 7-point scale ranging from 1 (*highly negative*) to 7 (*highly positive*). Because the correlation between the two judges' ratings was high ($r = .78$), these ratings were also averaged to form a single score. We then computed a total score for each participant by averaging the ratings of his or her five narratives (alpha = .82). The higher the score, the higher the positivity of the memories a participant retrieved to support or exemplify the adjectives used to describe his or her relationship with mother. Third, for each adjective we computed a discrepancy score between its positivity rating and the positivity of the corresponding narrative. We then computed a total discrepancy score for each participant by averaging discrepancies for the five adjective-narrative pairs (alpha = .73). The higher this score, the more positive the adjectives were in comparison with the supposedly supporting narratives.

Table 2.1 displays Pearson correlations between participants' self-reports of attachment anxiety and avoidance, on the one hand, and the description of their relationship with mother during childhood, on the other. Attachment anxiety but not avoidance was significantly associated with the generation of less positive adjectives describing the childhood relationship with mother, but both anxiety and avoidance were significantly associated with retrieval of less positive memories of this relationship. As a result, only attachment avoidance was significantly associated with the

TABLE 2.1. Pearson Correlations between Self-Report Attachment Scores and the Description of Relationship with Mother during Childhood

Description of relationship with mother during childhood	Attachment avoidance	Attachment anxiety
Positivity of semantic description	−.08	−.31*
Positivity of narrative description	−.38**	−.33**
Discrepancy of semantic–narrative levels	.39**	.09
Time for retrieving episodic memories	.36**	−.05

*$p < .05$; **$p < .01$.

discrepancy between the adjectival and narrative descriptions of the relationship with mother. That is, the higher the self-report of avoidance, the more positive the discrepancy between adjectival and narrative descriptions, a pattern that AAI researchers interpret as indicating defensive idealization of the relationship with mother.

A second AAI coding scale used to define the dismissing state of mind is "lack of memory for childhood" (Main et al., 1985). According to Hesse (1999), "this scale assesses the speaker's insistence upon her inability to recall her childhood, especially as this insistence is used to block further queries or discourse" (p. 403). Using methods borrowed from cognitive psychology (e.g., memory retrieval times, forgetting curves), researchers who use self-report measures of attachment style have found that self-reports of avoidance are related to poor memory of childhood experiences and attachment-related information. For example, Mikulincer and Orbach (1995) found that people who characterized themselves as avoidant took longer than other people to retrieve childhood memories of sadness and anxiety. Mikulincer (1998b) found that avoidant people took longer to recall personal experiences in which attachment figures (mother, father, and romantic partner) behaved in a trustworthy manner. In the study described in the preceding paragraph, we measured the time participants took to retrieve each of the five narratives concerning the childhood relationship with mother. As expected, there was a significant correlation between self-reported attachment avoidance and longer retrieval times (see Table 2.1). Similarly, Fraley, Garner, and Shaver (2000) found that self-reports of attachment avoidance were associated with poor immediate recall of information about attachment-related threats of separation and loss.

A third AAI coding scale that defines the dismissing state of mind is "active derogating dismissal of attachment-related experiences and/or relationships." In Hesse's (1999) words, "this scale deals with the cool, contemptuous dismissal of attachment relationships or experiences and their import" (p. 403). Relevant to this scale, there is extensive evidence that self-reports of attachment avoidance are related to derogating, negative evaluations of close relationships and partners (e.g., Bartholomew & Horowitz, 1991; Collins & Read, 1990; J. A. Feeney & Noller, 1991). In a diary study in which married couples rated the quality of their relationship each day for a period of 3 weeks, Mikulincer, Florian, and Hirschberger (2002) found that self-reports of attachment avoidance were associated with daily negative appraisals of, and feelings about, the relationship. More important, even on days when a spouse's behavior indicated availability and supportiveness, avoidance was still associated with less positive appraisals and feelings toward the relationship. That is, self-reports of attachment avoidance seemed to reflect derogative dismissal of attachment-related experiences, which may have encouraged people to divert attention from attachment-related cues and ignore their spouse's positive behavior.

A similar derogative dismissal was noted by Rom and Mikulincer (2003) in their study of attachment-related group processes. In this study, self-reports of attachment avoidance were associated with poor socioemotional functioning in small groups (as assessed by external observers) and negative attitudes and feelings toward the group. Interestingly, group cohesiveness—a group-level construct reflecting the extent to which a group serves safe-haven and secure-base functions—was found to improve the socioemotional functioning of its members and foster more positive attitudes and feelings toward the group. However, whereas group cohesion tempered the negative impact of attachment anxiety, it failed to moderate the negative manifestations of attachment avoidance. That is, even in highly cohesive groups, which provided support, comfort, and emotional security to members, self-reports of attachment avoidance were still associated with poor socioemotional functioning and negative group-related attitudes and feelings. Again, self-reports of attachment avoidance seemed to be fairly accurate indicators of a person's dismissal of security-enhancing experiences.

Adult attachment research also provides consistent evidence that self-reports of attachment anxiety are associated with one of Main and colleagues' (1985) defining characteristics of the preoccupied state of mind—experience and expression of dysfunctional anger toward attachment figures. For example, Mikulincer (1998a) reported that self-reports of attachment anxiety were associated with (1) proneness to experience anger toward attachment figures, (2) uncontrollable access to and expression of anger feelings, (3) excessive rumination on anger-related thoughts, (4) hostile attitudes toward relationship partners, and (5) the experience of overwhelming distress during anger-eliciting episodes. Moreover, Woike, Osier, and Candela (1996) found that self-reported attachment anxiety was associated with a tendency to write more violent stories in response to projective Thematic Apperception Test (TAT) cards, implying a pattern of hostile fantasies. It seems that self-reports of attachment anxiety reflect the underlying action of hyperactivating strategies and the dysfunctional experience of what Bowlby (1973) called the "anger of despair."

Two observational studies of actual interactions between romantic relationship partners also provide strong evidence for the ability of self-report measures of attachment anxiety to predict dysfunctional anger toward attachment figures (Rholes, Simpson, & Orina, 1999; Simpson, Rholes, & Phillips, 1996). In Simpson and colleagues' (1996) study, anger reactions were observed during conflictual interactions in which romantic partners were asked to identify an unresolved problem in their relationship, discuss it, and try to resolve it. Self-reports of attachment anxiety were associated with the display and report of more anger, hostility, and distress during the conversation. In Rholes and colleagues' (1999) study, overt manifestations of anger were assessed among women who interacted with their romantic partners while waiting to engage in an anxiety-provoking activity. In this study, self-reports of attachment anxiety were associated with more intense anger toward partners after the couples were told that the women would not have to perform the stressful activity. This association was particularly strong when women were more upset during the waiting period or when they sought more support from their partners. Overall, the two studies indicate that self-reports of attachment anxiety are a fairly accurate indicator of anger and hostility toward a close relationship partner during conflictual interactions and in stressful situations.

The studies reviewed in this section support our contention that self-report measures of avoidance and anxiety are related to some of the most important defining characteristics of dismissing and preoccupied states of mind assessed with the AAI. Only with regard to "passivity and vagueness of discourse concerning attachment issues," one indicator of the preoccupied state of mind (Hesse, 1999), is there no study examining its association with self-reports of attachment anxiety. Further studies should examine this association by asking participants to provide verbal accounts of attachment experiences and relationships and by analyzing structural aspects of their discourse (e.g., quality, vagueness, clarity). We predict that an association with self-reported attachment anxiety will be found.

NARRATIVES ABOUT ATTACHMENT FIGURES, INTERACTIONS, AND RELATIONSHIPS

Some critics argue against the use of self-report measures because of their inability to evoke the rich, multifaceted material that appears in people's narratives about attachment experiences and relationships (e.g., Crowell & Treboux, 1995; Hesse, 1999). In their view, self-report attachment scales cannot probe a person's defenses or idiosyncratic attachment history, and researchers who use self-report measures fail to acknowledge that attachment-related processes are woven into contexts, experiences, and memories that differ importantly from person to person. We agree, of course, that the scores people receive on self-report attachment-style scales are not generated from detailed descriptions of their attachment figures and relationships or from their idiosyncratic construal of attachment experiences. We acknowledge that coded interviews, such as the AAI and the Current Relationship Interview (CRI), are more useful than simple questionnaires in characterizing a person's unique narratives and specific mental representations. This does not mean, however, that attachment-style scales are unrelated to such narratives and cannot serve as fairly accurate indicators of the way adults spontaneously recount attachment-relevant descriptions and stories. In fact, there is accumulating evidence of theoretically coherent associations between attachment-style scales and the thematic content and structure of narratives about significant others and interpersonal experiences.

Two adult attachment studies (Levy, Blatt, & Shaver, 1998; Priel & Besser, 2001) explored the contents and structure of people's open-ended descriptions of their primary attachment figures using a scoring procedure developed by Blatt and his colleagues (e.g., Blatt, Chevron, Quinlan, Schaffer, & Wein, 1992). Whereas Levy and colleagues (1998) assessed mental representations of both mother and father in a sample of American undergraduates, Priel and Besser (2001) assessed representations of mother in a sample of pregnant Israeli women. Despite the differences between the studies, their findings were extremely consistent. In line with attachment theory, self-reports of attachment anxiety and avoidance were related to negative, diffuse, and undifferentiated representations of primary attachment figures. Specifically, people who scored high on attachment anxiety or avoidance tended to view their parents as less benevolent and more punitive and to describe them in more ambivalent terms. In addition, their narratives were scored as less conceptually complex and less differentiated than those of more securely attached people. That is, attachment-style scales were able to predict theoretically significant variations in the way people represented their attachment figures in their own words.

Feeney and Noller (1991) focused on romantic relationships and examined the association between people's self-reported attachment styles and their open-ended descriptions of their current romantic relationships. The narrative descriptions were coded for spontaneous references to attachment-related issues and relationship quality. The findings indicated that self-report measures are associated with valuable information about people's unique representations of their romantic relationships and partners. The relationships described by avoidant individuals were characterized by emotional distance and lack of mutuality and intimacy, whereas the relationships described by anxious individuals were characterized by overinvolvement, dependence, and lack of enjoyment and friendship. Interestingly, people with self-reported secure styles tended to describe their romantic relationships in more balanced terms. "Secure persons tended to emphasize the importance of openness and closeness in their relationships, while at the same time seeking to retain their individual identity" (Feeney & Noller, 1991, p. 208). This result fits well with Main and colleagues' (1985; Hesse, 1999) characterization of secure AAI respondents as "free and autonomous with respect to attachment."

The correspondence between self-reports of attachment style and interpersonal narratives was also documented in a recent study by Raz (2002), who coded the Core Conflictual Relationship Themes (CCRT; Luborsky & Crits-Christoph, 1998) contained in people's narratives. Study participants completed the Relationship Questionnaire (RQ; a measure of attachment style; Bartholomew & Horowitz, 1991) and performed the Relationship Anecdotes Paradigm (RAP; Luborsky & Crits-Christoph, 1998). Specifically, participants were asked to recall three meaningful interactions with significant others and describe in each case what happened, including what they and their partner said and did. The narratives were analyzed by two independent judges who used the CCRT coding scheme to extract the three main psychodynamic components of inner representations of relational episodes: (1) *wishes*—the underlying needs, motives, and intentions that guide a person's interactions with others; (2) *responses from others*—the way the person represents the significant other during the interaction; and (3) *responses from self*—the way the person represents himself or herself in the interaction. In addition, Raz (2002) scored the main conflictual feelings and emotions that were mentioned in each participant's narratives.

The narratives generated by more anxious individuals fit closely with Mikulincer and Shaver's (2003) theoretical description of anxious, hyperactivating strategies. Specifically, self-reports of attachment anxiety were associated with wishes for security and stability; to be loved, respected, and accepted by the significant other; and not to be hurt by the other. These are the defining goals of people with hyperactivating strategies. Characterizing oneself as anxiously attached was also associated with representations of significant others as hurtful, rejecting, distant, and disapproving and representations of oneself as anxious, weak, and unloved—the negative models of self and others that define hyperactivating strategies. Raz (2002) also found that the conflictual themes in anxious people's narratives centered on doubts about self-worth, excessive seeking of closeness and reassurance, dependence, and inability to deal with interpersonal conflicts and avoid conflict escalation—the main problematic outcomes of hyperactivating strategies.

The findings for avoidant individuals were congruent with Mikulincer and Shaver's (2003) conceptualization of avoidant, deactivating strategies. Specifically, self-reports of attachment avoidance were associated with two major wishes: (1) to assert oneself and be independent and (2) to be distant and avoid conflicts. These are the goals of deactivating strategies. Self-reports of attachment avoidance were also associated with representations of significant others as disgusting, hurtful, and rejecting, as well as representations of the self as unreceptive (distant, emotionally unexpressive)—the negative model of others and the model of oneself as detached that characterize deactivating strategies. The conflictual themes of the narratives of avoidant individuals mainly emphasized protecting oneself from emotional involvement in and commitment to the relationship and a tendency to avoid conflict escalation—the main outcomes of deactivating strategies.

Other studies have also yielded theoretically predictable associations between self-reports of attachment style and narratives generated in projective tests, such as the TAT and the Separation Anxiety Test (SAT). For example, Mikulincer, Florian, and Tolmacz (1990) found that anxious and avoidant people, as compared with securely attached people, expressed more anxiety, depression, and hostility in stories they wrote in response to TAT cards evoking death anxiety; and, as mentioned earlier, Woike and colleagues (1996) found that self-reported attachment anxiety was associated with writing more violent TAT stories. Furthermore, Mayseless, Danieli, and Sharabany (1996) found that people with self-reported anxious or avoidant attachment styles portrayed less constructive coping responses in stories they wrote in response to separation reminders (SAT cards). In this study, self-reports of attachment insecurity were associated with narratives reflecting lack of ability to handle the separation episode and inability to establish a balance between self-reliance and other-reliance. In addition, whereas self-reported attachment anxiety was predictive of narratives involving hyperactivation of negative emotions in response to separation episodes, the narratives associated with self-reported avoidance implied an underlying deactivating orientation and were characterized by failing to deal effectively with the threat of separation.

In a recent study, Gilad (2002) examined the extent to which self-reports of attachment style predict the way other people are portrayed in TAT stories. Israeli high school students completed the ECR attachment scales (Brennan et al., 1998) and wrote stories in response to six TAT cards. The resulting narratives were scored according to the Social Cognition and Object Relation Scales (SCORS; Westen, 1991). The SCORS measures four dimensions of object relations (i.e., mental representations of people and aspects of important social interactions and relationships) derived from TAT stories: (1) *complexity of representations of people*—the extent to which a person defines and differentiates the perspectives of self and others, seeing self and others as having complex motives and subjective experiences; (2) *affect tone of relationship paradigms*—the extent to which an individual represents relationships as safe, nurturant, and rewarding as opposed to destructive, harmful, or threatening; (3) *capacity for emotional investment*—the extent to which close relationships are portrayed as ends rather than means and are construed in terms of mutuality rather than need gratification; and (4) *understanding of social causality*—the extent to which causal attributions of interpersonal events reflect appreciation and understanding of the ways in which thoughts and actions are linked to complex conscious and unconscious psychological operations.

Gilad (2002) found that self-reports of attachment style predict important features of the structure and content of mental representations of others, as manifested in TAT narratives. First, self-reported attachment avoidance was associated with less positive "affect tone of relationships" and lower emotional investment. That is, the TAT narratives of more avoidant people contained more negative representations of close relationships (portraying them as threatening and harmful) and indicated relatively low emotional investment. These findings fit with Mikulincer and Shaver's (2003) conceptualization of avoidant people's deactivating strategies, which rely on negative representations of others and discourage emotional investment in close relationships. In contrast, self-reported attachment anxiety was associated with lower complexity of relationship representations, less positive "affect tone of relationships," and poor understanding of social causality. That is, anxious people's TAT narratives were marked by global and undifferentiated representations of others, negative representations of close relationships (as threatening and harmful), and distorted and egocentric causal attributions for interpersonal events. These findings fit with Mikulincer and Shaver's conceptualization of anxious people's hyperactivating strategies, which are based on negative (insecure) representations of others, discourage self–other differentiation, and create a chaotic, disorganized mental architecture that interferes with an accurate understanding of relationships.

Overall, this broad array of findings strongly confirms that attachment-style scales are appropriately associated with the content and structure of people's personal representations and narratives of attachment figures and attachment-relevant experiences. This confirmation is based on a variety of qualitative methods, such as coding descriptions of significant others (parents, romantic partners), coding narratives of interpersonal interactions, and coding stories generated in response to projective tests. Moreover, the findings are consistent and coherent across a variety of scoring systems, such as Blatt and colleagues' (1992) object-representation scales, the CCRT scoring system, and the SCORS, which measure substantive and structural aspects of a person's representations of self, significant others, and close relationships. These studies provide impressive evidence for the validity of self-report attachment scales in tests of theory-derived predictions about personal narratives and mental representations.

THE SOCIALLY OBSERVABLE NATURE
OF SELF-REPORTED DIFFERENCES IN ATTACHMENT STYLE

Another purported strike against self-report attachment scales is that scores derived from them are a long way from actual social behavior (e.g., Crowell, Treboux, & Waters, 1999). That is, self-reports of attachment style, being subjective and nonbehavioral, are unlikely to index actual behavior in close relationships. In contrast, AAI coders believe not only that they are classifying people's mental and behavioral responses but also that they are doing so in ways that the people themselves could not match and, in some cases, would not agree with. This argument is raised especially vigorously in relation to dismissingly avoidant people, who are believed "to distort, disorganize, or limit access to memories, feelings, intentions, and recognition of options" (Main, 1991, p. 146). According to this view, attachment avoidance can bias self-reports of attachment style and reduce the correspondence of these reports with actual behavior. For example, people who act avoidantly in close relationships may be unaware of their avoidance or may defensively deny their detachment and coolness, and therefore they may rate themselves lower than they should on self-report items meant to detect avoidance. A similar critique might apply in the case of anxiously attached individuals, who may be reluctant to answer honestly about their anxiety because it might be viewed as weak and socially undesirable.

This criticism is amplified by the fact that research on attachment style has been dominated by correlational studies examining associations between self-report measures of attachment and other self-report measures obtained from the same individual. As a result, some of the high correlations between attachment scales and other self-report measures may be attributable to shared-method variance, including shared social desirability bias and other response set biases. Despite the plausibility of this critique, evidence is accumulating that self-reports of attachment style are related to interpersonal behavior. Moreover, some adult attachment studies have included observer evaluations in addition to self-reports and have documented considerable correspondence between the two sources of information.

Several studies have included systematic observations of attachment-related behavior and have yielded theoretically coherent associations between these observations and self-report measures of anxiety and avoidance. For example, self-reports of attachment avoidance have been associated with less frequent engagement in actual support-seeking behavior in anxiety-provoking situations—one core manifestation of deactivating strategies (Collins & Feeney, 2000; Simpson, Rholes, & Nelligan, 1992; Simpson et al., 2002). Moreover, self-reports of avoidance have been associated with less frequent engagement in actual proximity seeking—another indicator of deactivation—during separation from a romantic partner at an airport (Fraley & Shaver, 1998). The distant and emotionally uninvolved stance of self-reportedly avoidant people has been associated with less frequent verbal and nonverbal expressions of intimacy and commitment during actual conversations with a relationship partner (e.g., Grabill & Kerns, 2000; Guerrero, 1996; Mikulincer & Nachshon, 1991) and also in less frequent engagement in actual caregiving behavior in response to a partner's distress (e.g., Collins & Feeney, 2000; Feeney & Collins, 2001; Simpson et al., 1992).

Self-reports of attachment anxiety are associated with attachment-specific behaviors that follow from hyperactivating strategies. As discussed earlier, these self-reports are associated with stronger actual expressions of anger and hostility during anxiety-provoking situations and conflictual interpersonal interactions (Rholes et al., 1999; Simpson et al., 1996). Moreover, self-reports of attachment anxiety are associated with more frequent expressions of distress and anxiety during separation from a romantic partner at an airport (Fraley & Shaver, 1998) and during discussions with a romantic partner about closeness and distance (Feeney, 1998). In a recent study of married couples, Feeney and Hohaus (2001) found that self-reports of attachment anxiety are associated with a demeaning or belittling tone of voice while talking about caring for a spouse in times of need.

Another set of studies revealed high levels of convergence between self-reported attachment styles and external observers' ratings of participants' traits (e.g., Banai, Weller, & Mikulincer, 1998; Bartholomew & Horowitz, 1991; Griffin & Bartholomew, 1994; Onishi, Gjerde, & Block, 2001). For example, Banai and colleagues (1998) compared a participant's own ratings of attachment style to those made about him or her by two same-sex friends, two opposite-sex friends, and a stranger who took part in a 5-minute getting-acquainted conversation with the participant. In this study, both discrete and continuous self-descriptions of a person's attachment anxiety and avoidance were significantly related to the same descriptions of the person provided by same-sex friends, opposite-sex friends, and a new acquaintance. Even more important, high correlations were also found among the five external observers' ratings. In addition, the strength of the correlations between self-descriptions and descriptions provided by other people was similar to those found in studies of other well-known traits (e.g., Funder & Colvin, 1988). These findings indicate that self-reports of attachment anxiety and avoidance reflect real and socially observable personal attributes and that their status is similar to that of other observable personality traits. Moreover, they suggest that a person's attachment orientation, as measured by self-report scales, is evident to interaction partners even in the very early stages of a relationship.

Overall, the findings reviewed in this section refute the argument that self-reports of attachment style are not manifested in actual behavior and instead are figments of a self-observer's biased imagination. Beyond this empirical evidence, the logic of the critics' argument against self-reports is at odds with the generally accepted conceptualization of attachment-related strategies of affect regulation (Cassidy, 1994). First, the contention that avoidant individuals are reluctant to endorse avoidant items because such items are socially undesirable is inconsistent with the documented goals of interpersonal distance and emotional detachment that guide deactivating strategies (Mikulincer & Shaver, 2003). For avoidant people, being distant and cool toward a relationship partner is not a problem but a desirable way to manage close relationships. In fact, there is evidence that people who score high on avoidance scales are satisfied with cool and low-involvement relationships and tend to represent ideal relationships in terms of adequate distance and detachment (e.g., Collins & Read, 1990; Feeney & Noller, 1990). Second, the contention that anxious individuals are reluctant to endorse items indicating anxious attachment is also at odds with theoretical accounts of hyperactivating strategies, which entail presenting the self as weak, distressed, and vulnerable so as to elicit relationship partners' love and support (Mikulincer & Shaver, 2003). Research has shown that people who score high on attachment anxiety scales overemphasize problems, doubts, and worries when interacting with relationship partners (e.g., Feeney & Ryan, 1994; Simpson et al., 1996).

THE DISCRIMINANT VALIDITY
OF SELF-REPORT MEASURES OF ATTACHMENT STYLE

Beyond delineating the "nomothetic net" (Cronbach & Meehl, 1955) of theory-consistent empirical associations that establish the construct validity of attachment-style scales, attachment researchers also need to be concerned about these scales' discriminant validity. Do they overlap too much with measures of constructs viewed as theoretically unrelated to attachment organization? If so, it could be argued (e.g., Waters et al., 2002) that self-report measures of attachment style actually measure something other than individual differences in attachment-system functioning. According to Bernier and Dozier (2002), "perhaps the most widespread concern regarding attachment research is that we are tapping into a general personality construct that does not need attachment theory's rich and nuanced developmental conceptualizations to be explained" (p. 176).

Fortunately, the issue of discriminant validity has received empirical attention in adult attachment research (e.g., Griffin & Bartholomew, 1994; Shaver & Brennan, 1992). Existing studies demonstrate clearly that self-reports of attachment anxiety and avoidance, although correlating with a broad network of cognitive, emotional, and behavioral manifestations of hyperactivating and deactivating strategies, are not simply redundant with these constructs. Correlations between self-reports of attachment style and constructs derived from other theoretical or descriptive frameworks rarely exceed .50 (indicating less than 25% shared variance). This conclusion holds for associations between self-reported attachment anxiety and measures of neuroticism, trait anxiety, global distress, emotional intensity, emotion-focused ways of coping, self-esteem, self-efficacy, threat appraisal, relationship quality and satisfaction, cognitive representations of others, and intergroup attitudes (for reviews, see Feeney, 1999; Shaver & Mikulincer, 2002). It also holds for associations between self-reported avoidant attachment and measures of defensiveness, social desirability, coping by distancing, support seeking, mental representations of self and others, relationship quality, reactions to others' needs, and exploration and cognitive openness (for reviews, see Feeney, 1999; Shaver & Mikulincer, 2002).

Several studies have also shown that self-reports of anxiety and avoidance explain theory-relevant cognitions, emotions, and behaviors even after controlling statistically for attachment-irrelevant constructs. For example, Shaver and Brennan (1992) found that self-reports of attachment style were associated prospectively with relationship variables, such as relationship length, satisfaction, and commitment, even after controlling for the contribution of the "Big Five" personality traits—extraversion, neuroticism, openness to experience, agreeableness, and conscientiousness. Other studies have shown that such associations were not explained by depression, dysfunctional beliefs, self-esteem, or sex-role orientation (e.g., Carnelley, Pietromonaco, & Jaffe, 1994; Jones & Cunningham, 1996; Whisman & Allan, 1996). Moreover, behavioral observation studies conducted by Simpson and Rholes's research team showed that the association between self-reports of attachment style and interpersonal behaviors such as support seeking, support giving, and conflict resolution are not explained by the Big Five traits, by self-esteem, or by relationship quality (e.g., Simpson et al., 1992, 1996, 2002).

In many of our own studies, associations between self-reports of attachment style and creative problem solving, intergroup hostility, reactions to others' needs, accessibility of mental representations of attachment figures, rejection sensitivity, and appraisal of interpersonal competencies are all significant even after controlling for positive mood, self-esteem, or trait anxiety (e.g., Mikulincer et al., 2001; Mikulincer, Gillath, & Shaver, 2002; Mikulincer & Shaver, 2001). These findings indicate that the nomothetic net of theory-consistent correlates of attachment style cannot be explained by other constructs that are theoretically distant from attachment processes and organization.

Our recent studies on the accessibility of representations of attachment figures (Mikulincer, Gillath, & Shaver, 2002) provide a powerful test of the discriminant validity of attachment-style scales. In these studies, we assessed the cognitive accessibility of names of people whom participants listed as serving proximity-seeking, safe-haven, and/or secure-base functions (i.e., the names of security-enhancing attachment figures), names of close others who were not nominated as serving any attachment functions (close persons), and names of people a participant knew but to whom the participant was not close (acquaintances). Accessibility of mental representations of attachment figures was assessed in cognitive tasks (lexical decision, Stroop color-naming) following priming with threatening and nonthreatening stimuli. We found that self-reports of attachment style significantly predicted accessibility of the names of security-enhancing attachment figures but not the names of close persons or acquaintances, *even when general anxiety was statistically controlled.* That is, attachment-style differences assessed via self-report measures were uniquely manifested in the accessibility of representations of specific attachment figures and could not be explained by nonattachment anxiety. Thus we believe that attachment-style scales tap attachment-specific personal attributes rather than global, general cognitions and emotions.

THE DEVELOPMENTAL ORIGINS
OF SELF-REPORTED ATTACHMENT STYLE

Another frequently mentioned criticism of self-report studies of attachment is that they fail to examine the developmental roots of individual differences in anxiety and avoidance (e.g., Belsky, 2002; Bernier & Dozier, 2002). That is, although these studies provide important information about the cognitive, emotional, and behavioral manifestations of self-reported attachment patterns in adulthood, they fail to examine whether variations in these self-reports are systematically associated with childhood experiences. We agree that Bowlby (1969/1982) was deeply interested in personality development and that a core proposition of attachment theory is that attachment patterns are a function of lived experiences, especially actual experiences within the family of origin in the first few years of life. Therefore, a rigorous test of the construct validity of attachment-style scales should trace adult differences in anxiety and avoidance to childhood experiences.

Adult attachment studies have not provided much data linking self-reports of adult attachment style to measures of attachment orientation in infancy or attachment-related experiences in early childhood. Although a few AAI studies include data going back to the first year of life (e.g., Hamilton, 2000; Waters, Merrick, Treboux, Crowell, & Albersheim, 2000; Weinfield, Sroufe, & Egeland, 2000), such studies are rare, their results are inconsistent, and they provide insufficient evidence about how adult attachment patterns emerge from childhood experiences (see Fraley, 2002, for a review and meta-analysis). This is an important issue, because Bowlby's theory is not just a theory of personality structure and functioning; it is also a theory of personality development.

Although there are no systematic data on the developmental trajectory of self-reports of attachment anxiety and avoidance, there are some longitudinal studies that examine continuity and change in these self-reports during adolescence and adulthood (see Fraley & Brumbaugh, Chapter 4, this volume, for a summary). For example, Kirkpatrick and Hazan (1994) found approximately 70% continuity in self-reported attachment types in a large, heterogeneous sample of adults over a period of 4 years. In addition, they found that instability in these self-reports was associated with changes in relationship status. Davila, Burge, and Hammen (1997) noted a similar degree of continuity in a sample of at-risk adolescent girls and showed that some of the discontinuity was theoretically explicable in terms of the experience of attachment-related events or personality dispositions. Klohnen and Bera (1998) examined longitudinal data from the Mills College sample at Berkeley—a group of women who were intensively studied from age 21 to age 52—and found that a simple self-report measure of attachment style at age 52 was systematically related to theoretically relevant variables going all the way back to age 21. Collins, Cooper, Albino, and Allard (2002) found that self-reports of attachment style during adolescence (average age = 16.8 years) predicted the nature and quality of romantic relationships 6 years later, in early adulthood. In a recent study, we followed up a sample of 85 mothers who completed attachment-style scales when their infants were diagnosed as suffering from congenital heart disease and asked them to complete the same scales 7 years later. The findings revealed considerable stability in self-reports of attachment style over the 7-year period—Pearson correlations of .58 and .56 for anxiety and avoidance, respectively.

Recent studies have also provided important information about the patterns of change in self-reports of attachment orientations during adulthood. For example, Simpson, Rholes, Campbell, and Wilson (2003) focused on the transition to parenthood and asked wives and husbands expecting their first child to report on their attachment orientations 6 weeks before and 6 months after childbirth. The findings indicated that women generally became less avoidant across the transition to parenthood and that prenatal appraisal of spousal support and anger explained the way self-reports of attachment orientations changed across this transition. Specifically, whereas women who perceived less spousal support and more spousal anger during pregnancy became more anxiously attached across the transition, women who sought less spousal support during pregnancy and whose husbands were higher in avoidance became more avoidant across the transition. In addition, husbands who perceived themselves as providing more spousal support during pregnancy became less avoidant across the transition to parenthood. These findings clearly indicated that changes in self-reports of attachment orientation are systematically and coherently related to the way people perceive themselves and their relationship partners during the encounter with attachment-relevant life events.

Davila and Cobb (Chapter 5, this volume) also emphasize the importance of a person's subjective construal of life events in explaining changes in self-reports of attachment orientation during adulthood. According to these authors, a life event can change self-reports of attachment orientation to the extent to which a person construes this event as disconfirming his or her attachment-relevant expectations. In support of this view, Davila and Cobb reported findings of an 8-week daily diary study, during which people reported on daily life events and daily levels of attachment security (Davila & Sargent, 2003). Although daily events and daily levels of attachment security covaried over time, this association was explained by the extent to which people appraised the events as involving interpersonal loss. As Davila and Cobb (Chapter 5, this volume) concluded, "this implies that it may not be life events per se that influence change but individuals' perceptions of changes in the interpersonal context that result in modifications of attachment models" (p. 144).

There are also a number of retrospective studies that assess the extent to which individual differences in self-reports of attachment style in adulthood are associated with specific attachment-relevant childhood experiences. These studies have consistently found, for example, that retrospective reports of sexual or physical abuse during childhood or adolescence are associated with heightened reports of attachment anxiety and avoidance in clinical and community samples (e.g., Mallinckrodt, McCreary, & Robertson, 1995; Roche, Runtz, & Hunter, 1999; Shaver & Clark, 1994; Swanson & Mallinckrodt, 2001). There is also evidence that heightened reports of attachment insecurity in adulthood are related to the occurrence of childhood experiences that are theoretically expected to have a long-term disturbing effect on the development of attachment security, such as parental drinking problems (Brennan, Shaver, & Tobey, 1991), parental death (Brennan & Shaver, 1998), and parental divorce (Brennan & Shaver, 1998; Lopez, Melendez, & Rice, 2000). However, other studies have failed to find an association between parental divorce and self-reported attachment style in adulthood (e.g., Brennan & Shaver, 1993; Tayler, Parker, & Roy, 1995).

Studies conducted in Mikulincer's laboratory in Israel revealed that young adults who experienced the deaths of their fathers or the divorces of their parents before age 4 reported higher attachment anxiety and avoidance than young adults who grew up in intact families or whose parents divorced after age 4 (see Table 2.2). In addition, young adults who were raised with communal sleeping arrangements in Israeli kibbutzim—an ecological factor that was found to disrupt secure attachment in childhood (Sagi, van IJzendoorn, Aviezer, & Donnell, 1994)—scored higher on scales of attachment anxiety and avoidance than young adults who grew up in kibbutzim where family sleeping arrangements were the norm (see Table 2.2). A similar pattern of findings was recently reported in a study of young Israeli women (Sharabany, Mayseless, Edri, & Lulav, 2001).

These studies are not sufficient to make a strong case for continuity, change, or developmental origins of self-reports of adult attachment patterns. They suggest, however, that prospective studies should turn up theoretically meaningful childhood antecedents of adult patterns. A recent conference paper (Sampson, 2003) provides an example: The author reported a 20-year correlation coefficient of .44 between observed parental

TABLE 2.2. Means and Standard Deviations of Self-Report Attachment Scores According to Study Groups

Study groups	n	Attachment avoidance		Attachment anxiety	
		M	SD	M	SD
Paternal death study					
Death of father before child's age 4	50	3.76	1.24	3.87	1.25
Intact family	50	3.02	1.27	3.09	1.24
$F(1, 98)$		8.57**		9.79**	
Parental divorce study					
Divorce before child's age 4	40	3.89	1.29	3.96	1.38
Divorce between ages 4 and 9	40	3.01	0.97	3.27	1.31
Divorce after age 10	40	2.88	1.20	3.18	1.32
Intact family	40	3.05	1.26	3.13	1.25
$F(3, 156)$		6.02**		3.53*	
Sleeping arrangement study					
Communal sleeping arrangement	55	3.58	1.32	3.79	1.17
Family sleeping arrangement	55	2.94	1.23	3.16	1.15
$F(1, 108)$		6.80*		8.12*	

*$p < .05$; **$p < .01$.

support at age 2 and self-reported comfort with depending on romantic partners in early adulthood, the latter being part of Collins and Read's (1990) self-report measure of nonavoidant attachment.

Nevertheless, even when additional longitudinal studies have traced self-reports of attachment anxiety and avoidance back to childhood experiences, we do not expect the developmental trajectories of these self-reports to be simple (see Fraley & Brumbaugh, Chapter 4, this volume, for systematic modeling and discussion of the dynamics of these trajectories). In our view, adult attachment patterns are likely to be affected by childhood experiences, adolescent experiences, recent experiences in adult relationships, and a broad array of contextual factors that can moderate or even override the effects of internalized representations of past experiences. In fact, Bowlby (1988) claimed that working models can be updated throughout life and that attachment relationships in adulthood can affect the organization and functioning of the attachment system. If this were not the case, psychotherapy—including the therapy conducted by Bowlby himself—would be useless. Individual longitudinal studies of the development of attachment style would be informative, but no single study is likely to reveal the numerous, complex determinants of this construct, especially as it is manifested under varying circumstances in adulthood.

CONCLUSION

There is substantial and growing evidence that criticisms of self-report attachment measures advanced by researchers from the AAI tradition are exaggerated, if not completely invalid. Our review of empirical data indicates that self-report measures are reasonably accurate indicators of (1) unconscious, implicit attachment-relevant processes, (2) dismissing and preoccupied strategies of information processing, and (3) thematic and structural properties of a person's narratives concerning attachment experiences and relationships. Our review also reveals that individual differences in self-report attachment scores are associated with observable interpersonal behavior, cannot be explained by alternative constructs and theories unrelated to the organization and functioning of the attachment system, and are predicted by relevant childhood experiences (e.g., abuse, losses). These findings add to the construct validity of self-report attachment measures and bolster our confidence in these measures as suitable instruments for exploring the psychodynamics and interpersonal processes addressed by attachment theory.

Despite the lack of empirical grounds for dismissing the self-report approach, further work is still needed to improve self-report measures. First, there is still some debate about the underlying dimensions of self-report attachment measures. Whereas most recent adult attachment studies are based on a two-dimensional model of anxiety (or model of self) and avoidance (or model of other), some studies suggest that it might be useful to rotate the axes of the measurement space and assess individual variations in security–insecurity and anxiety–avoidance (e.g., Asendorpf, Banse, Wilpers, & Neyer, 1997; Banse, 2004; Elizur & Mintzer, 2003). For example, Asendorpf and colleagues (1997) consistently found, for various samples including married couples, that the data fit a model in which a primary secure–fearful (security–insecurity) dimension was crossed by a secondary anxiety–avoidance (or preoccupied–dismissing) dimension. In this model, all of the insecure styles correlated negatively with the secure style. This 45-degree rotation of the measurement axes fits well with the process model proposed by Shaver and Mikulincer (2002; reproduced here in Figure 2.1), a model in which the appraisal of threat, attachment figure availability, and feasibility of hyperactivating and deactivating strategies occur in sequence. The rotated axes are also congruent with Kobak, Cole, Ferenz-Gillies, Fleming, and Gamble's (1993) and Fyffe and Waters's (1997) two-dimensional scoring systems for the AAI.

Second, researchers should attempt to assess both relationship-specific and generalized self-reports of attachment style and then examine the hierarchical arrangement of attachment working models first delineated by Collins and Read (1994). In a recent study, Overall, Fletcher, and Friesen (2003) provided initial evidence concerning the cognitive organization of attachment representations. They asked participants to complete self-reports of attachment style for three specific relationships within each of three domains—family, friendship, and romantic—and then examined whether all these measures were organized within (1) a single, global working model summarizing attachment orientations across relationships and domains; (2) three independent working models for the domains of family, friendship, and romantic relationships; or (3) a hierarchical arrangement of specific and global working models. Confirmatory factor analyses showed that the hierarchical model fit the data best, indicating that ratings of attachment orientations for specific relationships are nested within, or organized under, relationship-domain representations, which in turn are nested within, or organized under, a single, global attachment working model. Further studies should extend this pioneering work.

Third, it would be useful in future studies to examine the effects of different instructions on self-report ratings of attachment style. Should such instructions refer to a specific relationship, to one's history of romantic relationships, or to all close relationships? Some of our studies show that attachment style can be meaningfully measured at a fairly abstract level, with the resulting scores relating predictably to intergroup tolerance, responses to others' needs, and interpersonal behavior (e.g.,

Mikulincer & Nachshon, 1991; Mikulincer et al., 2001; Mikulincer & Shaver, 2001). Thus secure and insecure attachment orientations are relevant to much more than primary attachment relationships. This discovery seems to bother some attachment researchers (e.g., Waters et al., 2002) because they think of attachment as a feature of only a few very close relationships, but to us it opens the door to important conceptual links between attachment theory and other phenomena of interest to social psychologists.

Fourth, researchers should attempt to extend the use of self-report attachment measures to different age groups (children, elderly adults) and cultures and to adapt existing measures for use in different cultures. The applicability of infant–parent attachment theory to non-Western cultures has been documented and debated (e.g., Rothbaum, Weisz, Pott, Miyake, & Morelli, 2000; van IJzendoorn & Sagi, 1999), but cross-cultural studies of adult attachment are relatively rare.

Finally, researchers should look more carefully at detailed relations between AAI scores, including coder rating scales and secure–insecure and dismissing–preoccupied dimension scores, on the one hand, and self-reported avoidance and anxiety scores, on the other. Moreover, relations between these two kinds of measures and other experimental, physiological, and behavioral measures should be examined. In this way, we will learn more about the dynamics of the attachment system and the ways in which it can be revealed by various kinds of measures.

ACKNOWLEDGMENT

Preparation of this chapter was facilitated by a grant from the Fetzer Institute.

REFERENCES

Armsden, G. C., & Greenberg, M. T. (1987). The Inventory of Parent and Peer Attachment: Relationships to well-being in adolescence. *Journal of Youth and Adolescence, 16,* 427–454.

Asendorpf, J. B., Banse, R., Wilpers, S., & Neyer, F. J. (1997). Beziehungsspezifische Bindungsskalen fuer Erwachsene und ihre Validierung durch Netzwerk-und Tagebuchverfahren [Relationship-specific attachment scales for adults and their validation with network and diary procedures]. *Diagnostica, 43,* 289–313.

Baldwin, M. W., Fehr, B., Keedian, E., Seidel, M., & Thomson, D. W. (1993). An exploration of the relational schemata underlying attachment styles: Self-report and lexical decision approaches. *Personality and Social Psychology Bulletin, 19,* 746–754.

Baldwin, M. W., & Meunier, J. (1999). The cued activation of attachment relational schemas. *Social Cognition, 17,* 209–227.

Banai, E., Weller, A., & Mikulincer, M. (1998). Interjudge agreement in evaluation of adult attachment style: The impact of acquaintanceship. *British Journal of Social Psychology, 37,* 95–109.

Banse, R. (2004). Adult attachment and marital satisfaction: Evidence for dyadic configuration effects. *Journal of Social and Personal Relationships, 21,* 273–282.

Bartholomew, K., & Horowitz, L. M. (1991). Attachment styles among young adults: A test of a four-category model. *Journal of Personality and Social Psychology, 61,* 226–244.

Bartholomew, K., & Shaver, P. R. (1998). Methods of assessing adult attachment: Do they converge? In J. A. Simpson & W. S. Rholes (Eds.), *Attachment theory and close relationships* (pp. 25–45). New York: Guilford Press.

Belsky, J. (2002). Developmental origins of attachment styles. *Attachment and Human Development, 4,* 166–170.

Bernier, A., & Dozier, M. (2002). Assessing adult attachment: Empirical sophistication and conceptual bases. *Attachment and Human Development, 4,* 171–179.

Blatt, S. J., Chevron, S. E., Quinlan, D. M., Schaffer, C. E., & Wein, S. (1992). *The assessment of qualitative and structural dimensions of object representations.* Unpublished manuscript, Yale University.

Bowlby, J. (1973). *Attachment and loss: Vol. 2. Separation: Anxiety and anger.* New York: Basic Books.

Bowlby, J. (1982). *Attachment and loss: Vol. 1. Attachment* (2nd ed.). New York: Basic Books.

Bowlby, J. (1988). *A secure base: Clinical applications of attachment theory.* London: Routledge.

Brennan, K. A., Clark, C. L., & Shaver, P. R. (1998). Self-report measurement of adult attachment: An integrative overview. In J. A. Simpson & W. S. Rholes (Eds.), *Attachment theory and close relationships* (pp. 46–76). New York: Guilford Press.

Brennan, K. A., & Shaver, P. R. (1993). Attachment styles and parental divorce. *Journal of Divorce and Remarriage, 21,* 161–175.

Brennan, K. A., & Shaver, P. R. (1998). Attachment styles and personality disorders: Their connections to each other and to parental divorce, parental death, and perceptions of parental caregiving. *Journal of Personality, 66,* 835–878.

Brennan, K. A., Shaver, P. R., & Tobey, A. E. (1991). Attachment styles, gender, and parental problem drinking. *Journal of Social and Personal Relationships, 8,* 451–466.

Carnelley, K. B., Pietromonaco, P. R., & Jaffe, K. (1994). Depression, working models of others, and relationship functioning. *Journal of Personality and Social Psychology, 66,* 127–140.

Carpenter, E. M., & Kirkpatrick, L. A. (1996). Attachment style and presence of a romantic partner as moderators of psychophysiological responses to a stressful laboratory situation. *Personal Relationships, 3,* 351–367.

Cassidy, J. (1994). Emotion regulation: Influences of attachment relationships. *Monographs of the Society for Research in Child Development, 59,* 228–283.

Cassidy, J., & Kobak, R. R. (1988). Avoidance and its relationship with other defensive processes. In J. Belsky & T. Nezworski (Eds.), *Clinical implications of attachment* (pp. 300–323). Hillsdale, NJ: Erlbaum.

Chartrand, T. L., & Bargh, J. A. (2002). Nonconscious motivations: Their activation, operation, and consequences. In A. Tesser & D. A. Stapel (Eds.), *Self and motivation: Emerging psychological perspectives* (pp. 13–41). Washington, DC: American Psychological Association.

Collins, N. L., Cooper, M. L., Albino, A., & Allard, L. (2002). Psychosocial vulnerability from adolescence to adulthood: A prospective study of attachment style differences in relationship functioning and partner choice. *Journal of Personality, 70,* 965–1008.

Collins, N. L., & Feeney, B. C. (2000). A safe haven: An attachment theory perspective on support seeking and caregiving in intimate relationships. *Journal of Personality and Social Psychology, 78,* 1053–1073.

Collins, N. L., & Read, S. J. (1990). Adult attachment, working models, and relationship quality in dating couples. *Journal of Personality and Social Psychology, 58,* 644–663.

Collins, N. L., & Read, S. J. (1994). Cognitive representations of attachment: The structure and function of working models. In K. Bartholomew & D. Perlman (Eds.), *Advances in personal relationships: Vol. 5. Attachment processes in adulthood* (pp. 53–92). London: Kingsley.

Cronbach, L. J., & Meehl, P. E. (1955). Construct validity in psychological tests. *Psychological Bulletin, 52,* 281–302.

Crowell, J. A., Fraley, R. C., & Shaver, P. R. (1999). Measurement of adult attachment. In J. Cassidy & P. R. Shaver (Eds.), *Handbook of attachment: Theory, research, and clinical applications* (pp. 434–465). New York: Guilford Press.

Crowell, J. A., & Treboux, D. (1995). A review of adult attachment measures: Implications for theory and research. *Social Development, 4,* 294–327.

Crowell, J. A., Treboux, D., Gao, Y., Fyffe, C., Pan, H., & Waters, E. (2002). Assessing secure base behavior in adulthood: Development of a measure, links to adult attachment representations, and relations to couples' communication and reports of relationships. *Developmental Psychology, 38,* 679–693.

Crowell, J. A., Treboux, D., & Waters, E. (1999). The Adult Attachment Interview and the Relationship Questionnaire: Relations to reports of mothers and partners. *Personal Relationships, 6,* 1–18.

Crowell, J. A., Treboux, D., & Waters, E. (2002). Stability of attachment representations: The transition to marriage. *Developmental Psychology, 38,* 467–479.

Davila, J., Burge, D., & Hammen, C. (1997). Why does attachment style change? *Journal of Personality and Social Psychology, 73,* 826–838.

Davila, J., & Sargent, E. (2003). The meaning of life (events) predicts change in attachment security. *Personality and Social Psychology Bulletin, 29,* 1383–1395.

Dolev, T. (2001). *Adult attachment style and the suppression of separation-related thoughts in the Stroop task: The moderating effects of cognitive load.* Unpublished master's thesis, Bar-Ilan University, Ramat Gan, Israel.

Elizur, Y., & Mintzer, A. (2003). Gay males' intimate relationship quality: The roles of attachment security, gay identity, and social support. *Personal Relationships, 10,* 411–435.

Exner, J. E., Jr. (1993). *The Rorschach: A comprehensive system, Vol. 1. Basic foundations* (3rd ed.). Oxford, UK: Wiley.

Feeney, B. C., & Collins, N. L. (2001). Predictors of caregiving in adult intimate relationships: An attachment theoretical perspective. *Journal of Personality and Social Psychology, 80,* 972–994.

Feeney, B. C., & Kirkpatrick, L. A. (1996). Effects of adult attachment and presence of romantic partners on physiological responses to stress. *Journal of Personality and Social Psychology, 70,* 255–270.

Feeney, J. A. (1998). Adult attachment and relationship-centered anxiety: Responses to physical and emotional distancing. In J. A. Simpson & W. S. Rholes (Eds.), *Attachment theory and close relationships* (pp. 189–218). New York: Guilford Press.

Feeney, J. A. (1999). Adult romantic attachment and couple relationships. In J. Cassidy & P. R. Shaver (Eds.), *Handbook of attachment: Theory, research, and clinical applications* (pp. 355–377). New York: Guilford Press.

Feeney, J. A., & Hohaus, L. (2001). Attachment and spousal caregiving. *Personal Relationships, 8,* 21–39.

Feeney, J. A., & Noller, P. (1990). Attachment style as a predictor of adult romantic relationships. *Journal of Personality and Social Psychology, 58,* 281–291.

Feeney, J. A., & Noller, P. (1991). Attachment style and verbal descriptions of romantic partners. *Journal of Social and Personal Relationships, 8,* 187–215.

Feeney, J. A., Noller, P., & Hanrahan, M. (1994). Assessing adult attachment. In M. B. Sperling & W. H. Berman (Eds.), *Attachment in adults: Clinical and developmental perspectives* (pp. 128–152). New York: Guilford Press.

Feeney, J. A., & Ryan, S. M. (1994). Attachment style and affect regulation: Relationships with health behavior and family experiences of illness in a student sample. *Health Psychology, 13,* 334–345.

Fraley, R. C. (2002). Attachment stability from infancy to adulthood: Meta-analysis and dynamic modeling of developmental mechanisms. *Personality and Social Psychology Review, 6,* 123–151.

Fraley, R. C., Garner, J. P., & Shaver, P. R. (2000). Adult attachment and the defensive regulation of attention and memory: Examining the role of preemptive and postemptive defensive processes. *Journal of Personality and Social Psychology, 79,* 816–826.

Fraley, R. C., & Shaver, P. R. (1997). Adult attachment and the suppression of unwanted thoughts. *Journal of Personality and Social Psychology, 73,* 1080–1091.

Fraley, R. C., & Shaver, P. R. (1998). Airport separations: A naturalistic study of adult attachment dynamics in separating couples. *Journal of Personality and Social Psychology, 75,* 1198–1212.

Funder, D. C., & Colvin, C. R. (1988). Friends and strangers: Acquaintanceship, agreement, and the accuracy of personality judgment. *Journal of Personality and Social Psychology, 55, 149–158.*

Fyffe, C., & Waters, E. (1997, April). *Empirical classification of adult attachment status: Predicting group membership.* Poster presented at the meeting of the Society for Research in Child Development, Washington, DC.

Gal, Y. (2002). *Emotional and cognitive manifestations of adult attachment styles in the*

Rorschach test. Unpublished master's thesis, Bar-Ilan University, Ramat Gan, Israel.

George, C., Kaplan, N., & Main, M. (1985). *The Adult Attachment Interview* (2nd ed.). Unpublished manuscript, University of California, Berkeley.

George, C., & Solomon, J. (1999). Attachment and caregiving: The caregiving behavioral system. In J. Cassidy & P. R. Shaver (Eds.), *Handbook of attachment: Theory, research, and clinical applications* (pp. 649–670). New York: Guilford Press.

Gilad, G. (2002). *The integration of object relations theory and attachment theory: Object representations in the Thematic Apperception Test.* Unpublished master's thesis, Bar-Ilan University, Ramat Gan, Israel.

Grabill, C. M., & Kerns, K. A. (2000). Attachment style and intimacy in friendship. *Personal Relationships, 7,* 363–378.

Greenwald, A. G., McGhee, D. E., & Schwartz, J. L. K. (1998). Measuring individual differences in implicit cognition: The Implicit Association Test. *Journal of Personality and Social Psychology, 74,* 1464–1480.

Griffin, D. W., & Bartholomew, K. (1994). Models of the self and other: Fundamental dimensions underlying measures of adult attachment. *Journal of Personality and Social Psychology, 67,* 430–445.

Guerrero, L. K. (1996). Attachment-style differences in intimacy and involvement: A test of the four-category model. *Communication Monographs, 63,* 269–292.

Hamilton, C. (2000). Continuity and discontinuity of attachment from infancy to adolescence. *Child Development, 71,* 690–694.

Hazan, C., & Shaver, P. R. (1987). Romantic love conceptualized as an attachment process. *Journal of Personality and Social Psychology, 52,* 511–524.

Hesse, E. (1999). The Adult Attachment Interview: Historical and current perspectives. In J. Cassidy & P. R. Shaver (Eds.), *Handbook of attachment: Theory, research, and clinical applications* (pp. 395–433). New York: Guilford Press.

Jacobvitz, D., Curran, M., & Moller, N. (2002). Measurement of adult attachment: The place of self-report and interview methodologies. *Attachment and Human Development, 4,* 207–215.

Jones, J. T., & Cunningham, J. D. (1996). Attachment styles and other predictors of relationship satisfaction in dating couples. *Personal Relationships, 3,* 387–399.

Kirkpatrick, L. A., & Hazan, C. (1994). Attachment styles and close relationships: A four-year prospective study. *Personal Relationships, 1,* 123–142.

Klohnen, E. C., & Bera, S. (1998). Behavioral and experiential patterns of avoidantly and securely attached women across adulthood: A 31-year longitudinal perspective. *Journal of Personality and Social Psychology, 74,* 211–223.

Kobak, R. R., Cole, H. E., Ferenz-Gillies, R., Fleming, W. S., & Gamble, W. (1993). Attachment and emotion regulation during mother–teen problem solving: A control theory analysis. *Child Development, 64,* 231–245.

Levy, K. N., Blatt, S. J., & Shaver, P. R. (1998). Attachment styles and parental representations. *Journal of Personality and Social Psychology, 74,* 407–419.

Lopez, F. G., Melendez, M. C., & Rice, K. G. (2000). Parental divorce, parent–child bonds, and adult attachment orientations among college students: A comparison of three racial/ethnic groups. *Journal of Counseling Psychology, 47,* 177–186.

Luborsky, L., & Crits-Christoph, P. (1998). *Understanding transference: The Core Conflictual Relationship Theme method.* Washington, DC: American Psychological Association.

Lyons-Ruth, K., & Jacobvitz, D. (1999). Attachment disorganization: Unresolved loss, relational violence, and lapses in behavioral and attentional strategies. In J. Cassidy & P. R. Shaver (Eds.), *Handbook of attachment: Theory, research, and clinical applications* (pp. 520–554). New York: Guilford Press.

Main, M. (1991). Metacognitive knowledge, metacognitive monitoring, and singular (coherent) vs. multiple (incoherent) models of attachment: Findings and directions for future research. In C. M. Parkes, J. Stevenson-Hinde, & P. Marris (Eds.), *Attachment across the life cycle* (pp. 127–159). London: Tavistock/Routledge.

Main, M., Kaplan, N., & Cassidy, J. (1985). Security in infancy, childhood, and adulthood: A move to the level of representation. *Monographs of the Society for Research in Child Development, 50*(1 & 2, Serial No. 209), 66–104.

Mallinckrodt, B., McCreary, B. A., & Robertson, A. K. (1995). Co-occurrence of eating disorders and incest: The role of attachment, family environment, and social competencies. *Journal of Counseling Psychology, 42,* 178–186.

Mathews, A., & MacLeod, C. (1985). Selective processing of threat cues in anxiety states. *Behavior Research and Therapy, 23,* 563–569.

Mayseless, O., Danieli, R., & Sharabany, R. (1996). Adults' attachment patterns: Coping with separations. *Journal of Youth and Adolescence, 25,* 667–690.

Meyer, D. E., & Schvaneveldt, R. W. (1971). Facilitation in recognizing pairs of words: Evidence of dependence between retrieval operations. *Journal of Experimental Psychology, 90,* 227–234.

Mikulincer, M. (1998a). Adult attachment style and individual differences in functional versus dysfunctional experiences of anger. *Journal of Personality and Social Psychology, 74,* 513–524.

Mikulincer, M. (1998b). Attachment working models and the sense of trust: An exploration of interaction goals and affect regulation. *Journal of Personality and Social Psychology, 74,* 1209–1224.

Mikulincer, M., Birnbaum, G., Woddis, D., & Nachmias, O. (2000). Stress and accessibility of proximity-related thoughts: Exploring the normative and intraindividual components of attachment theory. *Journal of Personality and Social Psychology, 78,* 509–523.

Mikulincer, M., Florian, V., & Hirschberger, G. (2002, January). *The dynamic interplay of global, relationship-specific, and contextual representations of attachment security.* Paper presented at the annual meeting of the Society for Personality and Social Psychology, Savannah, GA.

Mikulincer, M., Florian, V., & Tolmacz, R. (1990). Attachment styles and fear of personal death: A case study of affect regulation. *Journal of Personality and Social Psychology, 58,* 273–280.

Mikulincer, M., Gillath, O., Halevy, V., Avihou, N., Avidan, S., & Eshkoli, N. (2001). Attachment theory and reactions to others' needs: Evidence that activation of the sense of attachment security promotes empathic responses. *Journal of Personality and Social Psychology, 81,* 1205–1224.

Mikulincer, M., Gillath, O., & Shaver, P. R. (2002). Activation of the attachment system in adulthood: Threat-related primes increase the accessibility of mental representations of attachment figures. *Journal of Personality and Social Psychology, 83,* 881–895.

Mikulincer, M., & Nachshon, O. (1991). Attachment styles and patterns of self-disclosure. *Journal of Personality and Social Psychology, 61,* 321–331.

Mikulincer, M., & Orbach, I. (1995). Attachment styles and repressive defensiveness: The accessibility and architecture of affective memories. *Journal of Personality and Social Psychology, 68,* 917–925.

Mikulincer, M., & Shaver, P. R. (2001). Attachment theory and intergroup bias: Evidence that priming the secure base schema attenuates negative reactions to out-groups. *Journal of Personality and Social Psychology, 81,* 97–115.

Mikulincer, M., & Shaver, P. R. (2003). The attachment behavioral system in adulthood: Activation, psychodynamics, and interpersonal processes. In M. P. Zanna (Ed.), *Advances in experimental social psychology* (Vol. 35, pp. 53–152). New York: Academic Press.

Morf, C. C., & Rhodewalt, F. (2001). Unraveling the paradoxes of narcissism: A dynamic self-regulatory processing model. *Psychological Inquiry, 12,* 177–196.

Onishi, M., Gjerde, P. F., & Block, J. (2001). Personality implications of romantic attachment patterns in young adults: A multi-method, multi-informant study. *Personality and Social Psychology Bulletin, 27,* 1097–1110.

Overall, N. C., Fletcher, G. J. O., & Friesen, M. (2003). Mapping the intimate relationship mind: Comparisons between three models of attachment representations. *Personality and Social Psychology Bulletin, 29,* 1479–1493.

Pottharst, K. (Ed.). (1990). *Explorations in adult attachment.* New York: Peter Lang.

Priel, B., & Besser, A. (2001). Bridging the gap between attachment and object relations theories: A study of the transition to motherhood. *British Journal of Medical Psychology, 74,* 85–100.

Raz, A. (2002). *Personality, core relationship themes, and interpersonal competence among young adults experiencing difficulties in establishing long-term relationships.* Unpublished doctoral dissertation, Haifa University, Haifa, Israel.

Rholes, W. S., Simpson, J. A., & Oriña, M. M. (1999). Attachment and anger in an anxiety-provoking situation. *Journal of Personality and Social Psychology, 76,* 940–957.

Roche, D. N., Runtz, M. G., & Hunter, M. A. (1999). Adult attachment: A mediator between child sexual abuse and later psychological adjustment. *Journal of Interpersonal Violence, 14,* 184–207.

Rom, E., & Mikulincer, M. (2003). Attachment theory and group processes: The association between attachment style and group-related representations, goals, memories, and functioning. *Journal of Personality and Social Psychology, 84,* 1220–1235.

Rorschach, H. (1942). *Psychodiagnostics: A diagnostic test based on perception* (P. Lenkau & B. Kroneberg, Trans.). New York: Grune & Stratton.

Rothbaum, F., Weisz, J., Pott, M., Miyake, K., & Morelli, G. (2000). Attachment and culture: Security in the United States and Japan. *American Psychologist, 55,* 1093–1104.

Sagi, A., van IJzendoorn, M. H., Aviezer, O., & Donnell, F. (1994). Sleeping out of home in a kibbutz communal arrangement: It makes a difference for infant–mother attachment. *Child Development, 65,* 992–1004.

Sampson, M. C. (2003, April). *Examining early correlates of self-report measures of adult attachment: A prospective longitudinal view.* Poster presented at the meeting of the Society for Research in Child Development, Tampa, FL.

Sharabany, R., Mayseless, O., Edri, G., & Lulav, D. (2001). Ecology, childhood experiences, and adult attachment styles of women in the kibbutz. *International Journal of Behavioral Development, 25,* 214–225.

Shaver, P. R., Belsky, J., & Brennan, K.A. (2000). The Adult Attachment Interview and self-reports of romantic attachment: Associations across domains and methods. *Personal Relationships, 7,* 25–43.

Shaver, P. R., & Brennan, K. A. (1992). Attachment styles and the "big five" personality traits: Their connections with each other and with romantic relationship outcomes. *Personality and Social Psychology Bulletin, 18,* 536–545.

Shaver, P. R., & Clark, C. L. (1994). The psychodynamics of adult romantic attachment. In J. M. Masling & R. F. Bornstein (Eds.), *Empirical perspectives on object relations theories* (pp. 105–156). Washington, DC: American Psychological Association.

Shaver, P. R., & Mikulincer, M. (2002). Attachment-related psychodynamics. *Attachment and Human Development, 4,* 133–161.

Simpson, J. A. (1990). The influence of attachment styles on romantic relationships. *Journal of Personality and Social Psychology, 59,* 971–980.

Simpson, J. A., Rholes, W. S., Campbell, L., & Wilson, C. L. (2003). Changes in attachment orientations across the transition to parenthood. *Journal of Experimental Social Psychology, 39,* 317–331.

Simpson, J. A., Rholes, W. S., & Nelligan, J. S. (1992). Support seeking and support giving within couples in an anxiety-provoking situation: The role of attachment styles. *Journal of Personality and Social Psychology, 62,* 434–446.

Simpson, J. A., Rholes, W. S., Orina, M. M., & Grich, J. (2002). Working models of attachment, support giving, and support seeking in a stressful situation. *Personality and Social Psychology Bulletin, 28,* 598–608.

Simpson, J. A., Rholes, W. S., & Phillips, D. (1996). Conflict in close relationships: An attachment perspective. *Journal of Personality and Social Psychology, 71,* 899–914.

Stroop, J. R. (1938). Factors affecting speed in serial verbal reactions. *Psychological Monographs, 50,* 38–48

Swanson, B., & Mallinckrodt, B. (2001). Family environment, love withdrawal, childhood sexual abuse, and adult attachment. *Psychotherapy Research, 11,* 455–472.

Tayler, L., Parker, G., & Roy, K. (1995). Parental divorce and its effects on the quality of intimate relationships in adulthood. *Journal of Divorce and Remarriage, 24,* 181–202.

van IJzendoorn, M. H. (1995). Adult attachment representations, parental responsiveness, and infant attachment: A meta-analysis on the predictive validity of the Adult Attachment Interview. *Psychological Bulletin, 117,* 387–403.

van IJzendoorn, M. H., & Sagi, A. (1999). Cross-cultural patterns of attachment: Universal and contextual dimensions. In J. Cassidy & P. R. Shaver (Eds.), *Handbook of attachment: Theory, research, and clinical applications* (pp. 713–734). New York: Guilford Press.

Waters, E., Crowell, J.A., Elliott, M., Corcoran, D., & Treboux, D. (2002). Bowlby's secure base theory and the social/personality psychology of attachment styles: Work(s) in progress. *Attachment and Human Development, 4,* 230–242.

Waters, E., Merrick, S., Treboux, D., Crowell, J., & Albersheim, L. (2000). Attachment security in infancy and early adulthood: A twenty-year longitudinal study. *Child Development, 71,* 684–689.

Wegner, D. M., & Smart, L. (1997). Deep cognitive activation: A new approach to the unconscious. *Journal of Consulting and Clinical Psychology, 65,* 984–995.

Weinfield, N. S., Sroufe, L. A., & Egeland, B. (2000). Attachment from infancy to early adulthood in a high-risk sample: Continuity, discontinuity, and their correlates. *Child Development, 71,* 695–702.

West, M. L., Sheldon, A. E. R., & Reiffer, L. (1987). An approach to the delineation of adult attachment: Scale development and reliability. *Journal of Nervous and Mental Disease, 175,* 738–741.

Westen, D. (1991). Clinical assessment of object relations using the TAT. *Journal of Personality Assessment, 56,* 56–74.

Whisman, M. A., & Allan, L. E. (1996). Attachment and social cognition theories of romantic relationships: Convergent or complementary perspectives? *Journal of Social and Personal Relationships, 13,* 263–278.

Woike, B. A., Osier, T. J., & Candela, K. (1996). Attachment styles and violent imagery in thematic stories about relationships. *Personality and Social Psychology Bulletin, 22,* 1030–1034.

Zayas, V., Shoda, Y., & Ayduk, O. N. (2002). Personality in context: An interpersonal systems perspective. *Journal of Personality, 70,* 851–900.

CHAPTER 3

What Does It Mean to Be Attached?

CINDY HAZAN
NURIT GUR-YAISH
MARY CAMPA

One of the many notable strengths of attachment theory is that it provides thorough accounts of both normative development and individual differences. Bowlby recognized early on that in order to fully understand maladaptive variations it first was necessary to explain normal attachment functioning. The ontogeny of normative attachment was the primary focus of the first volume in his trilogy (Bowlby, 1969/1982) and of early attachment research.

With the introduction of an experimental paradigm and the discovery of "secure," "ambivalent," and "avoidant" patterns of infant attachment (Ainsworth, Blehar, Waters, & Wall, 1978), the emphasis shifted to individual differences. This approach continues to dominate research on infant and child attachment. It has yielded an enormous body of findings that constitutes one of the most significant contributions to developmental psychology in the last century. However, as a result of this near-exclusive focus on individual differences, relatively little progress has been made on the normative front (Marvin & Britner, 1999).

The field of adult attachment grew more out of Ainsworth's research than out of Bowlby's theory. It was founded on self-report and interview measures designed to capture adult versions of the infant patterns (Bartholomew & Horowitz, 1991; Brennan & Shaver, 1995; Collins & Read, 1990; George, Kaplan, & Main, 1985; Hazan & Shaver, 1987; Levy & Davis, 1988; Simpson, 1990). Hundreds of studies have documented the correlates of adult attachment "styles," and the findings have led to significant theoretical advances (see Feeney, 1999, for a review). But, again, progress has been limited almost entirely to the domain of individual differences. Many basic questions surrounding normative adult attachment remain unanswered and unstudied—a limitation that several authors have pointed out (Berlin & Cassidy, 1999; Diamond, 2001; Fraley & Shaver, 2000; Hazan & Zeifman, 1994; Kobak, 1999; Main, 1999; Simpson & Rholes, 1998).

In considering new directions for adult attachment research, we agree that the field needs to address this imbalance by working toward the development of normative models. We share Bowlby's view that a full understanding of normative attachment formation and functioning is essential for interpreting variations on the norm. A logical starting point is to tackle the question of what it means to be attached. In describing the three major patterns of infant attachment, Ainsworth and colleagues (1978) emphasized that they reflect differences in kind, not degree. Avoidant and ambivalent infants are insecurely attached to their caregivers, but they are attached nonetheless. Even babies who suffer the misfortune of being born to neglectful or abusive caregivers nevertheless become attached to them (Crittenden, 1995). These observations suggest that there may be a fundamental answer to the question of what it means to be attached. In other words, it may be possible to define attachment in a way that captures its essence while simultaneously allowing for, and providing a context in which to interpret, individual differences.

To answer the question of what it means to be attached, and particularly what it means in adulthood, requires identifying attachment markers. In practical terms, it could prove useful for investigators to have a set of objective standards for determining whether participants in their research are attached or not. Finding such markers would help reveal the basic processes by which the endpoint of attachment is achieved, as well as any distinguishable transition points along the way. In addition, an emphasis on the processes of bond formation would redirect attention from intraindividual to interindividual aspects of attachment. The majority of adult attachment research is conducted within the broader field of interpersonal relationships, and thus greater emphasis on relational processes could facilitate integration of attachment theory and findings with other theoretical and research traditions in the area.

We feel obliged to state at the outset that this chapter does not provide a definitive answer to the title question. Although we consider it a fundamental and fruitful question for the field to address, the current state of knowledge does not allow for any conclusive answers. Instead, we draw on existing theory and research to explore various possibilities and suggest promising future directions. Our analysis rests on two assumptions: (1) that attachment is a process that unfolds over time, possibly in a sequence of identifiable phases, and (2) that it occurs and is manifested at multiple levels, including behavior, cognition, physiology, and emotion.

Our normative emphasis is not meant to discount the importance of individual differences. Their effects are well documented, and we expect that their influence will be significant at many, if not all, levels and in many, if not all, phases of attachment formation. Nevertheless, we think it important to understand individual differences within the context of a normative model. Consider, for example, a finding that avoidant adults appear undisturbed by brief separations from romantic partners. Does this finding reflect the quality of attachment to the current partner, the preexisting attachment style these individuals brought to their relationships, a normative change in separation reactions as relationships develop, or a combination of these factors? Without some means of determining whether an attachment has been established, observed differences in relationship functioning are difficult to interpret. Moreover, knowing how attachment bonds are formed and maintained will surely enhance understanding of how dispositional tendencies shape, and are shaped by, relationships.

In abstract terms, attachment results from the interaction of multiple intraindividual and interindividual processes operating at multiple levels over time. What needs to be better understood is *what* the relevant processes are and *how* they change over time. This is the approach taken here. We start with a brief theoretical background that focuses on Bowlby's definition of attachment and his normative model of bond formation. This is followed by four major sections corresponding to the different levels at which attachment has been studied—behavior, cognition, physiology, and emotion. Each section begins with representative research findings and ends with a discussion of what we see as the relevant processes and how they might change as attachment bonds develop.

THEORETICAL BACKGROUND

Bowlby (1982) defined attachment in terms of four distinct but interrelated classes of behavior: *proximity maintenance, safe haven, separation distress,* and *secure base.* These behaviors are readily observable in normal 1-year-old infants in relation to their primary caregivers (usually mothers). The infant continuously monitors the caregiver's whereabouts and makes any adjustments necessary for maintaining the desired degree of proximity, retreats to her as a haven of safety in the event of perceived threat, is actively resistant to and distressed by separations from her, and uses her as a base of security from which to explore the environment. Infants often direct one or more of these behaviors toward individuals to whom they are not attached. Importantly, it is the selective orientation of all these behaviors toward a specific individual that defines attachment.

In theory, this dynamic balance between the attachment and exploratory behavior systems is characteristic of humans at all stages of development, including adulthood. Nevertheless, with maturation, predictable changes occur. Separations of greater distance and duration are less distressing, and proximity-maintenance and safe-haven behaviors assume new and diverse forms. Such changes pose special challenges for researchers interested in identifying markers of attachment beyond infancy.

Bowlby (1969/1982) proposed that there are four phases in the development of an infant's attachment to a caregiver, which Ainsworth (1972) later elaborated on and labeled as follows: In the *preattachment* phase (approximately 0–2 months of age), infants are inherently interested in, responsive to, and adept at eliciting social contact and relatively open to interactions with and accepting of care from almost anyone. In the *attachment-in-the-making* phase (2–6 months), they begin to discriminate among caregivers by preferentially directing social signals (smiles, vocalizations, cries) and responding differentially (greeting more enthusiastically, settling more quickly) to certain individuals. In the *clear-cut attachment* phase (beginning at 6–7 months), all of the behaviors that define attachment are evident, but more important, they are organized around a particular caregiver. This is evident in an infant's active efforts to maintain proximity (differential following) and use of this individual as a safe haven (differential comfort seeking) and secure base (differential exploration) and being upset by separations (differential distress). By the final phase, *goal-corrected partnership* (around 36 months), children have less urgent needs for physical proximity and are able to negotiate with caregivers regarding separations and availability.

The separation-distress feature of attachment is centrally important for both theoretical and historical reasons. During the 1940s and 1950s, a number of reports (e.g., Burlingham & Freud, 1944; Robertson, 1953) suggested that infants and young children separated from primary caregivers for extended periods of time pass through an invariant sequence of reactions. At first, they actively resist the separation by crying, searching, and calling out in an attempt to regain contact. Eventually, agitation and anxiety subside, and they begin to evince deeper and more pervasive signs of distress, including lethargy, depressed mood, decreased appetite, and sleep disturbances. In time, they appear to recover. It is only when they are reunited with caregivers that otherwise invisible lingering effects of the separation show up in the form of anger mixed with anxious clinging or complete emotional withdrawal. This sequence of reactions is known as *protest, despair,* and *detachment.* Attachment theory was inspired by the need to explain why, even in relatively familiar environments and despite adequate surrogate care, separations from a specific attachment figure cause such distress.

Adult attachments differ in several respects from the complementary attachments of early life in which infants and children are the seekers, and caregivers the providers, of security and protection. According to Bowlby, the pair bond—a relationship in which sexual partners serve as mutual recipients and providers of care—is the prototypical instantiation of attachment in adulthood. Thus, in the course of normative development, the attachment, parental/caregiving, and reproductive/sexual systems become integrated (Ainsworth, 1990; Bowlby, 1969/1982; Hazan & Shaver, 1994; Shaver, Hazan, & Bradshaw, 1988). The earliest evidence that long-term mateships qualify as attachment bonds came from reports that adults grieving the death of a spouse proceed through a similar protest–despair–detachment sequence of reactions (Parkes, 1972; Weiss, 1975). Separation distress is the standard marker of attachment in infancy and childhood (Ainsworth et al., 1978; Sroufe & Waters, 1977a) and is thus a behavior that merits special attention in the search for adulthood markers.

Whether adult attachments develop in a manner that parallels attachment formation in infancy is an empirical question that awaits an answer, but Zeifman and Hazan (1997) proposed that Bowlby's four-phase model serve as a provisional research guide. They liken the adult counterpart of the infant preattachment phase to what Eibl-Eibesfeldt (1989) called the "proceptive program." Males and females of reproductive age are inherently interested in social interaction with potential mates and display flirtatious signals somewhat indiscriminately. It is likely that these playful, sexually charged exchanges continue when couples first become involved and are more characteristic of their interactions than attachment behaviors per se. In contrast, the behavior of couples in the throes of romantic infatuation show many resemblances to infant–caregiver interactions (Shaver & Hazan, 1988), including prolonged mutual gazing, cuddling, nuzzling, and "baby talk." Zeifman and Hazan suggested that these types of exchanges may be indicative of the second phase, attachment-in-the-making. This is consistent with Bowlby's view that "In terms of subjective experience, the formation of a bond is described as falling in love" (1979, p. 69). In infancy, the onset of the third phase, clear-cut attachment, is indicated by the emergence of new attachment behaviors and, specifically, their organization around a single caregiver who has become the reliably preferred target of proximity-maintenance and safe-haven behaviors and elicitor of secure-base and separation-distress behaviors. Zeifman and Hazan proposed that the selective orientation of these four behaviors toward a partner might signal clear-cut attachment in adulthood as well. The childhood indicators of the fourth phase, goal-corrected partnership, primarily reflect cognitive developmental changes over the first 3 years of life. Zeifman and Hazan hypothesized that there nevertheless may be a comparable final phase in adult attachment formation, characterized by a decline in overt displays of attachment behavior.

In the following sections we consider several behavioral, cognitive, physiological, and emotional processes likely to be important in the formation and maintenance of adult attachment bonds. We acknowledge the reality of fuzzy boundaries between and complex interrelations among levels but believe there is theoretical and practical value in parsing attachment processes in this way. At each level of analysis, we address the questions of what it means to be attached, how the process of becoming attached might unfold, and whether it is possible to identify markers of attachment that are not confounded with security or insecurity.

ATTACHMENT AT THE LEVEL OF BEHAVIOR

The near-exclusive focus on individual differences has meant that many basic tenets of attachment theory have never been empirically tested. Prominent among them is the claim that attachments are not just stronger than other social bonds but qualitatively different. If this is correct, it is important for attachment researchers to have some criteria by which to distinguish attachment from nonattachment relationships. As a first step in this direction, Hazan and Zeifman (1994) developed an instrument based on Bowlby's (1982) behavior-based definition. It asks respondents to name the individual they view as the *primary* target of each of the four defining behaviors: proximity maintenance (the person they most want to be close to, spend time with), safe haven (turn to when upset, feeling down), separation distress (hate being away from, miss when apart), and secure base (count on to be there, help when needed). The measure (WHOTO) was administered in interview or questionnaire format to hundreds of children, adolescents, and adults. We report only results for the adult sample, which were replicated by Fraley and Davis (1997) and later extended by Trinke and Bartholomew (1997).

On the proximity-maintenance and safe-haven scales, nearly all adults named a romantic partner or close friend as the primary target of these behaviors. In contrast, for the separation-distress and secure-base items, they tended to name either a romantic partner or a parent. Among the participants who reported having a romantic partner at the time of the study, the difference in whether they named their partner or a parent on separation-distress and secure-base items depended on length of romantic relationship. Over 80% of those whose romantic relationships met the definitional criteria of attachment (i.e., contained all four behavioral components) had been with their partners for 2 or more years, compared with 30% who had been with their partners for less than 2 years.

The findings are consistent with Bowlby's general claims regarding normative attachment. First, they provide initial support for the hypothesis that partners replace parents as primary attachment figures in adulthood. Second, they indicate that in adulthood, as in infancy, attachment bonds take time to form. And third, they serve as a cautionary reminder that the existence of attachment cannot be assumed solely from romantic involvement.

Although Hazan and Zeifman's (1994) study focused on the behaviors that Bowlby proposed to define attachment, their findings were based solely on self-reports. Two studies of adult attachment, one laboratory based and the other conducted in a naturalistic setting, included observations of actual behavior.

Simpson, Rholes, and Nelligan (1992) developed an experimental paradigm similar in several respects to the laboratory procedure created by Ainsworth and colleagues (1978) to assess infant attachment. Female undergraduates were separated from their male romantic partners and then led to expect a stressful experience. Reunions with partners were unobtrusively videotaped and later coded. The experimental manipulation was designed to elicit attachment behavior and, in secure females, it did. The more anxious they were, the more they sought contact with and comfort from their partners.

The Simpson and colleagues (1992) study is an excellent example of how attachment behaviors can be investigated in adulthood. In considering the specific behaviors they observed—proximity seeking and safe haven—as potential markers of adult attachment, it will be important to take relational and contextual factors into account. Simpson and colleagues created a context that should elicit attachment behavior toward an attachment figure. However, people of all ages have been shown to seek comfort even from relative strangers in situations that arouse anxiety (Shaver & Klinnert, 1982). In theory, what sets attachment figures apart is that they are reliably preferred over other targets of distress alleviation.

In a naturalistic study, Fraley and Shaver (1998) unobtrusively observed couples in an airport lobby awaiting either a joint trip or a separation (if only one member of the couple was traveling). In this study, the impending separation was expected to elicit attachment behavior. In general, the incidence of contact seeking (e.g., hugging, kissing, stroking, hand-holding) was significantly higher in couples facing a separation than in those traveling together. The incidence of these behaviors also varied as a function of relationship length. Overt displays of attachment behavior were less common in couples who had been together longer.

The Fraley and Shaver (1998) study represents another creative approach to studying attachment behaviors in adults. The results accord well with theoretical predictions that separations from attachment figures (whether actual or anticipated) activate contact-maintaining behaviors. And the lower incidence among longer term couples is reminiscent of the decline in attachment behavior seen in children during the fourth phase of attachment to caregivers. Such naturally occurring separations offer an ideal setting for investigating separation distress. Future studies could examine the reactions of partners following the separation to see whether these reactions, like preseparation behaviors, differ as a function of relationship length or separation length.

Recall that separation reactions in infancy and early childhood undergo qualitative change if separations are sufficiently protracted. The immediate (protest) response is anxiety, heightened activity, and agitation, whereas the later (despair) response is depression, diminished activity, and pervasive behavioral disturbance. In considering response to separation as a potential marker of adult attachment, it will be important to distinguish between acute and ensuing reactions. It will also likely be necessary to take into account how the nature and manifestations of separation distress change in the course of bond development. If children in the goal-corrected phase of attachment formation are able to tolerate short-term scheduled separations from attachment figures without undue upset, presumably adult partners can, too. It may require more than a few days of separation to elicit measurable distress in long-term couples.

Vormbrock's (1993) review of studies on marital separations revealed that reactions also differ depending on whether one is the leaver or the one left. It is important to note that these were not the usual 3- to 5-day partings for attendance at academic conferences or visits to ailing relatives that most couples have to contend with from time to time, but rather partner absences lasting weeks or months. Reactions of homebound spouses resembled many of the protest–despair–detachment behaviors seen in children, but responses to separation on the part of traveling spouses did not. Thus, in addition to relationship length and separation length, whether one is the partner who leaves or is left behind is yet another factor that can affect reactions to separation and, consequently, how such reactions should be interpreted.

What Behavioral Processes Are Important in Adult Attachment?

The most obvious candidates for behavioral markers of attachment are, of course, the ones that Bowlby used to define this special type of interpersonal bond. What are the behavioral indications that one individual is attached to another? Hypothetically, if person A maintains proximity to person B, uses B as a haven of safety and a base for exploration, and is distressed by separations from B, then person A is attached to person B. There are at least two major challenges that will have to be addressed if these behaviors are to be used as markers of adult attachment.

One challenge will be to determine the contexts in which they indicate the existence of an attachment bond. Experimental induction of anxiety was shown by Simpson and colleagues (1992) to be an effective elicitor of proximity-seeking and safe-haven behaviors. But as previously noted, these behaviors are, in certain situations, directed toward persons unlikely to be attachment figures. To be used as markers of attachment, it will be necessary to demonstrate that one or a few specific persons are the consistently preferred targets. Fraley and Shaver (1998) found that an impending separation evoked the same two types of attachment behavior. But the particular behaviors they noted (e.g., kissing, hand-holding) are not likely to be observed in interactions with strangers. Such physical intimacy clearly signals a special relationship, and presumably the anticipated separation was anxiety provoking because a special person was going to be temporarily absent. Still, it is unknown whether this can be interpreted as evidence of an attachment bond. Romantic partners tend to be much more physically affectionate at the beginning of their relationship than later on. Fraley and Shaver reported that the longer the couples in their study had been together, the less they exhibited various contact-mainte nance behaviors. If one assumes that longer term couples are more likely than shorter term couples to be attached, the dangers of inferring attachment solely on the basis of proximity-seeking and safe-haven behaviors— even when they take highly intimate forms—become clear. Were one to use these behaviors alone as markers of adult attachment, short-term couples would be more often classified as attached than long-term couples.

Are some attachment behaviors more indicative of an attachment bond than others? Hazan and Zeifman (1994) found that adults who named their romantic partners as the primary source of separation distress also tended to name them as primary targets of the other three types of attachment behavior. In infancy, separation distress is the standard marker of attachment, not because it is more important than other attachment behaviors but because it is uniquely displayed in relation to attachment figures. But of all the behavioral markers of adult attachment, separation distress is probably the most complicated. There is evidence that reactions to separations differ as a function of relationship length (Fraley & Shaver, 1998), separation length (Robertson, 1953), and status as the one who leaves or is left (Vormbrock, 1993). Although separation distress will likely be the most difficult to investigate empirically, it may be the most valid single marker of attachment.

A second major challenge will be to identify markers of adult attachment that are not confounded by relationship quality or attachment style. In the Simpson and colleagues experiment (1992), the behavior of avoidant females was the opposite of that of secure females. Instead of turning to their partners when they were most anxious and thus in greatest need of support, they exhibited less proximity-seeking and safe-haven behavior. This is reminiscent of the finding reported by Ainsworth and colleagues (1978) that avoidant infants are more likely to evade contact with caregivers under high- than low-stress conditions. It is also consistent with results from Fraley and Shaver's (1998) airport study. Avoidant women sought more contact with partners when the two were traveling together and less contact when a separation was imminent.

In the absence of an attachment indicator, it is impossible to determine whether the observed behaviors reflect the quality of the current relationship and/or the dispositional tendencies that individual participants brought to their current relationships. If one were to use distress alleviation via partner contact as a marker of adult attachment, secure people would be deemed attached more often than insecure people even though the differences in behavior might be more accurately attributed to attachment style.

Is there an attachment-style-free pattern of behavior that one could confidently point to as a marker of adult attachment? Infant and child attachment researchers continue to caution against confusing attachment quality with attachment quantity (Main, 1999). Again, insecure babies and children are differently, but no less, attached than their secure counterparts. So what do they have in common? It is that all of their attachment-defining behaviors are organized around a specific individual. This person may or may not be reliably responsive, may or may not be effective in alleviating distress, may or may not be approached for contact comfort in threatening situations. But she or he is nonetheless the selective target toward whom attachment behaviors are oriented. According to Bowlby (1969/1982), this is the hallmark of attachment.

Can similar patterns of selective orientation be found in adults, perhaps in style-adjusted, mean-level changes in attachment behavior? Avoidant adults would not be expected to share their concerns or request a reassuring hug as readily as secure adults, but when anxious they may nonetheless show an increase in their own version of safe-haven behavior (e.g., self-soothing in proximity to an attachment figure). Avoidant infants do not try to get as far away from their attachment figures as possible, but rather maintain a "safe" distance from them (Ainsworth et al., 1978). It is easy to imagine a comparable adult strategy of not overtly expressing anxiety or actively seeking contact comfort but instead engaging in more distal forms of communication (e.g., hanging around but not talking, calling but not disclosing). If attachment behaviors were conceptualized flexibly enough, they could potentially reveal markers that supersede attachment style.

How Does Behavior Change as Adult Attachment Bonds Develop?

To date, there have been no descriptive longitudinal studies of attachment behavior over the course of romantic relationship development. Based on Bowlby's (1969/1982) and Ainsworth's (1972) models of infant attachment formation, Zeifman and Hazan (1997) hypothesized that phases in the development of attachment bonds between romantic partners would manifest as changes in attachment behaviors. Specific-ally, they proposed that the process of becoming attached involves a log-ical progression in the emergence of specific attachment behaviors, as well as qualitative changes in their organization and expression over time.

In a hypothetical pair, the process might look something like the fol-lowing: In the preattachment phase, sexual attraction and/or romantic in-terest draw partners into flirtatious and arousing interactions. During this phase there is an increase in selective proximity seeking, but other forms of attachment behavior are not yet evident. If an exclusive relationship ensues and the two begin to fall in love, the stage is set for the attachment-in-the-making phase. During this phase, physical contact is at its highest level. In addition, the partners begin to display various forms of safe-haven behavior (i.e., increasing proximity when anxious). Although they continue to be stimulated by each other's presence, the balance begins to shift toward being calmed by each other's presence. Repeated instances of intimate physical and verbal exchanges that reduce arousal foster the de-velopment of an attachment bond. Partners come to be preferred over others as sources of comfort and anxiety alleviation. If the relationship survives the inevitable waning of romantic infatuation, they may find themselves in the phase of clear-cut attachment. They have habituated to and are thus no longer as excited by each other's presence. They have sex less often and experience less urgent needs for physical contact, but each has become sufficiently reliant on the other that separations are now dis-tressing. With growing confidence that the relationship will endure, they enter the final, goal-corrected phase of attachment formation. From the base of security that has been established, attention is redirected toward external obligations and opportunities. Interactions between partners take on a more mundane quality, with fewer overt displays of attachment behaviors.

ATTACHMENT AT THE LEVEL OF COGNITION

In the course of normative development, individuals become less depend-ent on the physical presence of attachment figures and increasingly reli-ant on mental representations of them. The final, goal-corrected phase of attachment formation, during which children begin to negotiate with care-givers regarding separations and availability, is made possible by advances in cognitive development. But the construction of attachment repre-sentations begins in infancy, on the foundation of daily interactions with caregivers. Indeed, the different patterns of attachment observed in the original "Strange Situation" experiments (Ainsworth et al., 1978) were at-tributed to differences in caregiver responsiveness that infants had internalized during the preceding 12 months. "In the working model of the world that anyone builds a key feature is his notion of who his attachment figures are, where they may be found, and how they may be expected to respond" (Bowlby, 1973, p. 203).

Some of the most exciting new work on adult attachment takes advantage of this normative shift to the level of representation. Borrowing methods from the field of cognitive psychology, researchers have begun to explore basic questions about affectional bonding and attachment dynamics. In this area of attachment research, Baldwin (1992, 1994) and colleagues (e.g., Baldwin, Fehr, Keedian, Seidel, & Thomson, 1993; Baldwin, Keelan, Fehr, Enns, & Koh-Rangarajoo, 1996) paved the way. Their findings confirmed that most adults have a "chronically accessible" attachment schema that influences social information processing in ways consistent with Bowlby's ideas, as well as subsidiary mental models that can be activated via priming. An equally important by-product of this research was the introduction of a novel method for investigating adult attachment phenomena.

Using a priming task, Mikulincer, Gillath, and Shaver (2002) tested the hypothesis that activation of the attachment system in response to threat increases the accessibility of mental representations of attachment figures. They had participants complete a shortened version (Fraley & Davis, 1997) of Hazan and Zeifman's (1994) WHOTO measure (to obtain names of attachment figures) and, in addition, provide lists of other persons (e.g., close but not attachment figures, known but not close). A lexical decision task similar to one that Baldwin and colleagues (1993) had found effective for investigating attachment representations was used. On a computer screen, participants were subliminally exposed to either a threat word ("failure," "separation") or a neutral word ("hat"). The prime was followed by either a name from individuals' lists or a nonword. The task for participants was to decide as quickly as possible whether the target letter string was a word or not, and they recorded their responses by a key press. The dependent measure was reaction time (RT).

The findings provided clear support for the main hypothesis. Following a threat but not a neutral prime, participants were quicker to recognize the name of a person they had listed on the WHOTO—that is, an attachment figure—than the names of persons from their other lists. This is a powerful demonstration that threats automatically activate mental representations of attachment figures, even when the threats are not consciously perceived and pose no real danger. Importantly, this effect was found across attachment styles. All individuals, whether secure or insecure, called attachment figures to mind in response to threat.

This combination of methods shows tremendous promise for enhancing our understanding of normative attachment formation. For example, they could be used to address the question of whether some attachment features are more indicative of an attachment bond than others. In the Mikulincer and colleagues (2002) study, persons named on any scale items of the WHOTO were counted as attachment figures, although most participants named the same person on more than one. It could be informative in future work to test whether the effects vary as a function of specific attachment features and whether, as Hazan and Zeifman (1994) argued, secure base and separation distress are more indicative of attachment than proximity seeking and safe haven.

This method could also be useful for addressing questions about the organization of attachment representations and, specifically, the unresolved issue of whether or not they are organized hierarchically (Pietromonaco & Feldman Barrett, 2000). For example, one could test whether participants are reliably quicker to recognize the names of some attachment figures than others, whether some attachment representations are activated more frequently than others, and whether reactions to the names of romantic partners change as relationships progress.

Another cognitive method that shows promise for investigating attachment phenomena comes from the work of Andersen and colleagues (e.g., Andersen & Glassman, 1996; Andersen, Reznik, & Chen, 1997). Their research program is based on the clinical concept of transference, the idea that mental representations of important interpersonal relationships affect how information about a new person is processed. To explore this concept, they have developed a paradigm that incorporates idiographic methods into a nomothetic experimental design. For instance, in a sentence-completion task, participants generate descriptions of known individuals with whom they have a "significant" relationship. In a follow-up, weeks later, they are presented with descriptions of several new target persons. The test set contains descriptions composed to resemble a significant other of each of the participants. Afterward, they complete a standard recognition memory task consisting of sentences taken (or not) from their own earlier descriptions that were (or were not) included in the test set, along with several filler sentences. Across a series of studies (reviewed in Andersen & Berk, 1998), the results are consistent with a transference hypothesis. A representative finding is that participants are more likely to falsely "remember" having seen a not-presented sentence if it was derived from a description of their own significant other.

This paradigm could be adapted for use in studies of adult attachment formation. For example, one might look for the point at which a romantic-partner representation becomes sufficiently "significant" to affect how information about an unknown person is processed. Comparisons might also be made between partners and other presumed attached figures, such as parents, as a way of investigating changes in the relative influence of partner representations and in the overall organizational structure of attachment hierarchies.

Social-cognitive methods have also been used creatively to investigate the secure-base component of attachment. In infancy, this feature of attachment is manifested in exploratory behavior. Once clear-cut attachment to a specific caregiver has been established, the proximity of that individual is what largely determines an infant's exploratory activity. For older children, the secure expectation that attachment figures can be found if needed and counted on to be responsive is enough to support full engagement in exploration.

In theory, the dynamic balance between attachment and exploration is essentially the same throughout life. For a recent pair of studies designed to investigate this link in adulthood, Green and Campbell (2000) developed a self-report "exploration index" on which participants rated their interest and likelihood of engaging in a variety of novel activities. In the first study, these ratings were evaluated in relation to a measure of attachment styles, and, as hypothesized, security predicted higher exploration scores. In the second study, a semantic priming task was used. The method was borrowed from Baldwin and colleagues (1993), and the procedure was based on their finding that most individuals, regardless of attachment style, have both secure and insecure representations that can be accessed. To prime secure representations, participants were asked to memorize a set of sentences derived from a prototypic description of adult attachment security in which characters express trust, offered comfort, shared feelings, and so forth.

The results were consistent with theoretical predictions. Primed attachment security was associated with greater reported openness to such novel and stimulating exploratory activities as traveling to new places, meeting new people, and trying new things (like bungee jumping). This method and procedure could be modified in a variety of ways to investigate basic questions about adult attachment. For example, one could test whether priming representations of attachment figures affects exploratory openness and, if so, at what point in attachment formation partner effects are observed.

What Cognitive Processes Are Important in Adult Attachment?

A cornerstone of attachment theory is the idea that attachment experiences are internalized. The inborn attachment system enhances survival not by regulating behavior in a fixed or rigid manner but rather in a way that is adapted to the local caregiving environment. Attachment representations are the mechanism by which such adaptation occurs. Through countless interactions over the first year of life, infants learn what to expect from caregivers and adjust their attachment behavior accordingly. These experience-based expectations form the foundation of attachment representations that, in theory, become the filters through which social information is processed. According to Bowlby (1973, 1988), they influence all aspects of processing, including what information is attended to or (defensively) excluded. Like all cognitive schemas, attachment representations are biased toward assimilating new information as opposed to accommodating it (Piaget, 1951).

Nearly all of the adult research on "internal working models" of attachment has been designed to explore individual differences in cognitive processes (see Pietromonaco & Feldman Barrett, 2000, for a review). Given that attachment representations are primarily the products of individual differences in experience, one would not expect all people to have similar memories or expectations or interpretive biases. Individuals' attachment representations differ, and therefore their effects surely differ. The challenge for researchers in developing normative models is to identify markers of attachment that are not confounded with individual differences. Is there any aspect of cognitive processing one could point to as evidence that one individual is attached to another?

This question already has a viable answer. Mikulincer and colleagues (2002) demonstrated that subliminal threats automatically make representations of attachment figures more accessible, regardless of individual attachment style. Had these researchers instead asked participants to report which persons they think of first in anxiety-provoking situations, the results would likely have replicated well-documented attachment style effects. The transference paradigm (Andersen & Berk, 1998) offers another promising research strategy. In this approach, participants are also unaware of the effects that representations of significant people in their lives have on how they process information.

These methods may be useful for discovering basic cognitive markers of adult attachment precisely because they circumvent conscious processing. From an individual-differences perspective, the contents of people's representations are of interest, such as whether or not others are perceived as available and responsive, but they are not conclusive evidence that an attachment bond exists. Simply knowing that an individual expects his or her partner to be rejecting is not enough to determine whether he or she is attached to the partner. From a normative perspective, of greater interest is whether or not partner representations are selectively activated under relevant conditions and whether or not they have selective effects on information processing.

How Does Cognition Change as Adult Attachment Bonds Develop?

Assuming that virtually all long-term partners have representations of each other that they did not have when they first met, it should be possible to track the development of such representations. Deciding whether partner representations are cognitive markers of attachment formation is a separate issue. To our knowledge, studies on the development of mental representations of romantic partners have not yet been conducted, and so it may be useful to think through a plausible scenario.

In the preattachment phase, the construction of partner representations begins. At this point, one would not expect to observe any of the priming or schema-activation effects described previously. In the attachment-in-the-making phase, the nature of couple interactions is highly conducive to schema building. Partners spend long hours studying each other's faces and bodies, behaviors and reactions. They have ample opportunities to develop expectations about partner availability and responsiveness. At some point, partner representations begin to be selectively activated in attachment-relevant situations and to selectively influence information processing. The emergence of these effects might be an indication that a couple has entered the phase of clear-cut attachment. Partner representations may undergo further elaboration and/or organizational changes that would signal a goal-corrected phase, such as quicker activation or more pervasive processing influence.

ATTACHMENT AT THE LEVEL OF PHYSIOLOGY

Attachment theory specifies a broad range of ways that infants are affected, in both the short and long term, by relationships with primary caregivers. What the theory underestimates, in the view of some, are the effects of attachment figures on infant physiology (Kraemer, 1992; Polan & Hofer, 1999; Reite & Capitano, 1985). Interest in this issue has grown in recent years such that there is now a large body of empirical work on the psychophysiology of infant–caregiver attachment (reviewed in Fox & Card, 1999). The main focus of this research has been on individual differences, primarily temperament and attachment pattern differences in infant reactivity.

A few studies of adult attachment have incorporated physiological measures (e.g., Feeney & Kirkpatrick, 1996; Mikulincer, 1998), and here, too, the emphasis has been on individual differences, mainly on how attachment style affects arousal under various experimental conditions. In the field of health psychology, hundreds of studies have examined the physiological correlates of social interaction (reviewed in Uchino, Cacioppo, & Kiecolt-Glaser, 1996), and although many of the findings are relevant to questions about affectional bonding, the studies were not designed to address them. Missing from the human literature as a whole are systematic investigations of the physiological underpinnings of normative attachment (Diamond, 2001).

In contrast, animal researchers have made significant strides in identifying the neurobiological and neuroanatomical substrates of normative attachment in a variety of mammalian species (see Carter, Lederhendler, & Kirkpatrick, 1997, for a review). Several of these investigators have explicitly discussed the implications of their findings for research on human attachment (e.g., Carter, 1998; Hofer, 1994; Reite & Boccia, 1994; Suomi, 1999).

Prominent among them is Hofer, who, in 1987, summarized his research on separation distress in rat pups. The work was motivated by the question of what, exactly, the pups missed about their mother during separations from her. To find out, Hofer and his colleagues designed a series of experiments in which they introduced specific features of the absent mother, one at a time, and then measured the effect of each on the pups' distress. They devised ways of mimicking the mother's odor, touch, and movements, added furry mats resembling her soft coat, heated the cage to her body temperature, administered her milk via a gastric canula, and so on. These studies revealed that each of the pups' distress symptoms was tied to a specific maternal feature. For example, in the mother's absence, the pups became listless and inactive, but warming the cage normalized activity; the pups' heart rate returned to normal when their stomachs were filled with mother's milk; by imitating mother's grooming behavior with rhythmic stroking, sleep disturbances were corrected. The major discovery was that each maternal feature alleviated a single distress symptom but had no effect on the others.

Hofer saw the findings as evidence that specific features of the mother regulate the pups' physiological systems. In his view, the reason pups showed the constellation of symptoms that in human infants and children is called despair was because in the mother's absence all of these "hidden" regulators were also absent. Surprisingly, the findings regarding the acute, protest phase of separation distress were quite different. The presence of nearly any maternal feature reduced overall protest to some degree, and the presence of litter mates effectively precluded it. Eliminating protest, however, did not prevent the behavioral and physiological disruptions that characterize despair.

Bowlby (1973) conceptualized protest and despair as interdependent responses. Vigorous crying and active searching are adaptive as immediate reactions to separation, but when they fail to achieve the goal of bringing the attachment figure back, it then becomes more adaptive to quiet down, conserve energy, and avoid attracting predators. Hofer's (1987) experimental results provide strong support for an alternative conceptualization of protest and despair as manifestations of two independent processes, the latter involving physiological coregulation. The fact that extended separations cause behavioral and physiological disorganization is widely accepted as evidence that an attachment exists. The flip side, according to Hofer, is that attachment is what keeps these systems organized and regulated.

The superficial (behavioral) symptoms of protest and despair in rats are virtually identical to the symptoms observed in human infants and children separated from caregivers and to those seen in bereaved adults (Hofer, 1984). This raises the intriguing possibility that the underlying physiology is also similar. In other words, across species and ages, physiological coregulation may be an inherent part and reliable marker of attachment.

Extrapolating findings from one species to another can be risky, but cross-species comparisons can also be an invaluable source of new ideas. In formulating attachment theory, Bowlby drew inspiration from Harlow's experiments on affectional bonding in rhesus monkeys and from research by Lorenz on imprinting behavior in goslings, both of which led him to postulate an innate system to regulate attachment behavior.

It is easy to accept that the physiology of helpless newborn rats is regulated by the mother who nurses, licks them clean, and keeps them warm. But is this a plausible model of attachment in our species, especially beyond infancy? In fact, there is much evidence for the social entrainment of biological rhythms in human adults. Biological systems have a 24-hour functional rhythm run by two pacemakers in the hypothalamus. These pacemakers require daily synchronization, and for every species there are certain aspects of the environment that entrain the rhythms (known as *Zeitgebers*, from the German for timekeepers). In insects, timekeepers are ambient temperature and light–dark cycles. A major *Zeitgeber* for humans is social interaction.

The field of chronobiology is replete with examples of this phenomenon. Vernikos-Danellis and Winget (1979; cited in Hofer, 1984) found that adults removed from their normal environments and housed together show circadian rhythm synchronization and, if shifted to a different group, quickly become entrained to the new group rhythm. Examples from other literatures include evidence of menstrual synchrony among coresident women (McClintock, 1971), earlier pubertal onset for girls living in households with unrelated adult males (Moffitt, Caspi, & Belsky, 1992; Surbey, 1990), and more regular ovulation in women with steady male sexual partners (Veith, Buck, Getzlaf, Van Dalfsen, & Slade, 1983). Thus even as adults our physiological systems remain "open" to external social influences. And given the centrality of romantic partners in individuals' social environments and the extraordinary duration of exposure to them, it follows that they would be major physiological regulators.

A different kind of coregulation is suggested by evidence that, across a variety of mammalian species, bonds between infants and parents and between adult reproductive partners involve the same psychoneuroendocrine core: the hypothalamic–pituitary–adrenocortical (HPA) axis and the autonomic nervous system (ANS; Carter, 1998; Carter et al., 1997; Hennessy, 1997). The primary function of this core is to up-regulate system activity to prepare an organism to take action in potentially harmful situations and then down-regulate system activity to restore homeostasis after the threat has passed. Evidence that this physiological core is involved in attachment comes from both human and animal research (reviewed in Carter, 1998).

In a sample of couples, all married or cohabiting, Gump, Polk, Kamarck, and Shiffman (2001) used blood pressure as an index of ANS activity (specifically, the sympathetic nervous system). All participants wore ambulatory monitors during waking hours for 1 week. Every 45 minutes, blood pressure was recorded, and diary entries were made to report what they were doing and feeling and whether anyone was with them at the time. Blood pressure was found to be significantly lower when partners were present than during one-on-one interactions with others or during periods of solitary activity. Although exchanges with partners were rated as more intimate, this did not mediate the association with blood pressure. The results suggest that attachment figures may have unique effects on physiological indices of arousal that are not dependent on relationship closeness.

Mason and Mendoza (1998) have found evidence of physiological markers of attachment in titi monkeys, one of the rare pair-bonding species. Titi mates maintain close proximity, often sitting shoulder-to-shoulder for hours with their long tails intertwined, and show extreme agitation and distress if separated. Like humans, titi parents do not direct attachment behaviors toward their infants; unlike humans, titi infants tend to be primarily attached to their fathers. Differences in HPA responses to separation correspond to these social structural differences. Specifically, mates show increased HPA activation when separated from each other, but not when separated from offspring; titi infants show increased HPA activation in response to separations from their fathers, but not their mothers.

The subjects in Carter's (1998; Carter et al., 1997) studies are prairie voles, small rodents native to the midwestern United States. Prairie voles display attachment behaviors toward their mates and form enduring bonds with them. Pairs simply housed in the same cage eventually become attached, but the process is speeded if they have sexual contact or undergo stressful experiences together.

Carter's work focuses on the hormones oxytocin and vasopressin, which are closely associated with the parasympathetic branch of the ANS and, as such, have a down-regulating effect on arousal. Through a series of experiments (Carter 1998; Carter et al., 1997), she and her colleagues have demonstrated that oxytocin and vasopressin play central roles in the formation and maintenance of pair bonds. Prairie voles typically display proximity maintenance and separation distress in relation to mates and reliably prefer them to novel sexual partners, but these normal behavioral tendencies are precluded by administration of an antagonist (see also Insel, 2000). The distribution of synthesizing cells for both hormones is sexually dimorphic, and initial results suggested that oxytocin mediated pair bonding in females, whereas vasopressin served this function in males. However, it was subsequently found that administration of either hormone in relatively high doses induces pair bonding in both sexes. Thus the difference seems to be one of relative sensitivity.

Based on these findings, Carter (1998) has proposed a normative model of attachment formation: It begins with sustained proximity, sexual contact, and/or stress, all of which trigger HPA activation and social approach. HPA activation signals the hypothalamus, which in turn signals the posterior pituitary to release oxytocin or vasopressin. The ensuing hormone-induced state of calm is thus experienced in the context of social contact. When contact and calming coincide with sufficient frequency and/or intensity, conditioning occurs. That is, a specific individual becomes associated with feelings of security.

In humans, oxytocin is best known for triggering the contractions of labor in pregnant women and milk letdown in nursing mothers and is thought to foster infant bonding via a similar mechanism—a conditioned association between the mother and feelings of security (Uvnas-Moberg, 1994, 1998). Oxytocin is sometimes referred to as the "cuddle chemical" because intimate physical contact is sufficient to stimulate its release, and its presence enhances the desire for close contact. Importantly, its effects are not limited to infants or caregivers or perinatal experiences. The oxytocin system remains active throughout life. In fact, adult levels are highest in both men and women at the moment of sexual orgasm (Uvnas-Moberg, 1997). This suggests that the effects of intimate physical contact on adult attachment formation may also be hormonally mediated and involve a similar conditioning mechanism.

What Physiological Processes Are Important in Adult Attachment?

Animal research on the neurobiology of pair bonding has resulted in normative models of mammalian mate attachment that have tremendous potential for human application. In addition, research on the physiological effects of human social interaction offers clues and methods that should prove useful in the development of normative models in our species. These literatures highlight two processes that appear to be especially good candidates for markers of romantic attachment, each of which involves a different type of coregulation. One type is evident when individuals modulate each other's physiological arousal in specific situations. Most pertinent to attachment is the attenuation of arousal responses to various stressors. In considering this form of coregulation as a possible marker of adult attachment, two issues must be addressed. One is the inconsistency of findings from studies comparing the effectiveness of (presumed) attachment figures versus others in buffering stress reactivity. In the Gump and colleagues (2001) study, participants had significantly lower blood pressure in the presence of partners than in the presence of friends, whereas other studies (e.g., Fontana, Diegnan, Villeneuve, & Lepore, 1999) found that supportive strangers were just as effective as close friends in attenuating physiological responses to stress.

The other issue concerns the complicating effects of individual differences. In one study (Carpenter & Kirkpatrick, 1996), undergraduate females experienced a psychological stressor on two separate occasions, once in the presence of their romantic partners and once alone. For secure women, whether their partners were present or not made no difference in their physiological responses. In contrast, avoidant women had higher blood pressure with their partners than when alone. The findings are consistent with results from a study in which the heart rates of 1-year-old infants were monitored during separations from and reunions with their mothers (Sroufe & Waters, 1977b). All infants, whether secure or insecure, appeared to be distressed by the separations, as evidenced in accelerated heart rate. But there were striking individual differences in reactions to reunion. Secure infants' heart rates returned to preseparation levels after less than 1 minute of contact with their mothers. Avoidant infants, who by definition tend to avoid contact when highly stressed, continued to show increases in heart rate well into the reunion.

In light of such findings, is there any basis for seeking a normative marker of adult attachment formation in the way partners regulate each other's stress reactivity? There may be. In the Sroufe and Waters (1977b) study, avoidant infants were distressed in both their mother's absence and presence. We suspect that these reactions would not have been observed in relation to nonattachment figures. In the Carpenter and Kirkpatrick (1996) study, avoidant women were more stressed in their partners' presence than absence. Again, we wonder whether they would have shown the same reaction in relation to others. The nonreaction of secure women to the presence of their partners may have been due to the use of a relatively low-stress task (i.e., mental arithmetic). Recall that in the Simpson and colleagues (1992) study, secure women sought comfort only if they were highly anxious.

To return to the question of whether there are normative attachment markers to be found in physiological stress reactivity, the answer may lie not in *how* partners regulate each other but rather in the fact that they *do*. In situations of high stress, whether a partner's presence has a soothing or additionally arousing effect may be less revealing of attachment status than whether he or she has a significant effect of any kind.

The second type of coregulation that may be useful as an attachment marker involves long-term reciprocal influences on a wide variety of physiological systems. The idea that adult partners become attached at a physiological level has yet to be empirically tested, but there is indirect evidence consistent with it. As Hofer (1984) noted, the cardiovascular, endocrine, and immunological changes that occur in adults grieving the loss of a long-term partner are similar to the physiological symptoms found in rat pups and rhesus infants during prolonged separations. In his view, if the extended absence of attachment figures reliably leads to dysregulation in multiple physiological systems, it implies that attachment figures play a major role in regulating these systems. His experiments have convincingly demonstrated that such coregulation occurs in rats. In a recent set of recommendations for future directions in attachment research, Main (1999) urged investigators to begin searching for hidden physiological regulators in human attachment bonds.

How might these regulatory processes manifest in adult couples, and what degree or form of coregulation would be necessary to qualify as a marker of attachment? It has been shown that, in some circumstances, mere proximity induces synchronization of biological rhythms among virtual strangers. Hence, physiological synchrony alone would be insufficient evidence of attachment. But as Hofer (1984, 1987) emphasized, the human capacity for mental representation means that biobehavioral regulation in our species can, over the course of development, become increasingly internalized and decreasingly dependent on immediate sensorimotor input. Thus one possibility is that physiological coregulation between attached pairs would extend and be evident beyond actual interactions. An obvious alternative is to examine reactions to separation for signs of physiological dysregulation, which presumably would ensue only if coregulation had been established. If attachment at this level results primarily from close physical proximity and interaction over an extended period of time, and if it occurs outside of conscious awareness, it may serve as a marker of bond formation that crosses all attachment style categories.

Finding hidden physiological regulators in adult attachment bonds will not be easy. At this point, it is unclear what specific processes should be targeted for investigation and what form coregulation may take. But the potential for research on this issue to advance our understanding of attachment phenomena is too great to allow difficulty to serve as a deterrent. (For more on the physiology of attachment, see Diamond & Hicks, Chapter 8, this volume.)

How Does Physiology Change as Adult Attachment Bonds Develop?

If physiological coregulation is inherent to attachment bonds, it presumably follows a developmental course that could be tracked. Romantic partners may ultimately achieve such a state, but how do they get there? Is cohabitation for a long period sufficient? What, if any, measurable transitions occur in the interim? Because research on this issue is currently nonexistent, we can offer only a speculative possibility.

In the preattachment phase, romantic partners would not be expected to show any signs of physiological coregulation beyond what has been observed among acquaintances and strangers. In the attachment-in-the-making phase, they interact frequently and engage in the kinds of physically intimate and arousal-modulating exchanges that foster the development of coregulation in multiple physiological systems, including those related to distress alleviation. At some point, they begin to have a significant and selective effect on one another's reactions to stress and also achieve a broader state of physiological coregulation. These context-specific and general effects mark the onset of clear-cut attachment. In the goal-corrected phase, they may be further consolidated and internalized.

ATTACHMENT AT THE LEVEL OF EMOTION

Emotions occupy a central place in attachment theory and attachment bonds. "Many of the most intense emotions arise during the formation, the maintenance, the disruption, and the renewal of attachment relationships" (Bowlby, 1979, p. 130). The affective responses that both reveal and sustain attachments are thought to have resulted from evolutionary pressures. Infants who experienced positive emotions in the company of protectors and negative emotions in their absence were motivated to maintain proximity to them and, as a result, were more likely to survive.

In the first volume of his trilogy, Bowlby (1969/1982) emphasized the importance of physical proximity to attachment figures. In the second volume (1973), Bowlby placed greater emphasis on the child's appraisal of attachment figure availability. The idea was that feelings of security or insecurity derive less from the physical presence or absence of particular individuals than from the sense of their availability or unavailability. "Whether a child or adult is in a state of security, anxiety, or distress is determined in large part by the accessibility and responsiveness of his principal attachment figure" (Bowlby, 1973, p. 23). This new way of thinking about the set goal of the attachment system was well captured by Sroufe and Waters (1977a) in the concept of "felt security."

The proximal function of attachment bonds, at any age, is to modulate individuals' emotional states and reactions in a manner that is conducive to effective coping and full exploratory engagement—that is, to reduce anxiety and induce felt security. The primary source of felt security is the perception that attachment figures are accessible and responsive; maintaining proximity to them is the primary strategy for achieving it.

Adult attachment researchers have increasingly focused on affect regulation as a core feature of romantic relationships (e.g., Brennan & Shaver, 1995; Feeney, 1995; Simpson & Rholes, 1994).

Several findings described earlier are relevant here. In the Simpson and colleagues (1992) experiment, secure females whose behavior indicated anxiety about an impending stressor sought contact with their partners, presumably in the service of anxiety reduction. In the Fraley and Shaver (1998) airport study, couples awaiting a separation, which was assumed to be anxiety provoking, sought contact with their partners. The observed behaviors were taken as efforts to modulate anxiety. In the Mikulincer and colleagues (2002) experiment, representations of attachment figures became more accessible following a subliminal threat, presumably as a means of attenuating anxiety. In the Gump and colleagues (2001) study, participants' blood pressure dropped during interactions with partners, indicating that contact with them had a calming effect.

All of these studies provide support for Bowlby's conceptualization of attachment relationships as having an affect regulation function. Note that in each case internal feeling states, and changes in them, were inferred from behavior, cognition, or physiology. This approach is consistent with modern theories of emotion (Ekman, 1994; Frijda, 1986; Izard, 1994).

Emotions are inherently multilevel, multicomponent processes (Frijda & Mesquita, 1998). A small number of stimuli have privileged emotional associations, such as darkness or looming objects and a fear response, but most involve a greater degree of *cognitive* appraisal—though not necessarily deliberative or conscious. Emotions in general are usually triggered by events appraised as having personal relevance (primary appraisal); the specific type of emotion that is elicited is determined by a secondary appraisal of viable options for responding to triggering events. Emotions also have a *physiological* component. Arousal is a common feature of emotions, but so far no clear link has been established between specific emotions and particular patterns of physiological response (Cacioppo, Klein, Berntson, & Hatfield, 1993). Another component of emotions is *behavioral* tendencies or "action readiness," although frequently such inclinations (e.g., to run away in fear, strike out in anger) are inhibited. Of course, emotions are also associated with facial expressions. There is strong evidence that facial expressions of emotion are hard-wired, universal, and difficult to feign (Ekman, 1994; Izard, 1994). Yet there is considerable cross-cultural variation in the social rules regarding emotional displays (Ekman & Friesen, 1969), such as public expressions of joy over personal success or grief surrounding bereavement. And as has been noted (Russell, 1994), the same facial expression may in one situation reflect an internal feeling state and in another context be used as a social signal with a very different intent (e.g., smiling out of happiness vs. to appease).

The frequent lack of correspondence across behavioral, cognitive, and physiological levels of emotion make it extremely difficult to draw specific inferences about internal feeling states from any single level. But given the theorized centrality of affect regulation in attachment relationships, emotional processes must nevertheless be a major focus of adult attachment research. Fortunately, it may be possible to explore the emotion-related issues of greatest relevance to attachment without having to confront or resolve the problems faced by emotion researchers. For instance, they tend to struggle with questions about criteria for deciding whether an emotion is "basic" and whether there is a specific physiological profile associated with each emotion. What attachment researchers want to know, first and foremost, is how emotions are influenced by a specific type of interpersonal relatedness.

What Emotional Processes Are Important in Adult Attachment?

The fact that affect regulation is occupying an increasingly central place in adult attachment research represents a shift in emphasis that will bring the field into closer alignment with Bowlby's theory and into a better position from which to explore normative attachment phenomena. The emotional markers of attachment are likely to be found in the unrivaled ability of attachment figures to regulate affect. And given the multidimensional nature of emotions, these regulatory effects can be investigated using behavioral, cognitive, and/or physiological methods. Thus all of the processes highlighted herein are relevant to this level of analysis. How could one determine, on the basis of emotions, whether two individuals are attached? The answer lies in how they behave toward, think about, and/or respond physiologically to each other.

How Do Emotions Change as Adult Attachment Bonds Develop?

In the preattachment phase, one would not expect to observe affect regulation between romantic partners except in the form of mutual arousal due to novelty and sexual attraction. In the attachment-in-the-making phase, partners continue to find one another stimulating but also increasingly experience down-regulation of arousal in each other's presence. During this phase, couples direct attachment behaviors toward one another, construct mental representations of each other, and interact in a manner that fosters physiological coregulation. The onset of clear-cut attachment is marked by emotion regulation—at the levels of behavior, cognition, and physiology—that is selectively oriented toward and organized around partners. Further internalization of partner-directed affect regulation may constitute a final, goal-corrected phase of attachment formation.

CONCLUSION

After two decades of research on individual differences, it is time for the field of adult attachment to begin developing normative models and seeking answers to such basic theoretical questions as what it means to be attached and how attachment bonds are established. Implicit in our proposals for addressing these issues is a call for longitudinal studies. In light of the logistical problems associated with longitudinal investigations, it is not surprising that researchers would opt for other approaches. But there is a limit to how much can be learned from the correlates of individual differences in the absence of a normative theoretical framework, and the field may be nearing that limit. The good news is that documenting attachment formation may not require long-term longitudinal research. Conspicuous changes in the way romantic partners relate to one another over the first year or two of a relationship suggest that attachment-related developments take place within a relatively short time span. This makes it feasible to track attachment processes from the time of initial romantic involvement, but longitudinal designs also would be useful for examining how couples negotiate relationship junctures predicted to have especially powerful influences on attachment processes, such as the decline in romantic infatuation or the transition to cohabitation. It is an unavoidable fact that attachment formation takes time. Thus a complete understanding of the processes must be based on observations of how they change over time.

Our review of attachment research at the levels of behavior, cognition, physiology, and emotion and our proposals regarding possible markers of and phases in attachment formation at each level generate more questions than answers. This is reflective of the current state and exciting future of the adult attachment field, a future we think will be enhanced by exploring the many new issues and topics that a normative, developmental, process-oriented approach has to offer.

REFERENCES

Ainsworth, M. D. S. (1972). Attachment and dependency: A comparison. In J. L. Gewirtz (Ed.), *Attachment and dependency* (pp. 97–137). Washington, DC: Winston.

Ainsworth, M. D. S. (1990). Some considerations regarding theory and assessment relevant to attachments beyond infancy. In M. T. Greenberg, D. Cicchetti, & E. M. Cummings (Eds.), *Attachment in the preschool years: Theory, research, and intervention* (pp. 463–488). Chicago: University of Chicago Press.

Ainsworth, M. D. S., Blehar, M. C., Waters, E., & Wall, S. (1978). *Patterns of attachment: A psychological study of the Strange Situation.* Hillsdale, NJ: Erlbaum.

Andersen, S. M., & Berk, M. S. (1998). The social-cognitive model of transference: Experiencing past relationships in the present. *Current Directions in Psychological Science, 7,* 109–115.

Andersen, S. M., & Glassman, N. S. (1996). Responding to significant others when they are not there: Effects on interpersonal inference, motivation, and affect. In R. M. Sorrentino & E. T. Higgins (Eds.), *Handbook of motivation and cognition: Vol. 3. The interpersonal context* (pp. 262–321). New York: Guilford Press.

Andersen, S. M., Reznik, I., & Chen, S. (1997). The self in relation to others: Cognitive and motivational underpinnings. *Annals of the New York Academy of Sciences, 818,* 233–275.

Baldwin, M. W. (1992). Relational schemas and the processing of social information. *Psychological Bulletin, 112,* 461–484.

Baldwin, M. W. (1994). Primed relational schemas as a source of self-evaluative reactions. *Journal of Social and Clinical Psychology, 13,* 380–403.

Baldwin, M. W., Fehr, B., Keedian, E., Seidel, M., & Thomson, D. W. (1993). An exploration of the relational schemata underlying attachment styles: Self-report and lexical decision approaches. *Personality and Social Psychology Bulletin, 19,* 746–754.

Baldwin, M. W., Keelan, J. P. R., Fehr, B., Enns, V., & Koh-Rangarajoo, E. (1996). Social-cognitive conceptualization of attachment working models: Availability and accessibility effects. *Journal of Personality and Social Psychology, 71,* 94–109.

Bartholomew, K., & Horowitz, L. M. (1991). Attachment styles among young adults: A test of a four-category model. *Journal of Personality and Social Psychology, 61,* 226–244.

Berlin, L. J., & Cassidy, J. (1999). Relations among relationships: Contributions from attachment theory and research. In J. Cassidy & P. R. Shaver (Eds.), *Handbook of attachment: Theory, research, and clinical applications* (pp. 688–712). New York: Guilford Press.

Bowlby, J. (1973). *Attachment and loss: Vol. 2. Separation: Anxiety and anger.* New York: Basic Books.

Bowlby, J. (1979). *The making and breaking of affectional bonds.* London: Tavistock.

Bowlby, J. (1982). *Attachment and loss: Vol. 1. Attachment* (2nd ed.). New York: Basic Books.

Bowlby, J. (1988). *A secure base: Clinical applications of attachment theory.* London: Routledge.

Brennan, K. A., & Shaver, P. R. (1995). Dimensions of adult attachment, affect regulation, and romantic relationship functioning. *Personality and Social Psychology Bulletin, 21,* 267–283.

Burlingham, D., & Freud, A. (1944). *Young children in wartime.* London: Allen & Unwin.

Cacioppo, J. T., Klein, D. J., Berntson, G. G., & Hatfield, E. (1993).The psychophysiology of emotion. In M. Lewis & J. M. Haviland (Eds.), *Handbook of emotions* (pp. 119–142). New York: Guilford Press.

Carpenter, E. M., & Kirkpatrick, L. A. (1996). Attachment style and presence of a romantic partner as moderators of psychophysiological responses to a stressful laboratory situation. *Personal Relationships, 3,* 351–367.

Carter, C. S. (1998). Neuroendocrine perspectives on social attachment and love. *Psychoneuroendocrinology, 23*, 779–818.

Carter, C. S., Lederhendler, I. I., & Kirkpatrick, B. (Eds.). (1997). *The integrative neurobiology of affiliation.* Cambridge, MA: MIT Press.

Collins, N. L., & Read, S. J. (1990). Adult attachment, working models, and relationship quality in dating couples. *Journal of Personality and Social Psychology, 58,* 644–663.

Crittenden, P. M. (1995). Attachment and psychopathology. In S. Goldberg, R. Muir, & J. Kerr (Eds.), *Attachment theory: Social, developmental, and clinical perspectives* (pp. 367–406). Hillsdale, NJ: Analytic Press.

Diamond, L. M. (2001). Contributions of psychophysiology to research on adult attachment: Review and recommendations. *Personality and Social Psychology Review, 5,* 276–295.

Eibl-Eibesfeldt, I. (1989). *Human ethology: Foundations of human behavior.* Hawthorne, NY: Aldine de Gruyter.

Ekman, P. (1994). Strong evidence for universals in facial expressions: A reply to Russell's mistaken critique. *Psychological Bulletin, 115,* 268–287.

Ekman, P., & Friesen, W. V. (1969). Nonverbal leakage and clues to deception. *Psychiatry: Journal for the Study of Interpersonal Processes, 32,* 88–106.

Feeney, B. C., & Kirkpatrick, L. A. (1996). Effects of adult attachment and presence of romantic partners on physiological responses to stress. *Journal of Personality and Social Psychology, 70,* 255–270.

Feeney, J. A. (1995). Adult attachment and emotional control. *Personal Relationships, 2,* 143–159.

Feeney, J. A. (1999). Adult romantic attachment and couple relationships. In J. Cassidy & P. R. Shaver (Eds.), *Handbook of attachment: Theory, research, and clinical applications* (pp. 355–377). New York: Guilford Press.

Fontana, A. M., Diegnan, T., Villeneuve, A., & Lepore, S. J. (1999). Nonevaluative social support reduces cardiovascular reactivity in young women during acutely stressful performance situations. *Journal of Behavioral Medicine, 22,* 75–91.

Fox, N. A., & Card, J. A. (1999). Psychophysiological measures in the study of attachment. In J. Cassidy & P. R. Shaver (Eds.), *Handbook of attachment: Theory, research, and clinical applications* (pp. 226–245). New York: Guilford Press.

Fraley, R. C., & Davis, K. E. (1997). Attachment formation and transfer in young adults' close friendships and romantic relationships. *Personal Relationships, 4,* 131–144.

Fraley, R. C., & Shaver, P. R. (1998). Airport separations: A naturalistic study of adult attachment dynamics in separating couples. *Journal of Personality and Social Psychology, 75,* 1198–1212.

Fraley, R. C., & Shaver, P. R. (2000). Adult romantic attachment: Theoretical developments, emerging controversies, and unanswered questions. *Review of General Psychology, 4,* 132–154.

Frijda, N. H. (1986). *The emotions.* Cambridge, UK: Cambridge University Press.

Frijda, N. H., & Mesquita, B. (1998). The analysis of emotions: Dimensions of variation. In M. F. Mascolo & S. Griffin (Eds.), *What develops in emotional development? Emotions, personality, and psychotherapy* (pp. 273–295). New York: Plenum Press.

George, C., Kaplan, N., & Main, M. (1985). *The Adult Attachment Interview* (2nd ed.). Unpublished manuscript, University of California at Berkeley.

Green, J. D., & Campbell, W. K. (2000). Attachment and exploration in adults: Chronic and contextual accessibility. *Personality and Social Psychology Bulletin, 26,* 452–461.

Gump, B. B., Polk, D. E., Kamarck, T. W., & Shiffman, S. M. (2001). Partner interactions are associated with reduced blood pressure in the natural environment: Ambulatory monitoring evidence from a healthy, multiethnic adult sample. *Psychosomatic Medicine, 63,* 423–433.

Hazan, C., & Shaver, P. (1987). Romantic love conceptualized as an attachment process. *Journal of Personality and Social Psychology, 52,* 511–524.

Hazan, C., & Shaver, P. R. (1994). Attachment as an organization framework for research on close relationships. *Psychological Inquiry, 5,* 1–22.

Hazan, C., & Zeifman, D. (1994). Sex and the psychological tether. In K. Bartholomew & D. Perlman (Eds.), *Advances in personal relationships. Vol. 5. Attachment processes in adulthood* (pp. 151–177). London: Kingsley.

Hennessy, M. B. (1997). Hypothalamic–pituitary–adrenal responses to brief social separation. *Neuroscience and Biobehavioral Reviews, 21,* 11–29.

Hofer, M. A. (1984). Relationships as regulators: A psychobiologic perspective on bereavement. *Psychosomatic Medicine, 46,* 183–197.

Hofer, M. A. (1987). Early social relationships: A psychobiologist's view. *Child Development, 58,* 633–647.

Hofer, M. A. (1994). Hidden regulators in attachment, separation, and loss. In N. Fox (Ed.), The development of emotion regulation: Biological and behavioral considerations. *Monographs of the Society for Research in Child Development, 59*(2–3, Serial No. 240), 192–207.

Insel, T. R. (2000). Toward a neurobiology of attachment. *Review of General Psychology, 4,* 176–185.

Izard, C. E. (1994). Innate and universal facial expressions: Evidence from developmental and cross-cultural research. *Psychological Bulletin, 115,* 288–299.

Kobak, R. (1999). The emotional dynamics of disruptions in attachment relationships: Implications for theory, research, and clinical intervention. In J. Cassidy & P. R. Shaver (Eds.), *Handbook of attachment: Theory, research, and clinical applications* (pp. 21–43). New York: Guilford Press.

Kraemer, G. W. (1992). A psychobiological theory of attachment. *Behavioral and Brain Sciences, 15,* 493–541.

Levy, M. B., & Davis, K. E. (1988). Lovestyles and attachment styles compared: Their relations to each other and to various relationship characteristics. *Journal of Social and Personal Relationships, 5,* 439–471.

Main, M. (1999). Epilogue: Attachment theory: Eighteen points with suggestions for future studies. In J. Cassidy & P. R. Shaver (Eds.), *Handbook of attachment: Theory, research, and clinical applications* (pp. 845–887). New York: Guilford Press.

Marvin, R. S., & Britner, P. A. (1999). Normative development: The ontogeny of attachment. In J. Cassidy & P. R. Shaver (Eds.), *Handbook of attachment: Theory, research, and clinical applications* (pp. 44–67). New York: Guilford Press.

Mason, W. A., & Mendoza, S. P. (1998). Generic aspects of primate attachments: Parents, offspring and mates. *Psychoneuroendocrinology, 23,* 765–778.

McClintock, M. K. (1971). Menstrual synchrony and suppression. *Nature, 229,* 244–245.

Mikulincer, M. (1998). Adult attachment style and individual differences in functional versus dysfunctional experiences of anger. *Journal of Personality and Social Psychology, 74,* 513–524.

Mikulincer, M., Gillath, O., & Shaver, P. R. (2002). Activation of the attachment system in adulthood: Threat-related primes increase the accessibility of mental representations of attachment figures. *Journal of Personality and Social Psychology, 83,* 881–895.

Moffitt, T. E., Caspi, A., Belsky, J., & Silva, P. A. (1992) Childhood experience and the onset of menarche: A test of a sociobiological model. *Child Development, 63,* 47–58.

Parkes, C. M. (1972). *Bereavement studies of grief in adult life.* New York: International Universities Press.

Piaget, J. (1951). *Play, dreams and imitation in childhood.* New York: Norton.

Pietromonaco, P. R., & Feldman Barrett, L. (2000). The internal working models concept: What do we really know about the self in relation to others? *Review of General Psychology, 4,* 155–175.

Polan, H. J., & Hofer, M. A. (1999). Psychobiological origins of infant attachment and separation responses. In J. Cassidy & P. R. Shaver (Eds.), *Handbook of attachment: Theory, research, and clinical applications* (pp. 162–180). New York: Guilford Press.

Reite, M., & Boccia, M. L. (1994). Physiological aspects of adult attachment. In M. B. Sperling & W. H. Berman (Eds.), *Attachment in adults: Clinical and developmental perspectives* (pp. 98–127). New York: Guilford Press.

Reite, M., & Capitano, J. P. (1985). On the nature of social separation and social attachment. In M. Reite & T. Field (Eds.), *The psychobiology of attachment and separation* (pp. 3–49). New York: Academic Press.

Robertson, J. (1953). *A two-year-old goes to hospital* [Motion picture]. London: Tavistock Child Development Research Unit.

Russell, J. A. (1994). Is there universal recognition of emotion from facial expression? A review of the cross-cultural studies. *Psychological Bulletin, 115,* 102–141.

Shaver, P. R., Hazan, C., & Bradshaw, D. (1988) Love as attachment: The integration of three behavioral systems. In R.J. Sternberg & M.L. Barnes (Eds.), *The psychology of love* (pp. 68–99). New Haven, CT: Yale University Press.

Shaver, P. R., & Hazan, C. (1988). A biased overview of the study of love. *Journal of Social and Personal Relationships, 5,* 473–501.

Shaver, P. R., & Klinnert, M. (1982). Schachter's theories of affiliation and emotions: Implications of developmental research. In L. Wheeler (Ed.), *Review of personality and social psychology* (Vol. 3, pp. 37–71). Beverly Hills, CA: Sage.

Simpson, J. A. (1990). Influence of attachment styles on romantic relationships. *Journal of Personality and Social Psychology, 59*(5), 971–980.

Simpson, J. A., & Rholes, W. S. (1994). Stress and secure base relationships in adulthood. In K. Bartholomew & D. Perlman (Eds.), *Advances in personal relationships: Vol. 5. Attachment processes in adulthood* (pp. 181–204). London: Kingsley.

Simpson, J. A., & Rholes, W. S. (1998). Attachment in adulthood. In J. A. Simpson & W. S. Rholes (Eds.), *Attachment theory and close relationships* (pp. 3–21). New York: Guilford Press.

Simpson, J. A., Rholes, W. S., & Nelligan, J. S. (1992). Support seeking and support giving within couples in an anxiety-provoking situation: The role of attachment styles. *Journal of Personality and Social Psychology, 62,* 434–446.

Sroufe, L. A., & Waters, E. (1977a). Attachment as an organizational construct. *Child Development, 48,* 1184–1199.

Sroufe, L. A., & Waters, E. (1977b). Heart rate as a convergent measure in clinical and developmental research. *Merrill-Palmer Quarterly, 23,* 3–27.

Surbey, M. K. (1990). Family composition, stress, and the timing of human menarche. In T. E. Ziegler & F. B. Bercovitch (Eds.), *Monographs in primatology: Vol. 13. Socioendocrinology of primate reproduction* (pp. 11–32). New York: Wiley-Liss.

Suomi, S. J. (1999). Attachment in rhesus monkeys. In J. Cassidy & P. R. Shaver (Eds.), *Handbook of attachment: Theory, research, and clinical applications* (pp. 181–197). New York: Guilford Press.

Trinke, S. J., & Bartholomew, K. (1997). Hierarchies of attachment relationships in young adulthood. *Journal of Social and Personality Relationships, 14,* 603–625.

Uchino, B. N., Cacioppo, J. T., & Kiecolt-Glaser, J. K. (1996). The relationship between social support and physiological processes: A review with emphasis on underlying mechanisms and implications for health. *Psychological Bulletin, 119,* 488–531.

Uvnas-Moberg, K. (1994). Oxytocin and behaviour. *Annals of Medicine, 26,* 315–317.

Uvnas-Moberg, K. (1997). Physiological and endocrine effects of social contact. *Annals of the New York Academy of Sciences, 807,* 146–163.

Uvnas-Moberg, K. (1998). Oxytocin may mediate the benefits of positive social interaction and emotions. *Psychoneuroendocrinology, 23,* 819–835.

Veith, J. L., Buck, M., Getzlaf, S., Van Dalfsen, P., & Slade, S. (1983). Exposure to men influences the occurrence of ovulation in women. *Physiology and Behavior, 31,* 313–315.

Vernikos-Danellis, J., & Winget, C. M (1979). The importance of light, postural, and social cues in the regulation of the plasma corticel rhythms in man. In A. Reinberg & F. Halbert (Eds.), *Chronopharmacology* (pp. 101–106). New York: Pergamon.

Vormbrock, J. K. (1993). Attachment theory as applied to wartime and job-related marital separation. *Psychological Bulletin, 114,* 122–144.

Weiss, R. S. (1975). *Marital separation: Coping with the end of a marriage and the transition to being single again.* New York: Basic Books.

Zeifman, D., & Hazan, C. (1997). A process model of adult attachment formation. In S. Duck (Ed.), *Handbook of personal relationships* (2nd ed., pp. 179–195). Chichester, UK: Wiley.

CHAPTER 4

A Dynamical Systems Approach to Conceptualizing and Studying Stability and Change in Attachment Security

R. CHRIS FRALEY
CLAUDIA CHLOE BRUMBAUGH

In his 1973 volume, *Separation,* Bowlby analyzed the concept of developmental pathways by exploring the metaphor of a complex railway system. Bowlby asked his readers to consider a railway track that begins in a large metropolitan center. If a traveler were to begin his or her journey by selecting the main route, the traveler would eventually reach a point at which the railroad branches into a number of distinct tracks. Some of these tracks will lead to distant, unfamiliar lands; other tracks, although deviating from the main route, will run more or less parallel to it. As the traveler's journey progresses, he or she will be faced with new choices at each juncture. The choices that traveler makes will have important implications for his or her destination, making some locations more accessible and placing others further out of reach.

Bowlby believed that the railway metaphor was an apt one for characterizing personality development. Early in life, for example, there are a multitude of pathways along which people may develop and a variety of destinations at which they may arrive (see Sroufe & Jacobvitz, 1989). Some of these "destinations" may involve well-functioning relationships with family, peers, and partners, whereas others may not. As people navigate alternative pathways, they generate a certain degree of momentum, making their life trajectories more entrenched and increasingly difficult to transform. In Bowlby's view, one of the key goals of developmental science is to map the pathways by which people develop and, importantly, uncover the processes that either keep people on a specific developmental course or allow them to deviate from routes previously traveled.

Although developmental psychologists have made substantial progress toward documenting the life events that may lead a person to follow one route as opposed to another, they have yet to elucidate the dynamic processes that allow these life events to shape personality development. Our objective in this chapter is to take a novel step in this direction by exploring Bowlby's ideas on development, stability, and change from a dynamical systems perspective (see Smith & Thelen, 1993; van Geert, 1994). Briefly stated, a *dynamical systems approach* to development emphasizes the ways in which a system of coordinated variables evolves over time. One of the themes of this approach is that interesting properties of behavior can emerge from processes that are not explicitly represented in the system's "rules" per se. For example, the global schematic properties of memory systems appear to emerge from the local interactions among interconnected neurons, none of which is designed to behave in a schematic manner (Rumelhart, McClelland, & the PDP Research Group, 1986). Understanding the rules that underlie the global and emergent properties of such systems is one of the major objectives of a dynamical approach.

By adopting a dynamical systems perspective, we hope to answer some unresolved questions in contemporary attachment theory and research. The first is, What are the dynamic mechanisms that contribute to both stability and change in attachment organization? We focus less on the *specific kinds of events* (e.g., divorce) that may lead to change in security and emphasize instead the more *general processes* that allow such events to sustain and contribute to personality dynamics. In doing so, we hope to provide a general framework within which future researchers can conceptualize the ways that specific life events influence the dynamics of attachment. The second question we address is, What are the implications of these dynamic mechanisms for how we understand the stability of attachment patterns over time? The issue of how much stability exists in attachment patterns is a hotly debated one in contemporary research (e.g., Lewis, Feiring, & Rosenthal, 2000; Waters, Merrick, Treboux, Crowell, & Albersheim, 2000). One of the arguments that we make in this chapter is that, when Bowlby's ideas about stability and change are formalized, they do not necessarily lead to the prediction that attachment patterns will be highly stable across different developmental periods. Although Bowlby's ideas have some fascinating implications for how we should conceptualize stability, these implications are much more complex and nuanced than has been previously assumed.

We begin this chapter by reviewing Bowlby's ideas on development, stability, and change. As we discuss, many of Bowlby's thoughts were shaped by the writings of C. H. Waddington, a developmental embryologist whose work has had an enormous impact on developmental science and the study of biological systems. We review Waddington's ideas in some depth and summarize the relationship between his ideas and Bowlby's thinking on continuity, change, and personality development. Next, we use simulation techniques and mathematical analysis—the common methodological tools of dynamical systems approaches—to model the theoretical mechanisms that Bowlby discussed. As we illustrate, the forms of stability that emerge from the formalization of these mechanisms have important implications for the way attachment researchers should conceptualize and measure attachment stability across the life course. Finally, we review empirical data on stability and change and discuss the implications of those data for Bowlby's ideas about the role of early experiences in shaping adult relationships. It is our hope that this chapter will help clarify attachment theory's predictions about the degree of stability that should (and should not) be observed over the life course, as well as highlight some innovative avenues for research that may lead to advances in our understanding of attachment and human development.

THE CONCEPTS OF DEVELOPMENTAL PATHWAYS AND CANALIZATION

Bowlby's railway metaphor was inspired by C. H. Waddington's (1957) discussion of the cybernetics of cell development. Because Waddington's ideas had a profound influence on Bowlby, as well as on other developmentalists, we explore them in some depth in this chapter. Waddington, an esteemed developmental embryologist writing in the middle of the 20th century, was trying to understand how a cell may maintain a specific developmental trajectory in the face of external disturbances. Waddington and others had observed that, once a cell begins to assume specific functions (e.g., it becomes integrated into a structure that will become part of the visual system), weak experimental interventions are unlikely to alter the cell's developmental trajectory. Although a cell has the potential to assume many different fates early in its development, once a developmental trajectory becomes established, Waddington argued that the trajectory becomes *canalized* or buffered to some degree, making it less and less likely that the cell will deviate from that developmental course.

   To illustrate these dynamics more concretely, Waddington compared them to the behavior of a marble rolling down a hill (see Figure 4.1). In Waddington's well-known analogy, the marble represents a cell, and the various troughs at the end of the landscape represent alternative developmental functions or "fates" that the cell can assume. Waddington considered the specific shape of the landscape to be controlled by the complex interactions among genes, hence leading Waddington to refer to it as the *epigenetic landscape*.

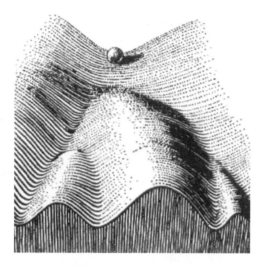

FIGURE 4.1. Waddington's (1957, p. 29) epigenetic landscape.

After the marble begins its descent, it settles into one of several pathways defined by the valley floors of the epigenetic landscape. A slight push may force the marble away from its course, but the marble will eventually reestablish its trajectory. As the marble continues along the basin of a specific valley, it becomes increasingly unlikely that external forces will cause it to jump from one valley to the next. Certain features of the marble, such as its smoothness and momentum, help to keep the marble moving along the previously established path. Features intrinsic to the landscape itself also help to maintain the marble on its original pathway. The steepness and curvature of the hills, for example, serve to cradle the marble and buffer it from external forces.

Waddington (1957) considered the tendency for the marble to maintain its initial course in the face of external pressures to be an analogue to a fundamental self-regulatory process in cell development, one he called *homeorhesis*. Homeorhesis refers to the tendency of a system to maintain a specific developmental trajectory—or a course toward a specific developmental outcome—despite external perturbations. Although many biologists had discussed a similar concept, *homeostasis*, Waddington considered homeostasis to be an inadequate concept for understanding certain features of development. In Waddington's view, the concept of homeostasis placed too much emphasis on the steady state being regulated by the system. For example, in the physiological regulation of body temperature, there may be a tendency for the nervous system to activate or terminate certain physiological processes that function to minimize the discrepancy between a "desired" temperature and the current body temperature. Although Waddington recognized that the dynamic quality of homeostatic processes was critical to understanding certain features of physiological functioning, Waddington argued that self-organizing developmental processes function to maintain a *pathway* or *trajectory* toward a specific *end state* rather than a steady state per se: "We are not dealing with the maintenance of a steady state but with the attainment of some particular end-state in spite of temporary deviations on the way there" (Waddington, 1957, p. 42).

Waddington (1957) argued that the specific pathways available to the cell early in development are determined by the way the genes interact to initiate and control biochemical reactions. Moreover, as symbolized in Figure 4.1, he believed that these reactions operate in a manner that leads the valleys of the epigenetic landscape to become more entrenched over time. Thus, once a cell settles into one of several available pathways, it becomes increasingly likely to follow that specific pathway.

The notion that the cell's development might be buffered or canalized to some extent was a critical aspect of Waddington's (1957) analogy. Waddington, however, also recognized that different kinds of physiological systems may require a stronger degree of canalization than others. For some systems, external influences are critical for organizing the system in a way that will allow it to function appropriately. For example, cortical cells in the visual system may not develop appropriately without specific forms of feedback from the external world (O'Leary, Schlaggar, & Tuttle, 1994). Other systems, however, develop in a fairly specific way despite external perturbations (Geary & Huffman, 2002; Rakic, 1988).

Homeorhetic Mechanisms in Personality Development

The concept of "degree of canalization" was highly influential in Bowlby's thinking, and he often wrote of "environmentally labile" traits to refer to properties that were less subject to canalization. For example, Bowlby (1969/1982) argued that the development of the attachment behavioral system was highly canalized, in the sense that the rudimentary set of control mechanisms and behavior programs needed to allow a child to regulate his or her proximity to a caregiver effectively would emerge despite a diverse range of environmental experiences. Bowlby believed, however, that the *specific way* a child comes to regulate his or her attachment behavior is highly influenced by interpersonal experiences and that, for the system to function appropriately in a specific caregiving environment, it needs to be calibrated, more or less, to that environment. Bowlby believed that early experiences within the family—especially those concerned with separation or threats of loss—were particularly influential in shaping the way the attachment system would become organized for an individual. According to his railway metaphor, early experiences in the family help to determine which of many possible routes the individual may travel.[1]

In the context of personality development, Bowlby believed that once an initial pathway has been established, a number of homeorhetic processes keep an individual on that pathway. Bowlby separated these homeorhetic processes into two broad kinds. The first is concerned with the *caregiving environment* itself. To the extent to which the individual's environment is stable, he or she is unlikely to experience interactions that challenge his or her representations of the world. The powerful nature of this variable was emphasized by Bowlby's (1973) observation that a child is typically born into a family in which he or she has the same parents, same community, and the same broad ecology for long periods of time. It is during periods of transition (e.g., parental divorce, relocating to a new town, tragedy, or good fortune), Bowlby believed, that an individual is most likely to be forced off of one developmental track and onto another.

Bowlby (1973) also discussed *intraindividual* or *psychodynamic* homeorhetic processes that may promote continuity. Bowlby noted that people often select their environments in ways that maximize the overlap between the psychological qualities of the situation and the expectations and preferences that the individual holds. Moreover, the mind, Bowlby argued, operates in a way that is likely to assimilate new information into existing schemas (see Collins & Read, 1994, for an excellent discussion of this point in the context of theory and research on social cognition). Consistent with these ideas, empirical research has shown that people's working models influence the kinds of reactions they elicit from others (Arend, Gove, & Sroufe, 1979; Troy & Sroufe, 1987; Waters, Wippman, & Sroufe, 1979) and the kinds of inferences they make about people's intentions during experimental contexts (Brumbaugh & Fraley, 2004; Collins, 1996; Pierce, Sarason, & Sarason, 1992; Pietromonaco & Carnelley, 1994). Such dynamics allow working models to shape the kinds of interactions the person experiences and, in concert, help to maintain the individual on the pathway that is already being traveled. To the extent to which the individual diverges from that pathway, it would seem unlikely that he or she would wander far.

MODELING THE DYNAMICS OF STABILITY AND CHANGE

One of the challenges of trying to understand psychological development is the recursive, iterative nature of the dynamics involved. Bowlby, for example, believed that a child's working models are constructed on the basis of the early experiences he or she has in the family environment but that the nature of those experiences is based, in part, on the working models that the child holds. In this view, the child's beliefs and the social environment in which he or she is situated have reciprocal influences on one another. Although it is possible to speculate on the implications of such dynamics for the way attachment representations evolve over time, the feedback mechanisms entailed by such a process may produce patterns that are difficult to anticipate on the basis of intuition alone (see van Geert, 1997, for an excellent discussion on the nature of recursion and theoretical modeling). In order to understand better the precise implications of such processes, we formalize Bowlby's ideas using dynamic modeling techniques and explore those models via computer simulation and mathematics.

Simulation of the Dynamics of Waddington's Epigenetic Landscape

We begin with a computational simulation of Waddington's epigenetic landscape because it provides the theoretical foundation for Bowlby's ideas on stability and change. As discussed previously, Waddington's analogy is often used to illustrate the ways in which homeorhetic processes can keep an individual on a specific developmental course despite the existence of perturbations. Unfortunately, the role of external influences on the behavior of the marble is often overlooked when considering Waddington's analogy. If we were to give the marble a strong push toward an alternative pathway, the marble would clearly jump over the valley wall and assume a new fate. When Waddington's analogy is invoked, however, it is often assumed that external factors rarely come into play and that, when they do, the forces they exert are weak or inconsequential. Although external factors may, in reality, be weak, it is necessary to recognize that, because the marble *can* be pushed into a new valley with an appropriate amount of force, the model may not *ensure* stability.

Why does this matter? Bowlby clearly believed that there was a strong tendency for working models, once constructed, to maintain an individual on a specific developmental trajectory. At the same time, however, Bowlby (1969/1982, 1973, 1980) emphasized that working models need to be open to change in order to be adaptive. In fact, according to many perspectives on psychopathology, the persistence of previously established beliefs and expectations in light of evidence to the contrary is a sign of poor psychological adjustment (e.g., Horowitz, 1991). The fact that the theory allows for people to change implies that, even if we postulate the existence of homeorhetic mechanisms, Bowlby's basic model, like Waddington's, does not ensure stability. If this is the case, the predictions that psychologists often derive from attachment theory regarding the long-term stability of attachment patterns may be oversimplified.

Whether this is the case or not, of course, needs to be demonstrated in a formal manner. In the following set of investigations, we explore a computer simulation of Waddington's epigenetic landscape to obtain a better understanding of the implications of this analogy for the way personality ebbs and flows over time. Our first step was to simulate an epigenetic landscape. We generated a landscape that was similar to the one illustrated by Waddington in several important respects. As can be seen in Figure 4.2, the simulated surface is placed on an incline, thereby compelling the marble to move downward in the direction depicted by the arrow. Moreover, the various valleys become deeper (i.e., the pathways become more canalized) as the marble moves from one end of the surface to the other.

Next, we programmed some physical rules to govern the behavior of the marble. Specifically, the simulation was constructed so that the marble's direction of travel at any one point in time was a function of three factors: (1) the slope of the local (i.e., immediately surrounding) landscape, (2) the direction of the marble's current motion and its momentum, and (3) the relative magnitude of those two forces (i.e., the slope of the landscape with respect to the momentum of the marble).

To see how the simulation works, consider Figure 4.2. If we place a simulated marble in the upper left side of the surface, the marble descends into the first or left-most valley and settles into a trajectory defined by that valley floor (see the left-hand panel of Figure 4.2). When we place the marble in other locations, the marble settles into other pathways (see the right-hand panel of Figure 4.2).

What are the implications of the basic "rules" of this dynamic system for understanding global or emergent patterns of continuity and change? To systematically explore this issue, we simulated numerous trials in which we dropped a marble on the surface and traced its pathway over time. We conceptualized the different tiles, moving from left to right in Figure 4.2,

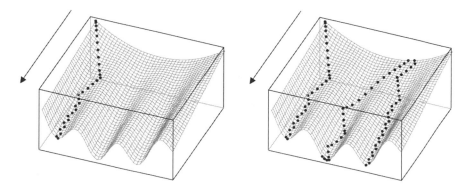

FIGURE 4.2. The canalization of developmental trajectories within Waddington's epigenetic landscape. The arrow depicts the flow of time.

as representing graded variation in a trait, such that marbles placed toward the left side of the surface exhibit less of the trait and marbles at the right side of the surface are better defined by the trait. By conceptualizing the surface in this manner, we could quantify the stability of the trait by computing the correlation between starting positions and ending positions for a population of marbles. The analogy to personality development should be clear: If we conceptualize the trait or property as being attachment security, the marble's trajectory over time represents the individual's developmental pathway with respect to attachment, and the correlation between the marble's position at Time 1 and the last time point represents the degree of stability in security from infancy to adulthood.[2]

In this example, the correlation between the starting positions and ending positions of the marbles is very high ($r > .90$). It is less than 1.00 because the shape of the landscape ensures that there are fewer viable ending positions than there are starting positions. In fact, this feature of the landscape creates a situation in which knowing the *precise* starting point of a marble (as opposed to the *general* vicinity of the marble's starting point) does not help us predict its fate. Because marbles that begin anywhere between the first and third tile all end up at the same point (the end of the first valley), information about the exact starting position is inconsequential. If we were to quantify the starting position with respect to the *bifurcations* imposed by the surface (i.e., if we were to classify an individual's starting position with respect to the developmental pathways afforded by the system rather than exact position), we would have perfect knowledge (i.e., $r = 1.00$) of the marble's end state simply by knowing its beginning state.

The fact that the surface has this *channeling effect* on the marble's pathway leads to an interesting pattern in the test–retest correlations. We have illustrated these patterns in Figure 4.3 through the use of *stability functions*. Stability functions provide an efficient way to portray graphically the information contained in a test–retest correlation matrix for a trait assessed over multiple points in time (see Fraley, 2002; Fraley & Roberts, in press). A Time k stability function characterizes the degree of stability observed between Time k and all points in time. For example, a Time 1 stability function describes the stability between Time 1 and Time 1, Time 1 and Time 2, Time 1 and Time 3, and so on. Similarly, a Time 25 stability function describes the stability between Time 25 and all time points (i.e., Time 1 through Time 50). Figure 4.3 illustrates the Time 1, Time 25, and Time 50 stability functions for the simulation described previously.

There are a couple of noteworthy features of these functions. First, the Time 1 stability function initially decreases rapidly but then levels off at a very high value ($r \cong .94$). This occurs because, once the marbles settle into their pathways, their position on the left-to-right axis does not

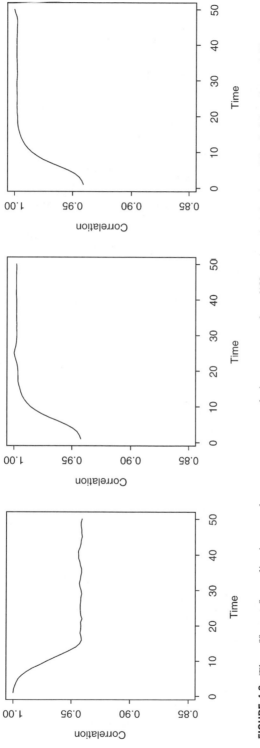

FIGURE 4.3. The effects of canalization on the test–retest correlations expected at different points in time. The left-hand panel illustrates the Time 1 stability function; the middle panel illustrates the Time 25 stability function; the right-hand panel illustrates the Time 50 stability function.

change. As a consequence, given knowledge of a marble's position at Time 1, it is possible to predict the position of a marble at Time 50 with the same degree of accuracy as at Time 25—despite the fact that the time span differs considerably. Another feature of the curves worth noting is the asymmetry involved in predicting a marble's position forward in time versus backward in time. At Time 25, for example, it is easier to predict where the marble will be at Time 50 ($r \cong .99$) than it is to infer where the marble was at Time 1 ($r \cong .94$; see the middle panel of Figure 4.3). Although both time points are exactly 25 units of time away from Time 25, the degree of predictability is not equivalent.

We elaborate on these findings in more detail in subsequent sections. For now, however, it should be noted that these distinctive *patterns* (but not necessarily the precise quantitative *values*) of stability should be observed in empirical research on attachment if, in fact, the abstracted dynamics of Waddington's system apply to personality development.

Up to this point, we have simulated the behavior of marbles on the epigenetic landscape in the absence of external influences. What happens when we introduce a disturbance to the system? As a single-trial illustration, consider the left-hand panel of Figure 4.4. This figure illustrates the trajectory of a marble that begins near the upper right side of the landscape. About halfway through its journey, the marble is suddenly pushed up the valley wall. Nonetheless, the force is not powerful enough to cause the marble to reach the cusp of the wall, so the homeorhetic properties of the system guide the marble toward its original trajectory. The right-hand panel, in contrast, illustrates a case in which the external force was strong enough to force the marble over the hill and into a new valley. Once crossing the cusp, the marble establishes a new trajectory rather than return-

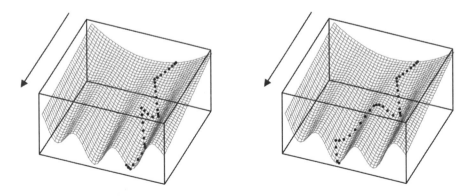

FIGURE 4.4. The effects of external influences on the trajectory of the marble across Waddington's epigenetic landscape. The arrow depicts the flow of time.

ing to its previous one. In Waddington's terms, the marble has established a new end state and, hence, a new developmental trajectory.

It should be clear from this simple illustration that whether homeorhetic processes allow for long-term stability will depend on how many times the marble is pushed around and with what degree of force it is pushed. If the marble is only gently nudged, homeorhetic forces will overcome the disturbance and return the marble to its original pathway. If, however, the marble is subject to the "slings and arrows of outrageous fortune," it may be impossible to determine the marble's fate in the long run.

To explore the impact of external perturbations more systematically, we conducted a simulation similar to the previous one, but this time we included external disturbances. To introduce disturbances to the system, we allowed the marble to be pushed in a random direction with variable force at varying points in time. We did, however, impose certain constraints on the nature of these disturbances. For example, we did not allow the marble to be pushed backward, and we never allowed the marble to be pushed off the epigenetic surface.

In Figure 4.5, we have plotted the Time 1, Time 25, and Time 50 stability functions resulting from a simulation in which the force of the perturbations was fairly strong. As can be seen from the Time 1 stability function, it is easy to determine where a marble will be at Time 2 from the simple knowledge of where it was at Time 1. However, *the further away in time we move from Time 1, the harder it is to predict a marble's fate.* In fact, in this simulation, our ability to predict a marble's final position is no better than chance; the limiting value of the correlation as time increases is 0.00.

It is noteworthy that, in comparison with the Time 25 stability function we observed in the previous simulation, the Time 25 stability function resulting from this simulation is much more symmetric. In this case, we can predict a marble's position from Time 25 with virtually the same degree of accuracy (or inaccuracy) regardless of whether we are looking forward in time (e.g., Time 30) or backward in time (e.g., Time 20).

We have deliberately presented two extreme situations (i.e., one in which there are no disturbances and one in which there are powerful disturbances) as a way of anchoring the range of dynamics exhibited by Waddington's system. As one might deduce, the patterning of the stability functions migrates between the two extremes previously illustrated, as we gradually manipulate the degree of disturbance (see Figure 4.6 for some example stability functions).

Implications of Waddington's Epigenetic Landscape Analogy for Personality Development

We believe that there are two important conclusions to be drawn from these simulations. First, the abstract processes described by Waddington

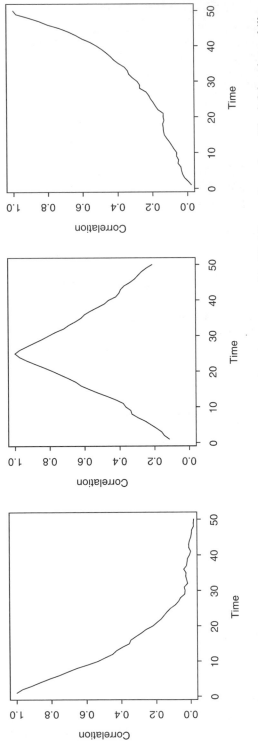

FIGURE 4.5. The effects of large external influences on the stability functions expected in Waddington's analogy. The left-hand panel illustrates the Time 1 stability function; the middle panel illustrates the Time 25 stability function; the right-hand panel illustrates the Time 50 stability function.

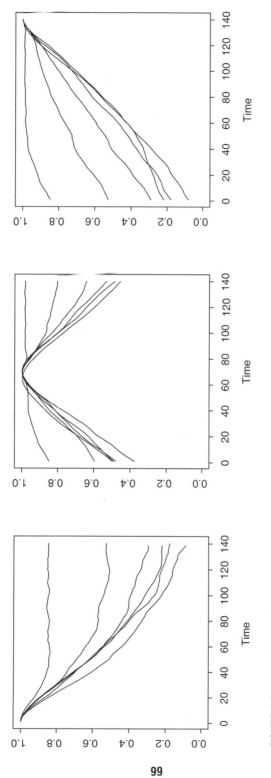

FIGURE 4.6. The effects of external influences of varying magnitude on the stability functions expected in Waddington's analogy. The left-hand panel illustrates the Time 1 stability function; the middle panel illustrates the Time 70 stability function; the right-hand panel illustrates the Time 140 stability function.

have concrete implications for the *pattern* of test–retest correlations that should be observed over time. This discovery is crucial because, if we did not have a way to translate the outcomes of Waddington's dynamics into a form that can be used to quantify stability in a variety of biological systems, the analogy loses its power as a theoretical tool. The fact that we can simulate the system and study the test–retest correlations observed in different conditions allows us to better understand the implications of the analogy for conceptualizing stability and change. Most important, it provides us with a means for determining the extent to which these dynamics manifest themselves in personality development. That is, by comparing empirical data on attachment against the patterns predicted by Waddington's model, we can begin to discern the extent to which homeorhetic processes underlie personality development. We return to this point later in the chapter.

The second key point to take away from these simulations is that, if we are to use the dynamics entailed by Waddington's analogy as a metaphor for those that underlie personality development, we must recognize that, *although these dynamics can give rise to stability, they do not ensure stability*. If we assume that the influence of external forces on the system is nontrivial, then the degree of stability predicted by the system in the long run will be zero. Of course, homeorhetic processes help to maintain the marble's pathway in the face of external influences, but they cannot do so if the force of the external influence is greater than the resistance provided by these processes. Once this theoretical threshold has been crossed, understanding the fate of the marble is more a matter of understanding the history of external influences that the marble has faced rather than of understanding the nature of homeorhetic processes per se.

MODELING HOMEORHETIC PROCESSES
IN PERSONALITY DEVELOPMENT

Thus far we have seen that Waddington's analogy—an analogy that has had a critical influence on the way Bowlby and others have conceptualized personality development—is much more complex in its implications than is generally recognized. In the absence of strong external forces, the analogy implies a high degree of stability in a marble's position over time. In the context of strong disturbances, however, the analogy implies not only that the degree of stability will be weaker but also that it will approach zero asymptotically over time. In short, Waddington's dynamics, although capable of providing an explanation for stability, do not necessarily predict a *high* degree of stability.

The next challenge is to take Bowlby's ideas about the specific processes giving rise to stability and change in attachment organization, formalize them, and determine whether they make the same predictions about continuity made by Waddington's analogy. We focus on two key questions: (1) What are the abstracted dynamic mechanisms that contribute to both stability and change in attachment organization? and (2) What are the implications of these dynamic mechanisms for how we understand the stability of attachment patterns over time?

The Mechanisms of Stability and Change in Attachment

Bowlby (1973) discussed three classes of homeorhetic mechanisms: (1) person–environment transactions, (2) the diminishing sensitivity over time of working models to environmental influences, and (3) the establishment of stable representations of attachment experiences (i.e., *prototypes*) early in life—representations that serve as a foundation for subsequent experiences. After briefly discussing each of these mechanisms of stability, we develop a mathematical model for each one and investigate the implications of those theoretical models for the patterns of stability and change that should be observed over time.

Transactional Processes

According to Bowlby, one reason that attachment patterns may be relatively stable over time is that there are reciprocal influences between the representational models constructed by an individual and the quality of his or her caregiving environment. Although working models are constructed on the basis of social experiences, those models eventually come to influence the quality of the social interactions the child has. This general theme—that people and their environments mutually constrain one another—is common to many contemporary perspectives on personality development (for reviews, see Caspi & Roberts, 1999; Fraley & Roberts, in press). The fact that the social environment is constrained by the working models that the individual holds suggests that working models are unlikely to be challenged over the course of development.

Decreasing Sensitivity

A second source of homeorhesis discussed by Bowlby (1973) was epigenetic sensitivity. Drawing on Waddington's ideas about "degrees of canalization," Bowlby argued that the attachment system is more sensitive to environmental influences early in development: "The model proposed postulates that the psychological processes that result in personality structure are endowed with a fair degree of sensitivity to environment, especially to family environment, during the early years of life, but a sensitivity that diminishes throughout childhood and is already very limited by the end of adolescence" (Bowlby, 1973, p. 367). Although Bowlby did not specify the precise mechanisms that may lead sensitivity to diminish (e.g., neural changes, social-cognitive mechanisms, environmental changes), his proposition implies that the social environment is less influential later in life.

Prototype Representations

A third homeorhetic mechanism that Bowlby discussed concerned the enduring nature of representations of early experiences:

> No variables . . . have more far-reaching effects on personality development than have a child's experiences within his family: for, starting during his first months in his relations with his mother figure, and extending through the years of childhood and adolescence in his relations with both parents, he builds up working models of how attachment figures are likely to behave towards him in any of a variety of situations; and on those models are based all his expectations, and therefore all his plans, for the rest of his life. (1973, p. 369)

According to Bowlby, a system of nonlinguistic representations, procedural "rules" of information processing, and behavioral strategies is constructed in early life that serves as an adaptation to the individual's early caregiving environment. As complex cognitive capacities emerge, however, representational models develop that are consciously accessible and more easily updated to reflect ongoing relationship experiences. However, the early representations themselves remain unchanged. These early "prototypes" remain autonomous yet continue to play an ongoing role in shaping the quality of the caregiving environment.

The prototype concept provides a powerful theoretical mechanism for explaining patterns of stability. If children are continuously drawing on patterns of behavior and belief acquired early in life, attachment patterns should be somewhat consistent across different developmental periods (Sroufe, 1979; Sroufe, Egeland, & Kreutzer, 1990). Sroufe and his colleagues (1990, p. 1364), for example, have argued that "earlier patterns may again become manifest in certain contexts, in the face of further environmental change, or in the face of certain critical developmental issues. While perhaps latent, and perhaps never even to become manifest again in some cases, the earlier pattern is not gone." The notion that some aspects of working models may be more primitive or have more priority than other attachment representations is consistent with contemporary perspectives on the organization of working models that emphasize the hierarchical structure of attachment representations (e.g., Collins & Read, 1994). In Collins and Read's (1994) hierarchical model, for example, relationship-specific representations, although influenced by existing representations, may be constructed and updated without affecting representations that have priority in the hierarchy. In short, although there may be a degree of coherence across the kinds of attachment representations that an individual develops, the representations that are constructed early in life may continue to be especially influential in later childhood and early adulthood (for further discussion of the prototype hypothesis, see Fraley, 2002; Owens et al., 1995; Sroufe et al., 1990; van IJzendoorn, 1996).

Modeling the Dynamics of Attachment Stability and Change

In the sections that follow, we explore formal mathematical models of each of these homeorhetic mechanisms. Although these processes could be construed as operating in concert, we begin by modeling and discussing each process separately in order to highlight the specific implications of each mechanism for understanding stability and change in attachment security. To model these dynamic processes, we use difference equations (see Haefner, 1996, and Huckfeldt, Kohfeld, & Likens, 1982, for a clear and concise introduction to the use of difference equations in behavioral science). In a *difference equation,* a variable at one point in time, t, is modeled as a function of itself at an immediately preceding time point, $t - 1$, and of any factors contributing to its change. For example, in the equation $P_t = P_{t-1} + \Delta P_{t-1}$, variable P, a personality trait, is modeled as a function of itself at an immediately preceding point in time $(t-1)$ and of all variables that cause it to change (ΔP_{t-1}). In the following sections, we show how the dynamics of these processes influence the patterns of stability and change that should be observed in attachment. Readers who are interested in the mathematical details of these analyses and simulations can find them in Fraley (2002) and Fraley and Roberts (in press).

Modeling Transactional Processes in Attachment Development

We begin by making explicit four assumptions previously discussed. First, on the basis of attachment theory and research, we assume that there is variability in the security of the working models held by individuals, such that some people are more secure than others (see Fraley & Spieker, 2003; Fraley & Waller, 1998). Although contemporary models of individual differences emphasize the two dimensions that underlie security (Fraley & Shaver, 2000; Griffin & Bartholomew, 1994), for the purposes of this chapter we assume that these dimensions exhibit the same dynamic properties. (Whether that is the case is open for future research and discussion.) Second, we assume that as an individual navigates his or her social environment, his or her working models are influenced by the quality of the social environment (i.e., whether others are sensitive and responsive to one's needs; see Ainsworth, Blehar, Waters, & Wall, 1978). In other words, if someone is treated in a cold or aloof manner, we expect that person's level of security to decrease to some extent. Conversely, if the individual experiences warm and responsive care or support from significant others, we expect his or her security to increase to some degree. Third, we assume that the responses solicited from significant others will tend to be consistent with existing working models. That is, working models not only reflect the quality of the caregiving environment but also play an active role in shaping the quality of the caregiving environment. This process may manifest itself in the way in which working models bias or color the interpretation of relational events (e.g., Collins, 1996) or in the kinds of interaction partners that people select (e.g., Frazier, Byer, Fischer, Wright, & DeBord, 1996). Fourth, we assume, as Lewis (1997) has argued, that there are some stochastic processes in these dynamics. In other words, working models are not 100% predictable from the quality of the caregiving environment, nor is the quality of the caregiving environment 100% predictable from the security of one's working models.

In the transactional model, the theoretical processes are fully interdependent: The person influences his or her relational context, and the relational context influences the person. What do these processes predict about the form and magnitude of stability over time? To explore this question, we studied the stability functions implied by the transactional model under a variety of parameter values. Figure 4.7 shows some typical stability functions implied by the transactional model under different parameter values. As can be seen, the age 1 stability function (left-hand panel) begins high (the correlation of a variable with itself is necessarily 1), decelerates rapidly, and gradually bottoms out at an expected test–retest correlation of zero. The age 30 and age 60 functions are similar; the curves decelerate quickly as the interval between the age in question and other ages increases, approaching zero in both directions for the age 30 function (i.e., going backward or forward in time) and approaching zero going back in time for the age 60 function.

Notice that the values chosen for different parameters in the model affect how rapidly the curves decelerate. When environmental factors are allowed to have a large impact on the person, for example, change occurs more quickly, and the curves decelerate rapidly. When environmental factors are allowed to have only a minor impact on the person, or, alternatively, when working models are allowed to have a powerful influence on the social environment that the person experiences, change in security is much more gradual. In each case, however, notice that the stability functions approach zero as the time interval increases. In other words, if transactional processes—coupled with stochastic forces—are the only processes affecting attachment development, the expected correlation between se-

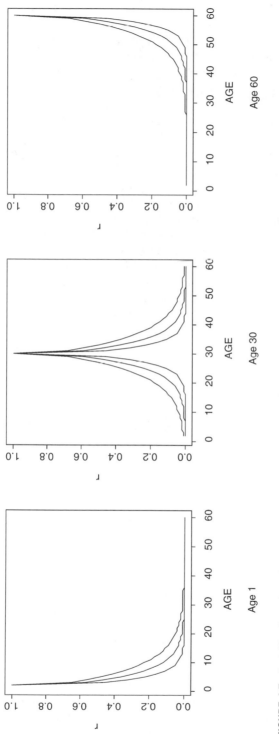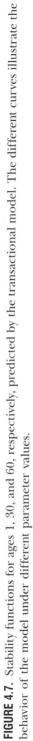

FIGURE 4.7. Stability functions for ages 1, 30, and 60, respectively, predicted by the transactional model. The different curves illustrate the behavior of the model under different parameter values.

curity in childhood and any sufficiently distant age is zero, regardless of how much or how little an effect the environment has on people.

In summary, according to the transactional model, the correlation between initial states of security and subsequent states of security gradually approaches zero. This is a critical finding because it demonstrates that, if transactional processes underlie attachment dynamics, we should not necessarily expect a high degree of stability from infancy to adulthood. Transactional processes promote stability in the sense that they affect the "decay rate" of the stability functions but do not alter the limiting value of those curves. Even if people play an active and powerful role in shaping their social environments, we expect the correlation between security early in life and later in life to approach zero over the long run.

Given that people are playing an active role in shaping their environments, why do transactional dynamics predict stability functions that approach zero over time? The answer to this question lies in the way the residuals affect the dynamics of the model. At each point in time, a portion of random variance contributes to security (see Fraley, 2002). To the extent that these stochastic factors play a role in shaping personality development, a person's developmental trajectory is guaranteed to get bumped around in unpredictable ways. Indeed, the individual developmental trajectories implied by the model could be described as *random walks*; it is nearly impossible to know where each person is going to end up in the long run from simple knowledge of where each person began (cf., our second Waddington simulation, Figure 4.5). The important point here is that nothing in the conjectured dynamics is "grounding" the person; there is no developmental tether, so to speak, keeping the person within a circumscribed region of developmental space. As such, a person's level of security, while influencing his or her environment, will tend to bounce around as random environmental events occur. Transactional dynamics can limit the magnitude of the influence of these random factors but do not remove them completely. If stochastic factors were removed from the model, transactional processes would imply perfect stability (i.e., $r = 1.00$ – measurement error) across all ages.

Modeling Decreasing Environmental Sensitivity

To incorporate Bowlby's ideas about the decreasing sensitivity of working models to environmental factors over time, we relaxed some of the constraints that were present in the previous simulation. Specifically, we allowed environmental factors to have less impact on security over time. Prototypical stability functions for the decreasing sensitivity model are depicted in Figure 4.8. As can be seen, the stability functions predicted by this model are similar to those observed before in that they all approach a zero asymptote. However, there is a noteworthy difference between these

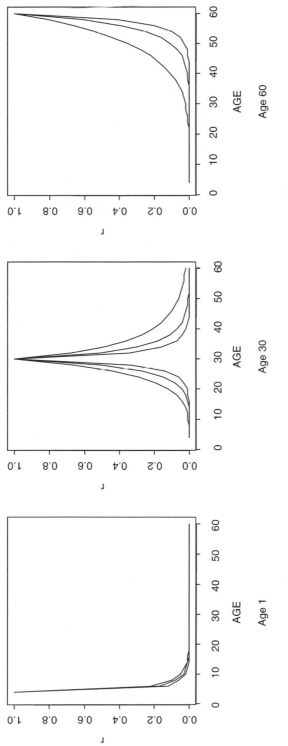

FIGURE 4.8. Stability functions for ages 1, 30, and 60, respectively, predicted by the decreasing-sensitivity model. The different curves illustrate the behavior of the model under different parameter values.

curves and those observed previously. Notice that the curves "decay" much more quickly going forward in time than backward in time. In other words, the rate of change for the age 1 stability function is faster than that of the age 30 stability function, whereas these curves were symmetric in the transactional model we studied previously.

The interesting implication of this finding is that, if one wanted to predict attachment security at any time from measurements taken at age 30, one would do much better making predictions about how people will turn out in the future as opposed to making inferences about what they were like in the past. Notice that the asymmetry in the stability functions is apparent under a variety of parameter values.

It is noteworthy that, despite the fact that environmental sensitivity decreases over time, the curves still approach 0.00 in the limit. Thus, although the decreasing sensitivity of working models may promote the stability of attachment from infancy to adulthood, this mechanism cannot do so in a way that ensures a high degree of stability over time. In other words, even if working models become increasingly resistant to change as people develop, it is still possible that an individual's attachment pattern in adulthood will be unpredictable from his or her attachment pattern in infancy. The exception to this rule occurs when the plasticity of working models is set to zero. In this case, there comes a point at which there is no change in working models, and they are perfectly stable.

In summary, the decreasing-sensitivity model implies that working models of attachment should become less responsive to environmental inputs over the course of development. When formalized, this model predicts an interesting asymmetry in the stability functions that should be observed at different points in the lifespan. For example, according to the model, it should be easier to predict how secure an adult will be across 5 years of adulthood than to predict how secure a child will be across 5 years of childhood.

Modeling the Dynamics of Prototype Processes

According to the prototype hypothesis, a latent factor (i.e., a representational prototype) exerts a consistent influence on attachment dynamics throughout the lifespan. We can represent this idea formally by modifying the transactional model that we discussed previously. Specifically, if we add a variable that represents early or primal representational models and allow it to influence working models at subsequent points in the lifespan, then the prototype will have both direct and indirect effects on the developmental dynamics of attachment (see Fraley, 2002). The mathematical structure of this model is an extension of the trait–state–error models explicated by Kenny and his colleagues (e.g., Kenny & Zautra, 2001; see Lemery, Goldsmith, Klinnert, & Mrazek, 1999, for a similar application).

What patterns of stability does this model imply? To explore this question, we varied the magnitude of the prototype effect and studied the resulting stability functions. Some examples of stability functions are depicted in Figure 4.9. As can be seen, the stability functions predicted by this model are dramatically different from those implied by the other models of development. Specifically, the stability functions have nonzero asymptotes. For example, in this particular simulation, the topmost age 1 stability function has a limiting value of .65. In other words, the predicted correlation between age 1 and age 11 (i.e., a 10-year span) is the same as the predicted correlation between age 1 and age 21 (i.e., a 20-year span). Notice that, as the influence of the prototype increases, the asymptote increases. The only condition in which the curves approach zero is when the influence of the prototype on attachment security is set to zero (see the lowest curve). (Under this parameter condition, however, the model cannot technically be considered a prototype model of development, and it reduces to the simpler transactional model.)

Why does this model predict nonzero asymptotes in the stability functions? The prototype constrains the range of possible security values the person can have. Because the prototype itself does not change, and because it exerts an effect on attachment dynamics over time, an unchanging constraint has been incorporated into the system. This constraint leads to some interesting predictions about the developmental trajectories of individuals. Specifically, changes in security appear to be deviations from a theoretical central tendency determined by the individual's prototype representations (this point is discussed in more depth by Fraley, 2002). In short, these processes give rise to a *dynamic equilibrium* for the individual—a point to which the individual gravitates despite statistical fluctuations in the caregiving environment. This dynamic equilibrium has clear homeorhetic properties because individuals will tend to return to the prototypical pathway even when interpersonal factors temporarily pull them in another direction. We elaborate on the implications of this finding later in the chapter.

In summary, the prototype model predicts a markedly different form of continuity when compared with that predicted by transactional and decreasing-sensitivity processes. Specifically, the predicted stability functions decrease to a nonzero asymptote. An important implication of the model is that stability need not be high when old representations continue to influence development. The key distinction between this model and the others is that this one implies that the degree of stability observed, whether large or small, will be the same over, for example, 10- and 30-year spans.

Notice also that, under certain parameter values, the prototype model predicts a dip in the backward stability functions between ages 1 and 5 (see Figure 4.9). This dip emerges when the initial (i.e., Time 1)

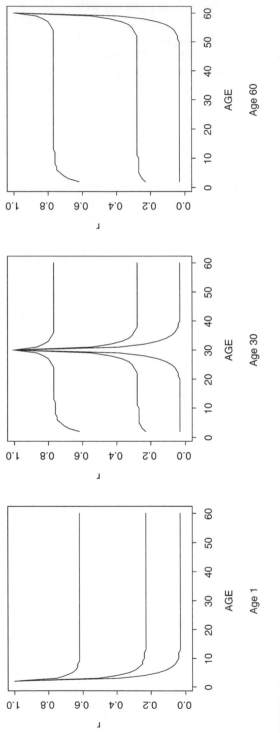

FIGURE 4.9. Stability functions for ages 1, 30, and 60, respectively, predicted by the prototype model. The different curves illustrate the behavior of the model under different parameter values.

covariances between persons, prototypes, and environments is smaller than what the dynamics of the system will naturally produce over time. In these particular simulations, the initial covariances were set to zero, so persons, prototypes, and environments were initially uncorrelated. However, the covariances among these variables increased as person–environment transactions took place because prototypes were affecting people, who were affecting their environments, which were, in turn, affecting people. As these indirect effects accumulate, the covariation among prototypical representations, environments, and security increases.

An interesting consequence of these dynamics is that this model, like the decreasing-sensitivity model, predicts an *asymmetry* in stability functions, such that the limiting value of the age 1 stability function is lower than that of the age 15 stability function. Importantly, the prototype model is capable of making this prediction without an explicit mechanism that increases or decreases plasticity. In the interest of parsimony, we do not explore decreasing-sensitivity mechanisms per se for the remainder of this chapter because such effects flow naturally from a prototype model of attachment dynamics.

Summary

In summary, analyses of the prototype model indicate that prototype-like processes are capable of predicting a nonzero degree of stability between early and later attachment patterns. If prototype processes exist, there should be evidence of stability from infancy to adulthood—even if early prototypes exhibit only a modest effect on social interactions. This prediction contrasts sharply with those made only on the basis of transactional and decreasing-sensitivity mechanisms, which indicated that the stability should always approach zero in the long run.

Although the prototype model does not explicitly suggest that working models should become less sensitive over time, analyses of the model revealed that such a phenomenon emerged naturally from the intrinsic dynamics of the model. This suggests that it may not be necessary to postulate explicit constructs to account for decreasing sensitivity over time. If we assume that the initial correlation between prototypes, environment, and security is low—but that that there is a causal relationship between these variables—prototypes, environment, and security will eventually come to covary positively together. If the initial covariation between these three variables is not as high as that implied by the dynamics between them, the stability of attachment will be weaker in early childhood than in later childhood or adulthood. It appears that resistance to change emerges in this model not because working models per se are becoming less flexible but because there is increased covariation among the variables that shape the expectations that people hold. *The interplay of these dy-*

namic forces causes the person's developmental pathway to become canalized over time.

On the basis of these simulations and analyses, we believe that Bowlby's theoretical ideas regarding the mechanisms that sustain and change attachment patterns *do not* necessarily imply that a high degree of stability will be observed between attachment patterns in infancy and attachment patterns in adulthood. Of the three homeorhetic mechanisms that Bowlby discussed, the first two—transactional dynamics and those that entail decreasing sensitivity over development—predict that degree of stability over long spans of time will be zero. Although these processes *do* serve to boost stability in comparison with situations in which they are not operating, these processes cannot be used to support the conjecture that attachment security will be highly stable across development. The one mechanism that does allow for nonzero degrees of stability in the limit (i.e., the prototype process) is neutral with respect to the *degree* of stability (i.e., high or low) that should be observed. In other words, although this mechanism implies that secure children may tend to grow up to be secure adults, it does not imply that this association must be high in magnitude.

Although each of the three homeorhetic processes discussed by Bowlby leads to higher levels of stability than would be observed in its absence, there is nothing intrinsic in the dynamics of these processes that ensures that an individual's developmental trajectory will be easy to predict on the basis of early caregiving experiences. The homeorhetic dynamics implied by the prototype model, like those implied by Waddington's marbles on epigenetic landscapes, "break down" if the degree of environmental influence is too large. Although the system is still "trying" to maintain a specific developmental pathway, the specific pathway maintained is changing too rapidly to give rise to developmental stability.

EMPIRICAL TESTS OF BOWLBY'S DYNAMIC MECHANISMS

How can Bowlby's ideas about the homeorhetic properties of human development be tested empirically? Although an increasing number of studies have addressed the stability of attachment patterns over time (see Fraley, 2002, for a review), the typical study on stability and change assesses security at only two points in time. Unfortunately, this kind of information does not allow us to evaluate the homeorhetic dynamics thought to underlie attachment development. To understand why, consider a hypothetical study that finds a test–retest correlation of .30 between security levels assessed over a period of 2 years. Do these data support or refute the notion that transactional processes, for example, play a key role in attachment dynamics? The question is difficult to answer for at least two reasons. First, no one writing about transactional dynamics—including Bowlby—has made a *point prediction* (i.e., a quantitative prediction) about the magnitude of test–retest coefficients that should be observed over 2 years if these processes are operating. One might assume that the prediction would be 0.00 based on our previous discussion, but, as can be seen from the decaying nature of the curves in Figure 4.7, that is not the case. Even if transactional dynamics were taking place, the test–retest correlation over 2 years may be quite high. Second, a coefficient of .30 clearly indicates *some* degree of stability, and it is not clear whether this particular value is more consistent with a perspective that emphasizes instability (e.g., Lewis, 1999) over stability (e.g., Waters et al., 2000). In short, simply knowing the magnitude of stability over two points in time is insufficient for determining whether attachment dynamics behave in the homeorhetic manner that Bowlby envisioned.

As our previous simulations illustrate, evaluating the homeorhetic nature of these theoretical mechanisms requires studying the *pattern* or *form* of test–retest coefficients observed over time, not the magnitude of a single test–retest coefficient (as is common in longitudinal research on attachment). In the following sections, we study patterns of stability by piecing together diverse longitudinal findings on the stability of attachment. Specifically, we summarize meta-analytic data originally reported by Fraley (2002) on the stability of attachment from infancy to adulthood. We supplement these data with data on the stability of attachment across adulthood, as culled from the empirical literature on adult attachment in the social–personality research tradition.

Data on Stability from Infancy to Adulthood

How stable are attachment patterns from infancy to adulthood? Although there are now an increasing number of longitudinal studies that are able to address this question, considerable diversity exists in the answers provided by these studies. Some studies suggest that, over the first 19 years of life, there is a strong degree of stability in attachment, such that secure children are highly likely to be secure as adults (see Waters et al., 2000). Other studies, in contrast, indicate that there is virtually no stability over such lengthy spans of time (e.g., Lewis et al., 2000).

Fraley (2002) adopted a meta-analytic approach to resolve the disparate results of alternative studies on stability. In 1999 he identified all studies containing test–retest data on attachment patterns between 12 months of age—as assessed with Ainsworth et al.'s (1978) Strange Situation procedure—and subsequent ages. Twenty-seven samples were obtained through PsycINFO computer searches, consultation with attachment researchers, and cross-referencing of articles as the database developed. Once the studies were identified, the stability results from each were transformed to a common metric. For studies in which attachment classifications, rather than continuous ratings of security, were employed, Fraley (2002) focused on the stability of secure–insecure classifications rather than the stability of three- or four-category classifications (e.g., A, B, C or A, B, C, D). One reason for doing so was that every study allowed an unambiguous secure–insecure distinction to be made across assessment times and methods (e.g., security manifests itself in functionally, if not in phenotypically, similar ways in infancy and adulthood). This distinction can be considered a rough approximation of a latent continuum of security. Also, two-category test–retest effects can be summarized conveniently as Pearson product-moment correlations—phi correlations, to be exact. This allows the stability findings across a variety of studies to be evaluated on the same Pearson correlation metric that we adopted in the simulations reported previously.

Table 4.1 reports the meta-analytic stability results for five temporal intervals: age 1 to age 1 (i.e., immediate test–retest), age 1 to age 2, age 1 to age 4, age 1 to age 6, and age 1 to age 19. Notice that the coefficients start off high (the age 1 test–retest correlation is 1.00) and, despite some variation, appear to decrease rapidly to a nonzero plateau. Because these data only reflect a single empirical stability function (i.e., the age 1 stability function), they cannot be used to evaluate the predicted asymmetrical properties of the stability functions. However, it should be clear from these data that the test–retest correlations do not approach zero in the limit. In fact, the data can be accounted for fairly well by the prototype model. If we use these data to calibrate the prototype model, we find an estimated asymptotic test–retest correlation of .39 (see Fraley, 2002). This suggests that, if the underlying model is correct, the expected correlation between security assessed at age 1 and security assessed at any other point later in the lifespan will be approximately .39.

What does this imply about the stability of attachment from infancy to adulthood? First, these data indicate that there is not a high degree of stability. A test–retest correlation of .39 suggests that, if we had a sample

TABLE 4.1. Meta-Analytic Data on Attachment Continuity from Infancy to Adulthood

Temporal group	r	Total n
Age 1–age 1	1.00	9
Age 1–age 1.5	.32	896
Age 1–age 4	.35	161
Age 1–age 6	.67	131
Age 1–age 19	.27	218

Note. These meta-analytic data were reported by Fraley (2002).

of secure children, approximately 70% of them would grow up to be secure adults, whereas 30% of them would grow up to be insecure as adults. Although this degree of stability is impressive when compared against the degree of stability observed in other personality traits ($r \cong .20$, see Fraley & Roberts, in press), one would not use such data to make the claim that early childhood experiences serve as a powerful foundation for the development of adult attachment patterns.

The second critical implication of these data is that a prototype-like process may underlie empirical patterns of stability and change in attachment. If this view is correct, then early attachment patterns, although not strongly influential in adult development, may exert a broad influence across different life periods. Because the empirical curve reaches its asymptote so quickly (around age 2), the degree to which early experiences shape attachment may be assumed to be the same at age 2 and at age 19. We expound on this implication in more depth later. For now, however, we note that, although early attachment is not a *strong* predictor of later attachment patterns, it is a *far-reaching* predictor of later attachment patterns in the sense that we can use it to predict attachment at age 4 with the same degree of precision as attachment at age 19.

Data on Attachment Stability in Adulthood

To further investigate empirical patterns of stability and change, we examined the ability of the prototype model to account for data on attachment stability among adults. A growing number of social and personality psychologists have conducted longitudinal investigations of attachment in adulthood (e.g., Baldwin & Fehr, 1995; Klohnen & Bera, 1998; Scharfe & Bartholomew, 1994). By collating the empirical data obtained in a diverse number of studies, we can take a small—but significant—step toward reconstructing the broader patterns of stability and change that exist in attachment security.

To identify longitudinal studies that included test–retest data on adult attachment patterns (i.e., those assessed after 18 years of age), we conducted PsycINFO computer searches and cross-referenced articles as the database developed. Twenty-four samples/datapoints were obtained. Many of the studies used categorical measures of attachment rather than continuous ratings. To transform the findings from such studies to a standard Pearson correlation metric, we computed the phi correlation for the test–retest stability of secure–insecure classifications. In cases in which base rate information was not reported and in which only the percent of the sample that retained the same classification was reported, we assumed that the base rate of security was 50% and used this base rate to compute phi. (Alternative assumptions do not have any noteworthy impact on the patterns of data we report.)

We have reproduced these data in Table 4.2. One thing to note about these data is that, for the most part, very few studies have examined the stability of attachment security over a period extending more than 1 year. One noteworthy exception is the study by Klohnen and Bera (1998), which examined the stability of attachment patterns in the Mills College sample at ages 27, 43, and 52.

Overall, the raw magnitude of the test–retest correlations tends to be higher than those observed in childhood. The correlations reported in Fraley (2002) average around .39, whereas the adult correlations average around .54. A second noteworthy feature of the data is that the correlations do not behave as if they are approaching zero in the limit. For example, the Klohnen and Bera (1998) data suggest that the stability of attachment is roughly the same from age 27 to age 43 ($r \cong .58$) as it is from age 27 to age 52 ($r \cong .55$).

In Figure 4.10 we summarize the data for studies that had test–retest intervals of one year or longer in order to illustrate the patterns of stability. We have also superimposed the stability functions implied by the prototype model. There are several noteworthy features of these graphs. First, notice that the prototype model predicts that the asymptotic value of the stability functions in adulthood (e.g., the age 30 stability function) is higher (i.e., $r \cong .50$) than that expected for the age 1 stability function ($r \cong .39$). Second, notice that the adult data points are well approximated by the theoretical curve. Although the data do not fall precisely on the predicted curve, the discrepancy between the theoretical values and the predicted values is remarkably small.

What do these patterns, in conjunction with the childhood data reviewed previously, imply about the mechanisms underlying stability and change? The fact that the correlations estimated over 1-year intervals tend to be somewhat higher in adulthood than in childhood (i.e., they exhibit the property of asymmetry predicted by the prototype model) indicates that some degree of canalization may be taking place. The fact that the correlations do not approach zero in the limit also suggests that prototype-like dynamics may underlie empirical patterns of stability and change.

We also examined, in a separate analysis, the stability of attachment security reported in studies that used test–retest intervals that were shorter than 1 year. We have plotted attachment stability as a function of the test–retest intervals in Figure 4.11. (Among these adult samples, age was uncorrelated with the length of the test–retest interval, so we have not presented these data by age per se. We have also excluded the Baldwin et al., 1993, sample from the figure.) Notice that the test–retest correlations approach their asymptotic values almost immediately (i.e., within a week). Notice also that the asymptote implied by these data is much larger than zero and very close to the asymptote entailed by the other studies that examined stability over periods of 1 year or more.

TABLE 4.2. Longitudinal Studies Including Adult Attachment Test–Retest Data

Study	n	Age at first assessment	Test–retest interval (weeks)	r (continuous measures)	Percent stable (categorical measures)	Phi (categorical measures)
Baldwin & Fehr (1995)	221	20.5	16.0		67.4	0.35
Baldwin, Fehr, Keedian, Seidel, & Thomson (1993)	16	20.9	16.0		43.7	−0.13
Barnes (1991)[a]	46	18.0	12.0		67.4	0.35
Benoit & Parker (1994)						
Test–retest 1	84	29.2	54.0		77	0.54
Test–retest 2	84	29.2	54.0		90	0.80
Collins & Read (1990)	101	18.8	9.0	0.64		
Cozzarelli, Karafa, Collins, & Tagler (2003)	442	24.1	108.0	0.38		
Davila, Burge, & Hammen (1997)						
Test–retest 1	155	18.0	27.0	0.52		
Test–retest 2	155	18.0	108.0	0.48		
Davila & Cobb (2003)	86	18.0	54.0	0.63		
Davila, Karney, & Bradbury (1999)						
Test–retest 1	344	26.8	27.0	0.68		
Test–retest 2	344	26.8	54.0	0.71		
Test–retest 3	344	26.8	81.0	0.58		
Test–retest 4	210	26.8	108.0	0.61		
Feeney & Noller (1992)	172	17.9	10.0	0.67		
Feeney, Noller, & Callan (1994)	70	23.7	40.5	0.62		
Fuller & Fincham (1995)	44	31.8	108.0	0.62		
Hammond & Fletcher (1991)	102	20.0	18.0	0.47		
Keelan, Dion, & Dion (1994)	101	19.0	18.0		80.2	0.60
Kirkpatrick & Hazan (1994)	172	39.1	216.0		70.0	0.40
Klohnen & Bera (1998)						
Test–retest 1	142	27.0	864.0	0.58		
Test–retest 2	142	27.0	1350.0	0.55		
Test–retest 3	100	43.0	486.0	0.71		
Levy & Davis (1988)	63	20.0	2.0	0.58		
Lopez & Gormley (2002)	207	18.0	31.5		57.0	0.14
Pistole (1989)	67	18.0	1.0		76.1	0.52
Ruvolo, Fabin, & Ruvolo (2001)	322	19.7	22.5	0.49		
Scharfe & Bartholomew (1994)	144	24.5	36.0	0.51		
Senchak & Leonard (1992)	335	23.8	52.0		74.2	0.48
Shaver & Brennan (1992)						
Test–retest 1	127	19.0	36.0	0.60		
Test–retest 2	242	19.0	36.0	0.68		
Smith, Murphy, & Coats (1999)	60	18.0	13.0	0.77		
Tinio (1992)[a]	12	18.0	16.0		83.3	0.67
Wieselquist et al. (1999)	130	32.5	54.0	0.56		

Note. For studies employing only categorical measures of adult attachment, we have reported the percent of the sample that retained the same attachment classification from time 1 to time 2 and a phi coefficient to express that information in a Pearson correlation metric (see text). For studies that included dimensional measures of adult attachment, we have reported the test–retest correlation, *r*. In cases in which the average age of the sample was not reported, we assumed an average value of 18.

[a]Unpublished studies reported by Baldwin and Fehr (1995).

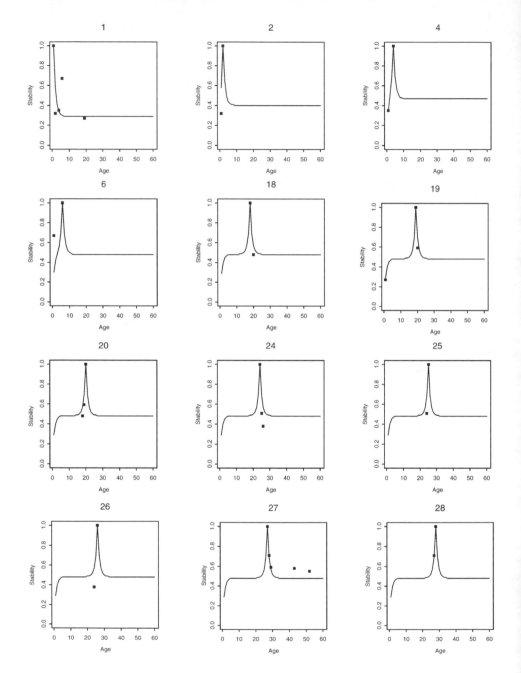

FIGURE 4.10. Stability functions for a variety of ages between 1 and 52. The points represent meta-analytic data points; the curves represent the stability functions predicted by the prototype model.

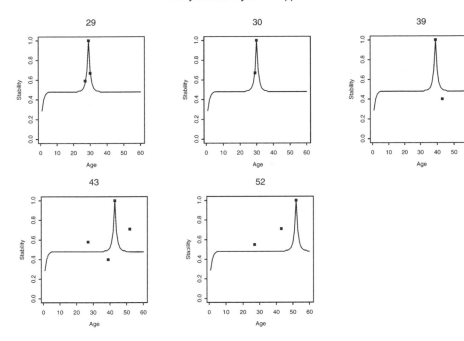

FIGURE 4.10. *(continued)*

CONCLUSIONS

In this chapter, we used dynamic modeling techniques to formalize Bowlby's ideas about the basic processes that may sustain attachment patterns over time. In the sections that follow, we discuss the implications of our simulations and analyses for (1) the assumptions researchers hold about how much stability should exist in attachment over the life course, (2) debates about within-person variation in attachment patterns, and (3) the methods that are used to study the dynamics of stability and change.

Assumptions about Stability

Many researchers are implicitly guided by the view that attachment theory predicts a strong association between early and later attachment patterns (e.g., Duck, 1994; Lewis, 1997; Westen, 1998). Indeed, one of the intriguing implications of attachment theory is that the way a person thinks, feels, and behaves in his or her romantic relationships is a reflection of the way in which that person's attachment system has become organized over the course of development—beginning with his or her earliest attachment relationships. The notion that early caregiving experiences influ-

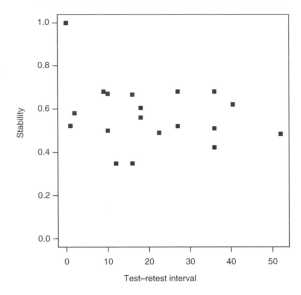

FIGURE 4.11. Stability of adult attachment in studies with test–retest intervals shorter than a year. Notice that the asymptote implied by these data is greater than zero and is reached within a few weeks.

ence the way we relate to others throughout the life course is compelling for a number of reasons. For one, it provides a straightforward explanation for why some people are relatively secure in their relationships, whereas others are more sensitive, defensive, or withdrawn. In addition, it raises the possibility that, if psychologists could intervene at an early stage in a child's life, it might be possible to foster permanent changes for the better in his or her psychological development.

Despite its allure, the assumption that early caregiving experiences foreshadow adult development is quite controversial in contemporary psychology (see Duck, 1994; Kagan, 1996; Lewis, 1997). If a person's style of regulating attachment-related feelings and behaviors in his or her romantic relationships is strongly influenced by his or her early caregiving experiences, it would seem that our relational fates are sealed within the first few years of life. This would appear to leave little room for psychological growth, change, or intervention beyond infancy (Lewis, 1997). In addition to these theoretical concerns, the assumption of stability has been challenged by a growing empirical database on the instability of attachment patterns (e.g., Baldwin & Fehr, 1995). If attachment patterns are only moderately stable across short spans of time, how is it possible for early attachment experiences to provide a solid foundation for subsequent development?

We believe that the model we have developed in this chapter provides a way to understand how early attachment patterns can exhibit continuing effects across the life span yet exhibit only a weak degree of stability over time. The empirical data that we reviewed indicate that there is a weak to moderate degree of stability from infancy to adulthood but that the stability that exists from age 1 to later ages does not decay as the length of the test–retest interval increases. According to our theoretical and empirical analyses, security is just as stable from age 1 to age 2 as it is from age 1 to age 20. Thus it is not the case that early attachment has a *strong* influence on later development but that the influence that exists appears to be *enduring*. According to Bowlby's ideas on the role of prototypical attachment representations and their homeorhetic effects on personality development, early attachment patterns manifest themselves in some shape or form across diverse developmental periods of the life course, even if the degree to which those patterns manifest themselves is minor.

Although Bowlby believed that early attachment patterns serve as the foundation for subsequent attachment relationships, he never made a quantitative prediction about the degree of stability that should be expected over long periods of time. The mechanisms he discussed, like Waddington's, offer an explanation for why stability may be observed, but they do not ensure that stability will be the rule rather than the exception. In light of these considerations, we believe that it may be inappropriate for researchers to predict high degrees of stability based on Bowlby's theory. It is of great theoretical interest, of course, to know how stable attachment patterns are over time, but the actual degree of stability, although it informs and constrains the way we conceptualize attachment dynamics, does not provide a test of the theory. As we explain later, testing the theory requires studying the *patterns* of stability and change across development, not appraising the *raw magnitude* of the stability coefficients.

Within-Person Variation in Attachment Patterns

In recent years an increasing number of researchers have documented substantial within-person variation in attachment patterns (see Baldwin & Fehr, 1995; La Guardia, Ryan, Couchman, & Deci, 2000; Pierce & Lydon, 2001). Baldwin and Fehr (1995), for example, reported that approximately 30% of research participants reported different attachment styles from one point in time to the next. This result raised the question of whether it was appropriate for attachment researchers to conceptualize attachment styles as trait-like properties of people or as phenomena exhibiting a more fluid, context-specific nature. Over the years, researchers have adopted a variety of perspectives on this issue. Fraley and Waller (1998), for example, argued for a trait-like approach and suggested that the instability observed by Baldwin and Fehr might be best explained by the kinds of measurement errors that are introduced when continuous data are categorized. La Guardia and her colleagues (2000) argued that a sizable proportion of the within-person variations in attachment could be attributed to ongoing interpersonal dynamics, such as variation in the extent to which people's basic needs for autonomy, competence, and relatedness are fulfilled. Although empirical and theoretical progress has been made toward exploring the extent to which attachment behaves in a trait-like manner, the field has yet to settle on a consensual interpretation of what this variation means and the implications it has for understanding attachment dynamics.

We believe that the homeorhetic processes discussed in this chapter provide a novel and compelling way to conceptualize both the within-person stability and the change that have been documented in attachment patterns. To illustrate how this may be the case, we explore one of the basic equations thought to underlie attachment dynamics (see Fraley, 2002): $dS/dT = \eta(E_t - S_t)$. According to this equation, the amount of change in working models at any time t is proportional to the discrepancy between security at Time t, S_t, and the quality of the caregiving environment at Time t, E_t. When E_t and S_t are equivalent, security will not change ($dS/dT = 0$). When the caregiving environment is harsher or more rejecting than expected, working models change in the direction of decreased security. Similarly, when the caregiving environment is more responsive than expected given one's working models, security increases. The parameter η controls the lability or plasticity of working models.

This basic equation has two important implications for the within-person dynamics of stability and change. First, if we conceptualize the environment as being a function of a stable representational prototype (P), the individual will tend to gravitate toward a value of security that corresponds to the security of that prototypical representation. To demonstrate this result, we can simply substitute P for E, set the derivative to zero, and solve for S (Huckfeldt et al., 1982). Simple algebraic manipulation shows that the attractor state of the system (i.e., the value toward which the system gravitates) is equal to P. In other words, an individual's security level will adjust itself in such a way that it eventually converges on the quality of the prototype. This is true regardless of how secure the individual is initially (see the left-hand panel of Figure 4.12).

Does this process exhibit the kind of homeorhetic stability discussed by Waddington and Bowlby? The middle panel of Figure 4.12 illustrates the security of an individual over time. At Time 390, the caregiving environment is temporarily disturbed so that it becomes substantially more rejecting than it was initially. (For example, it may be the case that the individual was rebuffed by a loved one.) At Time 391, the perturbation is removed. What happens to the security of the individual over time? The perturbation knocks the individual out of his or her pathway, but he or she quickly returns to the pathway previously established (and guided by his or her representational prototype). If there are a large number of environmental factors affecting the individual, then his or her trajectory will bounce around considerably from day to day, but those changes will tend to fluctuate around the same prototypical value (see the right-hand panel of Figure 4.12).

This very simple equation captures an important feature of the homeorhetic processes discussed by Waddington and Bowlby. Specifically, if we conceptualize the prototype as reflecting a critical component of the epigenetic landscape, we see that the individual will gravitate toward that end state despite disturbances from the external environment. Importantly, it is not the case that the person is unaffected by the environment. However, the effect of those experiences is only temporary, and the individual will eventually reestablish his or her original trajectory.

What does this imply about the nature of within-person variation? It suggests that attachment security can behave both as a trait-like and a contextual variable. In other words, it is not necessary to view trait-like and contextual interpretations of security as being in opposition. Although there may be considerable within-person variation in attachment patterns, that variation can be characterized as temporary deviations from a *dynamically* stable value. Although this conjecture flows naturally from the prototype model that we have discussed in this chapter, we are not aware of any existing empirical data that can be used to provide a rigorous test of this hypothesis. Testing this conjecture will require future research not only to demonstrate principled within-person variation, as La Guardia and colleagues (2000) and Pierce and Lydon (2001) have done, but to determine whether specific relational events, such as an argument with a significant other, lead to temporary, as opposed to enduring, changes in attachment security.

Baldwin and his colleagues (Baldwin & Fehr, 1995; Baldwin, Keelan, Fehr, Enns, & Koh-Rangarajoo, 1996) have made the argument that not only does within-person variation exist in attachment patterns but also one reason this variation exists is that people hold multiple working models of themselves in different relationships, each of which can be activated to varying degrees in any one context. Thus it is possible that people hold multiple prototypes based on different significant others in their lives. When this idea is incorporated into the basic model we have discussed, it has some interesting implications for the way the homeorhetic dynamics of the system manifest themselves. To expand the previous equation to accommodate this possibility, we simply added multiple prototypical states to the dynamic equation: $dS/dT = \eta(P_1 - S)(P_2 - S)(P_3 - S)$. Algebraically, this equation is cubic, and, therefore, it has three attractor states given by

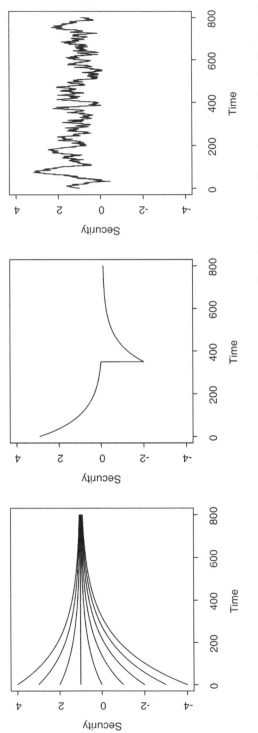

FIGURE 4.12. The dynamics of stability and change from a within-person perspective. The left-hand panel shows how people who begin with different levels of security converge on the same value when they held moderately secure prototypes. The middle panel shows the temporary impact of a disturbance on a person's developmental trajectory. The right-hand panel illustrates the maintenance of the system's dynamic equilibrium despite stochastic disturbances.

the security of the three prototypical representations (see the left-hand panel of Figure 4.13). The first and third attractors are what are called *sinks* (Blanchard, Devaney, & Hall, 1996). Values that begin near a sink tend to converge on that point. Conceptually, a sink is much like the valley floor in Waddington's epigenetic landscape; marbles placed within a certain vicinity of the floor tend to gravitate toward it; they are attracted to it. The second attractor, in contrast, is what is called a *source*. Values that begin near a source tend to move away from that point (Blanchard et al., 1996). A source is much like the cusp between two valley walls in Waddington's analogy. If a marble were to be poised in just the right place on the cusp, it may come to a stop. However, as soon as it moves away from that position—even by a minuscule amount—it will be forced down the hill.

Like the first equation we discussed, this equation exhibits homeorhetic properties. Specifically, if we disrupt an individual's developmental trajectory, he or she will find a way back to his or her original pathway (see the topmost trajectory in the right-hand panel of Figure 4.13). However, the homeorhetic properties of this system are more complex than those discussed previously. If the disturbance is strong enough to push the individual over a cusp point, he or she will change pathways, and a new developmental trajectory will be established. This is illustrated by the bottommost trajectory in the right-hand panel of Figure 4.13. This individual was initially on a trajectory leading her toward extreme insecurity; however, at Time 200, an external force was introduced that temporarily boosted her security. This change brought the person's current level of security over a cusp in the dynamic surface, leading her to establish a new trajectory toward greater security.

If multiple prototypes exist in the mental system, it is possible that they may combine in the way captured by the previous equation to produce multiple attractor points in developmental space (i.e., multiple valleys in the epigenetic landscape). If this is true, then when an individual's current state of security is relatively close to a source point, even a minor environmental disturbance may create a situation in which the individual is pushed off his or her pathway and onto a new one. This suggests that, for some people, minor events may lead to dramatic changes in their personality organization, whereas those same events may lead to nothing more than temporary changes for other people.[3] Regardless of whether we conceptualize the system as having one or more attractor points, this basic conceptualization suggests that the same dynamic mechanisms can lead security to behave as *both* a trait-like variable and a contextual or state-like variable. As such, this model provides a possible resolution to ongoing debate about whether attachment styles represent one kind of variable as opposed to the other.

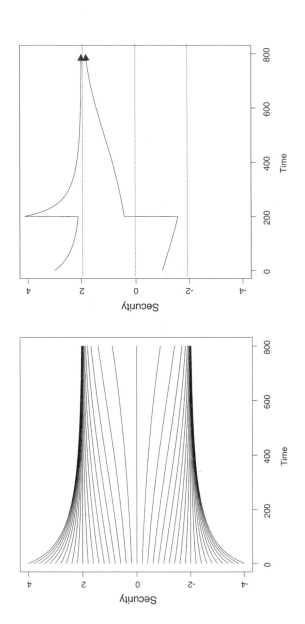

FIGURE 4.13. The dynamics of stability and change in a dynamic system involving multiple prototypes or multiple attractor states. The left-hand panel illustrates alternative developmental trajectories in a multiple attractor system. The right-hand panel demonstrates how the same kind of disturbance can have different effects for people with the same system.

126

Methods for Studying Change

Our analyses suggest that Bowlby's theory predicts that the degree of stability in attachment can fall anywhere between 0.00 and 1.00. In light of this derivation, one cannot empirically "test" attachment theory by studying the stability of attachment patterns between two points in time, as is often done in contemporary research. Theoretically, any test–retest correlation greater than zero would be consistent with the theory, thereby making such empirical tests extraordinarily weak and ambiguous. The power of Bowlby's theory lies not in the predictions that it makes about the *degree* of stability that should be observed from infancy to adulthood but in the *patterns* of stability that should be observed over time. Specifically, if the dynamics of stability and change can be characterized by homeorhetic, prototype-like processes, then we should expect (1) the correlation between security measured at age 1 and any other age to gradually decay to a nonzero value, (2) the test–retest correlations in childhood to be lower on average than those observed in adulthood, and (3) the stability functions later in the life course to decay to nonzero values.

We believe that a proper empirical test of attachment theory's assumptions about stability and change requires investigating these patterns of continuity. This will require a concerted effort on the part of investigators to develop methodological paradigms that allow individuals to be studied repeatedly over time. For example, it should be possible to test Bowlby's ideas by studying patterns of stability and change over brief periods of time in adulthood using Web-based technologies, diary studies, or event-sampling techniques. It is only through such work that the empirical patterns implied by Bowlby's theory can be documented and evaluated. We have tried to take a first step in uncovering such patterns by bringing together findings from a variety of studies that have examined the test–retest stability of attachment. Although these data seem to corroborate the dynamic processes entailed by Bowlby's theory, they are subject to obvious limitations (i.e., different measures, different samples). We hope future researchers will take advantage of the predictions outlined here in order to further evaluate Bowlby's ideas about human development.

NOTES

1. Although Bowlby (1973) didn't state exactly what he considered the railway destinations to represent in his analogy, it seems safe to assume that he considered them to represent alternative states of security or adjustment. For the purposes of this chapter, we assume that the railway destinations, as well as the valleys in Waddington's (1957) landscape, represent different degrees of security.
2. We use the term "trait" in its broadest sense to refer to any kind of biological or psychological quality, character, or property.

3. Davila and her colleagues have argued that some insecure people may be psychologically vulnerable and, consequently, exhibit less stability in their levels of security over time (Davila, Burge, & Hammen, 1997; Davila & Cobb, Chapter 5, this volume). There are a number of ways in which this observation can be accounted for by the prototype model. First, it is possible that, as Davila and Cobb (Chapter 5, this volume) discuss, highly insecure individuals hold multiple working models of themselves and their relationships. If this is true, insecure people will possess a greater number of potential equilibria in the dynamic space illustrated in Figure 4.13. An individual with a higher degree of such equilibria will be more likely to exhibit change, because minor fluctuations in the environment can easily knock the person out of one trajectory and into another. It is also possible that some people are more reactive to environmental fluctuations than others, and that this reactivity is correlated negatively with security. (See Fraley, Waller, & Brennan, 2000, for a psychometric interpretation of the association between insecurity and instability.)

REFERENCES

Ainsworth, M. D. S., Blehar, M. C., Waters, E., & Wall, S. (1978). *Patterns of attachment: A psychological study of the Strange Situation.* Hillsdale, NJ: Erlbaum.

Arend, R., Gove, F., & Sroufe, L. A. (1979). Continuity of individual adaptation from infancy to kindergarten: A predictive study of ego resiliency and curiosity in preschoolers. *Child Development, 50,* 950–959.

Baldwin, M. W., & Fehr, B. (1995). On the instability of attachment style ratings. *Personal Relationships, 2,* 247–261.

Baldwin, M. W., Fehr, B., Keedian, E., Seidel, M., & Thomson, D. W. (1993). An exploration of the relational schemata underlying attachment styles: Self-report and lexical decision approaches. *Personality and Social Psychology Bulletin, 19,* 746–754.

Baldwin, M. W., Keelan, J. P. R., Fehr, B., Enns, V., & Koh-Rangarajoo, E. (1996). Social cognitive conceptualization of attachment working models: Availability and accessibility effects. *Journal of Personality and Social Psychology, 71,* 94–104.

Barnes, M. (1991). *"I like your style": Effects of visualization and memory on relationship attachment styles.* Unpublished honors thesis, University of Winnipeg.

Benoit, D., & Parker, K. C. H. (1994). Stability and transmission of attachment across three generations. *Child Development, 65,* 1444–1456.

Blanchard, P., Devaney, R. L., & Hall, G. R. (1996). *Differential equations.* Boston: International Thomson.

Bowlby, J. (1973). *Attachment and loss: Vol. 2. Separation: Anxiety and anger.* New York: Basic Books.

Bowlby, J. (1980). *Attachment and loss: Vol. 3. Loss: Sadness and depression.* New York: Basic Books.

Bowlby, J. (1982). *Attachment and loss: Vol. 1. Attachment* (2nd ed.). New York: Basic Books. (Original work published 1969)

Brumbaugh, C. C., & Fraley, R. C. (2004). *Transference and attachment: How do attachment patterns get carried forward from one relationship to the next?* Manuscript submitted for publication.

Caspi, A., & Roberts, B. W. (1999). Personality continuity and change across the life course. In L. A. Pervin & O. P. John (Eds.), *Handbook of personality: Theory and research* (2nd ed., pp. 300–326). New York: Guilford Press.

Collins, N. L. (1996). Working models of attachment: Implications for explanation, emotion, and behavior. *Journal of Personality and Social Psychology, 71,* 810–832.

Collins, N. L., & Read, S. J. (1990). Adult attachment, working models, and relationship quality in dating couples. *Journal of Personality and Social Psychology, 58,* 644–663.

Collins, N. L., & Read, S. J. (1994). Cognitive representations of attachment: The structure and function of working models. In K. Bartholomew & D. Perlman (Eds.), *Advances in personal relationships: Vol. 5. Attachment processes in adulthood* (pp. 53–90). London: Kingsley.

Cozzarelli, C., Karafa, J. A., Collins, N. L., & Tagler, M. J. (2003). Stability and change in adult attachment styles: Associations with personal vulnerabilities, life events, and global construals of self and others. *Journal of Social and Consulting Psychology, 22,* 315–346.

Davila, J., Burge, D., & Hammen, C. (1997). Why does attachment style change? *Journal of Personality and Social Psychology, 73,* 826–838.

Davila, J., & Cobb, R. J. (2003). Predicting change in self-reported and interviewer-assessed adult attachment: Tests of the individual difference and life stress models of attachment change. *Personality and Social Psychology Bulletin, 29,* 859–870.

Davila, J., Karney, B. R., & Bradbury, T. N. (1999). Attachment change processes in the early years of marriage. *Journal of Personality and Social Psychology, 76,* 783–802.

Duck, S. (1994). Attaching meaning to attachment. *Psychological Inquiry, 5,* 34–38.

Feeney, J. A., & Noller, P. (1992). Attachment style and romantic love: Relationship dissolution. *Australian Journal of Psychology, 44,* 69–74.

Feeney, J. A., Noller, P., & Callan, V. J. (1994). Attachment style, communication and satisfaction in the early years of marriage. In K. Bartholomew & D. Perlman (Eds.), *Advances in personal relationships: Vol. 5. Attachment processes in adulthood* (pp. 269–308). London: Kingsley.

Fraley, R. C. (2002). Attachment stability from infancy to adulthood: Meta-analysis and dynamic modeling of developmental mechanisms. *Personality and Social Psychology Review, 6,* 123–151.

Fraley, R. C., & Roberts, B. W. (in press). Patterns of continuity: A dynamic model for conceptualizing the stability of individual differences in psychological constructs across the life course. *Psychological Review.*

Fraley, R. C., & Shaver, P. R. (2000). Adult romantic attachment: Theoretical developments, emerging controversies, and unanswered questions. *Review of General Psychology, 4,* 132–154.

Fraley, R. C., & Spieker, S. J. (2003). Are infant attachment patterns continuously or categorically distributed? A taxometric analysis of Strange Situation behavior. *Developmental Psychology, 39,* 387–404.

Fraley, R. C., & Waller, N. G. (1998). Adult attachment patterns: A test of the typological model. In J. A. Simpson & W. S. Rholes (Eds.), *Attachment theory and close relationships* (pp. 77–114). New York: Guilford Press.

Fraley, R. C., Waller, N. G., & Brennan, K. A. (2000). An item response theory analysis of self-report measures of adult attachment. *Journal of Personality and Social Psychology, 78,* 350–365.

Frazier, P. A., Byer, A. L., Fischer, A. R., Wright, D. M., & DeBord, K. A. (1996). Adult attachment style and partner choice: Correlational and experimental findings. *Personal Relationships, 3,* 117–137.

Fuller, T. L., & Fincham, F. D. (1995). Attachment style in married couples: Relation to current marital functioning, stability over time, and method of assessment. *Personal Relationships, 2,* 17–34.

Geary, D. C., & Huffman, K. J. (2002). Brain and cognitive evolution: Forms of modularity and functions of mind. *Psychological Bulletin, 128,* 667–698.

Griffin, D., & Bartholomew, K. (1994). Models of the self and other: Fundamental dimensions underlying measures of adult attachment. *Journal of Personality and Social Psychology, 67,* 430–445.

Haefner, J. W. (1996). *Modeling biological systems: Principles and applications.* New York: International Thomson.

Hammond, J. R., & Fletcher, G. J. O. (1991). Attachment styles and relationship satisfaction in the development of close relationships. *New Zealand Journal of Psychology, 20,* 56–62.

Horowitz, M. J. (1991) (Ed.). *Person schemas and maladaptive interpersonal patterns.* Chicago: University of Chicago Press.

Huckfeldt, R. R., Kohfeld, C. W., & Likens, T. W. (1982). *Dynamic modeling: An introduction.* Newbury Park, CA: Sage.

Kagan, J. (1996). Three pleasing ideas. *American Psychologist, 51,* 901–908.

Keelan, J. P. R., Dion, K. L., & Dion, K. K. (1994). Attachment style and heterosexual relationships among young adults: A short-term panel study. *Journal of Social and Personal Relationships, 11,* 201–214.

Kenny, D. A., & Zautra, A. (2001). Trait–state models for longitudinal data. In L. M. Collins & A. G. Sayer (Eds.), *New methods for the analysis of change: Decade of behavior* (pp. 243–263). Washington, DC: American Psychological Association.

Kirkpatrick, L. A., & Hazan, C. (1994). Attachment styles and close relationships: A four-year prospective study. *Personal Relationships, 1,* 123–142.

Klohnen, E. C., & Bera, S. (1998). Behavioral and experiential patterns of avoidantly and securely attached women across adulthood: A 31-year longitudinal perspective. *Journal of Personality and Social Psychology, 74,* 211–223.

La Guardia, J. G., Ryan, R. M., Couchman, C., & Deci, E. L. (2000). Within-person variation in security of attachment: A self-determination theory perspective on attachment, need fulfillment, and well-being. *Journal of Personality and Social Psychology, 79,* 367–384.

Lemery, K. S., Goldsmith, H. H., Klinnert, M. D., & Mrazek, D. A. (1999). Developmental models of infant and childhood temperament. *Developmental Psychology, 35,* 189–204.

Levy, M. B., & Davis, K. E. (1988). Lovestyles and attachment styles compared: Their relations to each other and to various relationship characteristics. *Journal of Social and Personal Relationships, 5,* 439–471.

Lewis, M. (1997). *Altering fate: Why the past does not predict the future.* New York: Guilford Press.

Lewis, M. (1999). On the development of personality. In L. A. Pervin & O. P. John (Eds.), *Handbook of personality: Theory and research* (2nd ed., pp. 327–346). New York: Guilford Press.

Lewis, M., Feiring, C., & Rosenthal, S. (2000). Attachment over time. *Child Development, 71,* 707–720.

Lopez, F. G., & Gormley, B. (2002). Stability and change in adult attachment style over the first-year college transition: Relations to self-confidence, coping, and distress patterns. *Journal of Counseling Psychology, 49,* 355–364.

O'Leary, D. D. M., Schlaggar, B. K., & Tuttle, R. (1994). Specification of neocortical areas and thalamocortical connections. *Annual Review of Neuroscience, 17,* 419–439.

Owens, G., Crowell, J. A., Pan, H., Treboux, D., O'Connor, E., & Waters, E. (1995). The prototype hypothesis and the origins of attachment working models: Adult relationships with parents and romantic partners. In E. Waters, B. E. Vaughn, G. Posada, & K. Kondo-Ikemura (Eds.), Caregiving, cultural, and cognitive perspectives on secure-base behavior and working models: New growing points of attachment theory and research. *Monographs of the Society for Research in Child Development, 60*(2–3, Serial No. 244), 216–233.

Pierce, G. R., Sarason, B. R., & Sarason, I. G. (1992). General and specific support expectations and stress as predictors of perceived supportiveness: An experimental study. *Journal of Personality and Social Psychology, 63,* 297–307.

Pierce, T., & Lydon, J. (2001). Global and specific relational models in the experience of social interactions. *Journal of Personality and Social Psychology, 80,* 613–631.

Pietromonaco, P. R., & Carnelley, K. B. (1994). Gender and working models of attachment: Consequences for perceptions of self and romantic relationships. *Personal Relationships, 1,* 63–82.

Pistole, M. C. (1989). Attachment in adult romantic relationships: Style of conflict resolution and relationship satisfaction. *Journal of Social and Personal Relationships, 6,* 505–510.

Rakic, P. (1988, July 8). Specification of cerebral cortical areas. *Science, 241,* 170–176.

Rumelhart, D. E., McClelland, J. L., & the PDP Research Group. (1986). *Parallel distributed processing: Explorations in the microstructure of cognition.* London: MIT Press.

Ruvolo, A. P., Fabin, L. A., & Ruvolo, C. M. (2001). Relationship experiences and change in attachment characteristics of young adults: The role of relationship breakups and conflict avoidance. *Personal Relationships, 8,* 265–281.

Scharfe, E., & Bartholomew, K. (1994). Reliability and stability of adult attachment patterns. *Personal Relationships, 9,* 51–64.

Senchak, M., & Leonard, K. E. (1992). Attachment styles and marital adjustment among newlywed couples. *Journal of Social and Personal Relationships, 9,* 51–64.

Shaver, P. R., & Brennan, K. A. (1992). Attachment styles and the "Big Five" personality traits: Their connections with each other and with romantic relationship outcomes. *Personality and Social Psychology Bulletin, 18,* 536–545.

Smith, E. R., Murphy, J., & Coats, S. (1999). Attachment to groups: Theory and measurement. *Journal of Personality and Social Psychology, 77,* 94–110.

Smith, L. B., & Thelen, E. (Eds.). (1993). *A dynamic systems approach to development: Applications.* Cambridge, MA: MIT Press.

Sroufe, L. A. (1979). The coherence of individual development: Early care, attachment, and subsequent developmental issues. *American Psychologist, 34,* 834–841.

Sroufe, L. A., Egeland, B., & Kreutzer, T. (1990). The fate of early experience following developmental change: Longitudinal approaches to individual adaptation in childhood. *Child Development, 61,* 1363–1373.

Sroufe, L. A., & Jacobvitz, D. (1989). Diverging pathways, developmental transformations, multiple etiologies and the problem of continuity in development. *Human Development, 32,* 196–203.

Tinio, E. J. (1992). *Career and relationship commitment in two university samples: The importance of self-efficacy.* Unpublished honors thesis, University of Winnipeg.

Troy, M., & Sroufe, L. A. (1987). Victimization among preschoolers: Role of attachment relationship history. *Journal of American Academy of Child and Adolescent Psychiatry, 26,* 166–172.

van Geert, P. (1994). *Dynamic systems of development.* New York: Harvester Wheatsheaf.

van Geert, P. (1997). Time and theory in social psychology. *Psychological Inquiry, 8,* 143–151.

van IJzendoorn, M. H. (1996). Commentary. *Human Development, 39,* 224–231.

Waddington, C. H. (1957). *The strategy of the genes: A discussion of some aspects of theoretical biology.* London: Allen & Unwin.

Waters, E., Merrick, S., Treboux, D., Crowell, J., & Albersheim, L. (2000). Attachment security in infancy and early adulthood: A 20-year longitudinal study. *Child Development, 71,* 684–689.

Waters, E., Wippman, J., & Sroufe, L. A. (1979). Attachment, positive affect, and competence in the peer group: Two studies in construct validation. *Child Development, 50,* 821–829.

Westen, D. (1998). The scientific legacy of Sigmund Freud: Toward a psychodynamically informed psychological science. *Psychological Bulletin, 124,* 333–371.

Wieselquist, J., Rusbult, C. E., Foster, C. A., & Agnew, C. (1999). Commitment, pro-relationship behavior, and trust in close relationships. *Journal of Personality and Social Psychology, 77,* 942–966.

CHAPTER 5

Predictors of Change in Attachment Security during Adulthood

JOANNE DAVILA
REBECCA J. COBB

Much of the literature on adult attachment security, including that contained in this book, focuses on the correlates and consequences of security for individual and interpersonal well-being. This literature rests on the assumption that attachment security in adulthood is a stable individual difference that guides thought, feeling, and behavior over time. Indeed, this is, in part, what Bowlby (1969) hypothesized. He suggested that early attachment relationships resulted in the development of internal working models that contain information about the self, others, and relationships. He proposed that these models guide functioning, particularly interpersonal functioning, over the life course and, in doing so, form the underpinnings of personality. A large body of literature supports these ideas, implicitly attesting to the stability of attachment security in adulthood.

However, Bowlby (1969) also proposed that, although people may be more likely to assimilate new information into their existing attachment models, people are also capable of accommodating new information by updating existing models. Hence people also should possess the capacity for change in levels and/or patterns of attachment security over time. It is this capacity for change that is the focus of our chapter. The goals of our chapter are to describe recent theory and research on whether and why attachment security changes during adulthood (specifically late adolescence and early and middle adulthood), to identify unresolved conceptual and methodological issues and provide suggestions for future research, and to discuss implications of the models of naturalistic change for change in attachment security through clinical intervention. Readers interested in change in attachment security also should see Fraley and Brumbaugh (Chapter 4, this volume), who present a framework for understanding patterns of change over time that complements the focus on predictors of change presented in this chapter.

There is a growing literature on change in attachment security during adulthood, as well as extant literatures on change in attachment security during childhood and from childhood to adulthood. As our chapter reveals, these literatures can be somewhat complex and have not always yielded consistent findings. As we review these literatures, a number of themes arise that may be useful in understanding why the inconsistencies emerged. In particular, we focus on a number of distinctions in the definition and measurement of the attachment construct that may have implications for how we understand change, including distinctions between trait and state components of security, conscious and latent components of security, security as a categorical versus a dimensional phenomenon, and security as a relationship specific or a general phenomenon.

CHANGE IN ATTACHMENT SECURITY DURING CHILDHOOD

Before discussing change during adulthood, we review the literature on change during childhood. This brief review is relevant to understanding the context in which research on adults emerged, and it offers important insights into change processes. As noted earlier, Bowlby (1969) suggested that people both accommodate and assimilate information into their working models, resulting in the opportunity for change over time. Two sets of findings regarding attachment during childhood are relevant to this hypothesis. First, in a series of longitudinal studies, children were observed as they separated from and reunited with caregivers, and their attachment behaviors were coded (i.e., they were assessed with Ainsworth's Strange Situation paradigm; Ainsworth, Blehar, Waters, & Wall, 1978) at two separate time points. The correspondence between attachment classifications at the two assessment times was measured. These studies showed that stability in attachment classification was evidenced when life circumstances remained stable but that change occurred when they did not (e.g., Egeland & Farber, 1984; Egeland & Sroufe, 1981; Vaughn, Egeland, Sroufe, & Waters, 1979).

For example, Egeland and Farber (1984) found that, in a sample of economically disadvantaged mothers, mothers of babies who changed from secure at 12 months to anxious–resistant at 18 months reported an increase in stressful life events during that period compared with mothers with stably secure babies who reported a decrease in life stress. Mothers of babies who changed from secure to anxious–resistant also reported more changes in living arrangements compared with mothers of stably secure babies. Specifically, 30% of the mothers of the babies who changed began living with a romantic partner during the change period. In addition, mothers of babies who changed from anxious–resistant at 12 months to secure at 18 months were less likely to have been separated from their babies during that time compared with mothers of babies who remained anxious–resistant. Using anecdotal evidence derived from interviews with the mothers in their study, Egeland and Farber reported that mothers of babies who changed from secure to an insecure classification tended to report increasing nervousness and dysphoria over time and a loss of interest in their babies. Mothers of babies who became more secure over time tended to report increasing confidence in being a mother. Therefore, changes in the mother's life circumstances, which likely corresponded with changes in the child's caregiving environment, covaried with changes in the child's level of security. This finding suggests that attachment patterns are not necessarily fixed during childhood but are responsive to environmental (typically interpersonal or caregiving) changes.

Second, another series of studies used the Strange Situation assessment procedure to examine whether children evidenced different attachment classifications with different caregivers (e.g., mothers and fathers). In fact, children did exhibit different attachment patterns with different people (Bridges, Connell, & Belsky, 1988; Lamb, 1977; Main & Weston, 1981). This finding also suggested that attachment patterns were responsive to specific aspects of the interpersonal environment, supporting the idea that attachment models can accommodate divergent interpersonal information, at least during childhood.

In sum, the childhood attachment literature supports the idea that during childhood some people do change attachment patterns or hold different attachment models over time and with different people and that this is largely due to experiences in their interpersonal environments. This suggests that the same might be true during adulthood. On the other hand, it could be that as people age and mature their attachment models become more set, less flexible, and less responsive to environmental input. In this case, adults might be less likely to show changes in their attachment models (Bowlby, 1973; for a discussion of these issues as they relate to personality more broadly, see Caspi & Roberts, 2001; Helson, Kwan, John, & Jones, 2002).

CHANGE IN ATTACHMENT SECURITY DURING ADULTHOOD

Empirical Evidence

Three sets of findings speak to the issue of change in attachment security during adulthood. The first comes from long-term longitudinal studies that have examined the correspondence between childhood attachment classification (assessed with the Strange Situation paradigm) and adult attachment classification (typically assessed with the Adult Attachment Interview [AAI]; George, Kaplan, & Main, 1985). A number of studies have been published, and they all show that change is possible. Two studies revealed very little correspondence between childhood and adult attachment classifications, suggesting that change is the predominant occurrence (Lewis, Feiring, & Rosenthal, 2000; Weinfeld, Sroufe, & Egeland, 2000). Two other studies showed significant, but not perfect, correspondence between childhood and adulthood, suggesting that some people change but many do not (Hamilton, 2000; Waters, Merrick, Treboux, Crowell, & Albersheim, 2000). A number of those studies examined predictors of change, such as major family life events (e.g., loss of a parent, parental divorce, parental psychopathology, child maltreatment) and found that change toward insecurity is associated with these negative life experiences (e.g., Waters et al., 2000; Weinfeld et al., 2000). Importantly, these studies typically focused on childhood life experiences and were not able to pinpoint when changes in attachment classifications took place (e.g., in childhood or adulthood), thereby leaving open the question of whether change *during* adulthood is possible.

The second set of findings comes from research on adult romantic attachment security, which uses self-report questionnaires to assess people's beliefs about their level of security. With these questionnaires, people can be classified as showing one of a number of attachment patterns or, more commonly, described along two dimensions of security thought to underlie the attachment patterns: avoidance of intimacy and anxiety about abandonment. In the attempt to assess the stability of these classifications and dimensions (and demonstrate the reliability of the measures), it became clear that, although there is moderate evidence of stability, many people (e.g., approximately 30%) *report* different attachment styles and many people show fluctuations on levels of security over time (e.g., Baldwin & Fehr, 1995; Baldwin, Keelan, Fehr, Enns, & Koh-Rangarajoo, 1996; Davila, Burge, & Hammen, 1997; Davila, Karney, & Bradbury, 1999). Whether this is evidence of a pervasive and lasting reorganization of attachment models and behavior is unclear. For some individuals it may be, but given evidence reviewed later that some people report frequent fluctuations in security, for some it may be more reflective of a transient change in self-perception.

The third set of findings comes from research on attachment security during late adolescence and adulthood, which uses interview assessments over relatively short time periods. This research also shows evidence of change. For example, in a 1-year longitudinal study of late adolescents, Davila and Cobb (2003) assessed attachment security using Bartholomew's interview procedure (Bartholomew, 1998; Bartholomew & Horowitz, 1991). Dimensional security ratings were only moderately correlated over the 1-year period (r = .53, p < .01), suggesting that people show change over time. Crowell, Treboux, and Waters (2002) examined stability of AAI classification over the transition to marriage. They found that 78% of spouses retained the same classification, suggesting that for most spouses, attachment security remains stable, but for some it does not. Of importance, among those showing change, the predominant change was toward greater security. Unlike the long-term longitudinal research described earlier, this short-term research does suggest that change can occur during adulthood and that people have the capacity to experience major changes in states of mind with regard to attachment.

In sum, although the long-term longitudinal research fails to locate the exact time of change, the short-term longitudinal research during late adolescence and adulthood suggests that self-reported and interviewer-assessed security has the capacity to change during these developmental periods. Therefore, at least some people, under some circumstances, show changes in their adult attachment models. Questions remain, however, about whether these changes represent a lasting reorganization of attachment models and behaviors.

Measurement Issues Affecting the Assessment and Conceptualization of Change

Researchers studying change in adult attachment security, particularly those using self-report measures, have faced a number of serious measurement issues. First, with regard to self-report questionnaires, researchers are concerned that the change being seen is due to measurement error. This possibility raises a number of important conceptual and assessment issues. From a conceptual standpoint, it raises the question of whether the change represents a "real" psychological phenomenon, that is, whether the change is psychologically meaningful and, if so, what its meaning is. What causes people to change? From an assessment standpoint, it raises the question of whether self-report measures are reliable.

In addition to these questions raised by the self-reported attachment stability findings, another concern has developed regarding the entire self-reported attachment enterprise. Many attachment scholars, particularly those who typically assess attachment security using interview or behavioral measures, are concerned about the construct validity of the self-report measures of adult attachment security (but see Shaver & Mikulincer, Chapter 2, this volume). The issue is whether the self-report measures tap the same construct as behavior- or interview-based measures. Research designed to answer this question is in an early phase and, at present, the controversy is largely unresolved.

For example, self-report and interview attachment measures tend not to correlate except when they assess the same relationship domain, and even then the correlations are only moderate (e.g., Bartholomew & Shaver, 1998; Crowell, Fraley, & Shaver, 1999; Shaver, Belsky, & Brennan, 2000; Simpson, Rholes, Orina, & Grich, 2002). On the other hand, research examining the correlates and consequences of adult attachment security often yields similar conclusions, regardless of which measure of attachment was used. However, evidence that attachment security can have different correlates depending on how it is assessed is also beginning to emerge. For example, Waters, Crowell, Elliot, Corcoran, and Treboux (2002) found, in a sample of married adults, that interview ratings were associated with observational measures of attachment-relevant behavior, whereas self-report measures were correlated with reports of relationship satisfaction and quality. Furman and Shaffer (2002) found similar results in a sample of adolescents in dating relationships. Simpson and colleagues (2002) found that both interview-assessed and self-reported security predicted support behaviors among couples but did so in different ways. For example, interview security was associated with sensitive providing of support (i.e., providing support when partners needed it most), whereas self-reported security was associated with increased providing of support in all circumstances. As we describe in more detail later, the literature on attachment change reflects similar inconsistencies. There is some evidence that changes in self-reported and interviewer-assessed security are associated with similar factors and some evidence that they are not. So, what are we to make of these findings? And what are the answers to the question posed previously regarding the reliability and validity of self-reported attachment security?

With regard to the related issues of the reliability of the self-report questionnaires and whether they capture psychologically meaningful change, a great deal of emerging research does suggest that change in self-reported adult attachment security is psychologically meaningful. A number of scholars have developed conceptual models of change (described later), and studies have shown that change can be reliably predicted from theoretically relevant variables (e.g., Baldwin et al., 1996; Davila et al., 1997, 1999; Davila & Cobb, 2003; Davila & Sargent, 2003; Simpson, Rholes, Campbell, & Wilson, 2003). However, answers to questions regarding the construct validity of the self-report measures are somewhat less clear. Although Shaver and Mikulincer (Chapter 2, this volume) present a strong case for the validity of self-report measures, a number of scholars, citing the inconsistent evidence described previously, have suggested that self-reported and interviewer-assessed attachment security assess different constructs, or at least different aspects of the attachment system. It will be critical for researchers to follow the lead of Shaver and Mikulincer and document precisely what self-report and interview measures assess, because to the extent that they do assess different constructs or different aspects of the attachment system, implications may exist for how change in attachment is interpreted for the different measures.

For example, proponents of interview measures, particularly the AAI, suggest that interviews assess conscious processes, such as cognitive, affective, and behavioral patterns, and also nonconscious processes, such as defensive strategies, and data about the organization and coherence of attachment information. Interviews are coded by raters who are trained to look across time and situation to examine the content of what people say, the coherence with which they say it, and the behaviors that they display in language and emotion. As such, codes from interview data reflect a great deal of information collected from a range of channels (both conscious and nonconscious) that has been synthesized by an objective coder. Therefore, assuming reliable coding of the interview, the types of variables that might lead to change over time in level or pattern of attachment security likely would need to be ones that could affect change in how people think about, feel about, and behave with regard to a particular attachment relationship at both conscious and nonconscious levels.

To the extent that self-reported attachment security assesses different aspects of the attachment system than do interviews, then different variables might lead to change. One way to conceptualize what self-report measures tap is to consider what we know about self-reported information more generally. Self-report measures can best be considered objective assessments because people provide descriptions of themselves using objectively defined standardized rating scales. One important quality of objective measures, at least according to many scholars, is that they largely rely on information that is consciously held. That is, people can report only on that information to which they have conscious access. Hence self-reported attachment security may be best considered to be a reflection of consciously held beliefs and feelings. If this is true, then it suggests that self-reports and interviews are tapping different types of attachment information and, consequently, that different types of attachment information are represented in their outcomes. It also suggests that different variables may be responsible for change. Specifically, change in self-reported beliefs likely would involve variables that can lead to change in consciously held ideas. Note, however, that we are not suggesting that self-reported security is not associated with nonconscious information—there is growing evidence that it is (e.g., see Shaver and Mikulincer, Chapter 2, this volume). Rather, we are suggesting that *change* in self-reported security must be conceptualized as involving factors that are most likely to affect self-reports. There may be many such factors, including nonconscious ones, as we describe subsequently.

Research in social and cognitive psychology has focused extensively on how people's consciously held attitudes, beliefs, and views change, and it suggests that change is, at least for some people, a regularly occurring experience. A good example of the changing nature of beliefs comes from work on priming, which shows that people can be made to think of almost anything without being aware of the process by which it came into consciousness (e.g., Nisbett & Wilson, 1977; see Wegner & Bargh, 1998). Hence the conscious content of thought may be constantly changing, even in response to things about which people are unaware. Conscious beliefs also fluctuate in response to mood (e.g., Bower, 1981). For example, a depressed mood leads to negative thoughts, which then become positive again once the depressed mood remits (see Segal, 1988). Consciously held self-views also change in response to the current social environment. Work on the spontaneous self-concept (e.g., McGuire, McGuire, Child, & Fujioka, 1978) shows this, as does work on social-comparison processes (e.g., Morse & Gergen, 1970). So there is a good deal of evidence that people's consciously held beliefs change regularly in response to various temporary internal and external circumstances. It is also the case that this change is not permanent—that consciously held beliefs may fluctuate quite a bit, even over relatively brief time periods.

Inherent in the preceding discussion is the possibility that adult attachment security has both conscious, explicit components and more latent, implicit components. Also inherent in the discussion is the possibility that adult attachment security has both trait and state components (see also Fraley & Brumbaugh, Chapter 4, this volume) and that it is the state component that may fluctuate more and in response to different events than the trait component does. Whether the trait and state components or the conscious and latent components map onto the different ways of measuring adult attachment security is unknown, but it might be useful to consider this possibility when conceptualizing change. We return to this issue later in the chapter when we discuss future research directions. At that time, we consider not only whether there are distinctions between trait–state and conscious–latent components of attachment security but also whether adult attachment security should be conceived of as categorical or dimensional in nature and as relationship specific or general. Different attachment measures tend to use different approaches. For example, interviews, such as the AAI, typically categorize people into attachment patterns, whereas self-report measures are typically dimensional in nature. Interviews such as the AAI also tend to be relationship specific, whereas self-report measures have used both relationship-specific and general approaches. These additional distinctions are important to bear in mind when considering whether change will be observed and what factors will predict it.

In sum, not only may self-reports and interviews assess different aspects of the attachment system and change in response to different types of variables, but also the duration and type of change may differ. Therefore, it may be worthwhile to take these issues into consideration in our models of change and stability of attachment security and to conduct empirical tests of the potential differences between change in the different aspects of adult attachment security and between change in self-reported and interviewer-assessed adult attachment security. These ideas will be revisited in later sections of this chapter, but first we turn to describing current models of predictors of change in adult attachment security.

CURRENT MODELS OF PREDICTORS OF CHANGE IN ADULT ATTACHMENT SECURITY

At present, there are three models of predictors of change in adult attachment security. We review each one in this section. Note that Fraley and Brumbaugh (Chapter 4, this volume) present a model of change. However, their model is not reviewed here, as it does not focus on predictors of change but rather on patterns of change over time (e.g., when in the life course change is most likely). Inherent in their model is the idea that changes in the interpersonal/caregiving environment facilitate changes in security—a model that we describe in the following section on life stress.

Life Stress Model

The life-stress or life-event model of change suggests that change in level or pattern of attachment security results in response to significant life events or significant changes in life circumstances. This model, although not named as such, was originally proposed by Bowlby (1969), who suggested that relatively lasting change in attachment models can come about as an adaptation to new, interpersonally relevant life circumstances that are ongoing and emotionally significant (see also Collins & Read, 1994). As described earlier, research on changes in attachment pattern during childhood, and from childhood to adulthood, using behavioral and interview measures of attachment security has borne this out. Children who had adverse life experiences were the most likely to show change, specifically to become more insecure (e.g., Waters et al., 2000; Weinfeld et al., 2000).

However, research on change in adult attachment security using self-report measures has not consistently shown change in response to life events. Thus far, only a few studies provide support for the life-stress model. Kirkpatrick and Hazan (1994) found that, over 4 years, people who experienced the breakup of a romantic relationship were more likely than others to become more insecure. Davila and colleagues (1999) found, in a 2-year longitudinal sample of newlyweds, that security increased over the course of the transition to marriage. Specifically, people became more comfortable with intimacy and less anxious about being abandoned. Simpson and colleagues (2003) found that wives (but not husbands) became more comfortable with intimacy (but not less anxious about being abandoned) over the transition to parenthood. On the other hand, others have failed to replicate these findings. For example, Baldwin and Fehr (1995), Scharfe and Bartholomew (1994), and Davila and colleagues (1997) all examined associations between interpersonal life stressors (broadly defined) and attachment change over periods ranging from 4 months to 2 years, but they found no evidence of such an association.

These inconsistent findings raise a number of important issues and questions, the most obvious being, Under what circumstances do life events predict or fail to predict change in self-reported attachment security and why? We discuss three possible answers that we have pursued in our own research.

First, it is possible that self-reported attachment security (or attachment security assessed in any manner, for that matter) will change only in response to certain types of events. As noted previously, events that are ongoing and interpersonally and emotionally significant may be the best candidates. In addition, adult romantic relationships are thought to be the primary attachment relationships in adulthood. As such, events that affect the romantic domain of life, particularly those that change the nature of a relationship or that affect relationship status, may be most relevant for change. It was these notions that drove our research on attachment change over the course of newlywed marriage (Davila et al., 1999). The transition to marriage is certainly an ongoing, emotionally significant change in relationship status. Other research has used various types of life events and has typically collapsed across them (e.g., to create general measures of the number of stressors), which may obscure the effects of the most meaningful events.

However, we have not been wholly successful in identifying those events that are relevant to self-reported change in attachment security. In a recent study, we examined the role of romantic stress, conflict events, loss events, and separation events in change in attachment security (Davila & Cobb, 2003). Based on attachment theory and on the criteria described previously, these events should be particularly relevant to levels of attachment security. However, although they did predict increases in insecurity using an interview measure of attachment security, they did not predict changes in self-reported attachment security over a 1-year period.

In another example, change in attachment security was investigated in a group of couples having their first child, another event that should be ongoing, emotionally significant, and relevant to the romantic relationship. As noted earlier, Simpson and colleagues (2003) found that wives reported more comfort with intimacy during this transition. Consistent with this finding, we expected that, given the significant changes in family structure and roles that occur during this period, spouses experiencing the transition to parenthood would show more changes in attachment security over the year following birth than would spouses who were not having babies. However, compared with voluntarily childless couples who were matched for duration of marriage, parent couples were no more likely to experience changes in levels of attachment security than were nonparent couples (Cobb, Davila, Rothman, Lawrence, & Bradbury, 2003). Differences in findings from these two studies may be accounted for by the inclusion of a nonparent control group in the Cobb and colleagues (2003) study. We compared whether attachment change was more likely for couples experiencing the stressful transition of parenthood than for those who were not and, further, whether the changes in attachment in the parent sample could be predicted by changes in social support. Although the rates of change are not significantly different for parents as compared with nonparents, there is evidence that attachment did change and that it covaried with social support received over the transition (discussed later in this chapter).

A second possibility regarding the circumstances in which life events are associated with change in self-reported security is that the link between self-reported attachment change and life events may be most evident over shorter, rather than longer, time periods. If it is true that self-reported attachment security reflects consciously held beliefs and that such beliefs change relatively easily, quickly, and regularly in response to environmental factors, then we would be less likely to be able to link change over relatively long periods of time to discrete and specific life events and more likely to show short-term, temporary changes in response to changing life circumstances. We evaluated this possibility in an 8-week daily diary study, during which people reported on daily life events and daily levels of security (Davila & Sargent, 2003). We found that daily events and daily levels of security covaried over time (controlling for the prior day's level of security), suggesting that peoples' self-reported beliefs about security were constantly fluctuating in response to life experiences. Therefore, the effect of life events on self-reported attachment security may be observed best when looking at short-term time periods and temporary changes.

A third possible answer to the question of when life events predict or fail to predict change in self-reported attachment security and why has to do with how people view events. To date, tests of life-event models of attachment change have considered only the direct effect of the objective features of the events (e.g., type, number) on change. However, it could be argued that inherent in Bowlby's construal of change is the notion of cognitive mediation. Bowlby suggested that life events would lead to change when they disconfirmed current attachment models. For that to happen, a person would need to experience the event as disconfirming. Therefore, whereas there might be objective features of events that contribute to whether they will disconfirm attachment models, a person would need to construe an event as providing evidence of disconfirmation. Hence, the effect of events on change in attachment models might be cognitively mediated through subjective perceptions. We found support for this prediction in the daily diary study described previously (Davila & Sargent, 2003). The association between daily events and daily levels of security was explained by the extent to which people viewed daily events as resulting in interpersonal loss. To the extent that people saw events as involving interpersonal loss (regardless of the type or number of events), they reported greater insecurity.

We also found support for the role of people's views of life events in the transition-to-parenthood study described earlier (Cobb et al., 2003). In the sample of parents, changes in perceptions about social support over the transition to parenthood were associated with changes in attachment security. Parents who perceived others as being more supportive and available for help and support over the transition demonstrated increases in security from prior to pregnancy to 1 year following birth. Simpson and colleagues (2003) reported similar findings. Perceptions of spousal support and anger were predictors of change in security over the transition to parenthood. Again, this implies that it may not be life events per se that influence change but individuals' perceptions of changes in the interpersonal context that result in modifications of attachment models.

Therefore, when we attempt to understand the role of life events in change in adult attachment security, it may be important to consider the specific type of event that may result in change (an objective feature), the time frame over which change is expected to occur and persist, and the way people view the events that happen to them, particularly the interpersonal meaning that they assign to events. Doing so may be most relevant for understanding change in self-reported attachment security, given the nature of self-reports, but it also may be relevant for understanding change in interviewer-assessed security. It may also be important when attempting to sort out potential differences between state changes in security and more pervasive, long-lasting reorganizations of attachment models. Assessing views of events may be a particularly promising avenue for further development, as it has the potential to shed light on the disconfirmation process that Bowlby described. It also has the potential to speak to another issue that has not been adequately addressed in the literature—the extent to which positive, as well as negative, events might lead to changes in attachment security.

Virtually all prior research other than the work on transitions to marriage and parenthood has examined the role of objectively defined negative events on attachment change. As such, we know very little about whether positive events play a role in attachment change or the extent to which people can become more secure, as well as more insecure, over time. Therefore, research needs to include both positive and negative events in an attempt to account for both positive and negative outcomes. By also including a focus on views of events, a broad range of attachment-related adaptations to stress can be examined. For example, it becomes possible to understand how an objectively defined negative event (e.g., a conflict between romantic partners), when resolved adaptively (e.g., when experienced by the partners as having a positive outcome), may be associated with positive experiences and growth. Hence examining views of self and others that result from events, rather than just the events themselves, allows for a more specific prediction of how an event may affect attachment change.

Social-Cognitive Model

This model was originally developed by Baldwin and colleagues (e.g., Baldwin & Fehr, 1995; Baldwin et al., 1996) as a way to explain why people report different attachment patterns at different times. The model suggests that change in level or pattern of attachment security is a result of changing states of mind. That is, people will report different levels or patterns of attachment security at different times depending on what is presently activated in their minds. According to this model, although people may have a chronically accessible attachment model that is stable over time, they also have a number of different attachment models, or relational schemas, that can be activated by specific circumstances (Baldwin et al., 1996; Davila et al., 1999). Attachment change is thus due to accessibility of different models at different times, depending on the person's current circumstances (e.g., environmental factors, what the person is cued/ primed to think about, etc.). Therefore, this model describes what are most likely to be temporary changes in security. As current circumstances change, so too should attachment security.

Initial tests of this model did not directly examine change in attachment security. Rather, different attachment experiences were primed, and people's behaviors were examined to see whether they differed depending on what was primed (Baldwin et al., 1996, Study 3). Indeed, they did. People responded differently to interpersonal information depending on the priming stimulus. Other priming studies, although not designed to study attachment change, also demonstrate that various types of attachment information can be made more or less salient and consequently influence thought, feeling, and behavior (e.g., Mikulincer & Arad, 1999; Mikulincer, Gillath, & Shaver, 2002).

A number of studies have examined change in attachment security directly, not experimentally, but with variables that could be construed as representing current states of mind about specific interpersonal experiences. For example, Davila and colleagues (1999) conceptualized marital satisfaction as a social-cognitive variable based on the idea that it represents people's states of mind about their marriage that can change relatively regularly, depending on marital circumstances. We demonstrated that, despite spouses' becoming more secure on average over the early years of marriage, marital satisfaction predicts changes in level of attachment security over time at the within-person level. Not surprisingly, when a spouse is happy in marriage, he or she feels more secure; when unhappy, he or she feels less secure. Our research on views of life events (Davila & Sargent, 2003), described earlier, could also be construed, at least loosely, as social-cognitive in nature. To the extent that daily life events result in bringing to mind feelings of loss, people feel more insecure than they previously did.

These findings highlight the relatively temporary changes in attachment security that are predicted by the social-cognitive model and highlight the ways in which attachment security can be state-like. Importantly, all of the research just described used self-report measures of adult attachment security, which, as we noted earlier, may have state-like properties. However, the extent to which the social-cognitive model applies only to self-reported security is unknown given that it has not been tested using other measures. It would be informative to examine, for example, whether interviewer-assessed attachment security would systematically differ among groups of people primed with different types of attachment-relevant information.

Individual-Difference Model

This model was also proposed as an explanation for why some people report different levels or patterns of attachment security at different times. Instead of focusing on normative cognitive activation processes that likely apply to everyone, this model focuses on more pathological individual differences that make a subset of individuals more likely than others to report different attachment levels and patterns. The model states that people who have certain vulnerability factors (e.g., parental divorce, parental psychopathology, personality pathology, personal psychopathology) will be more prone to change attachment levels and patterns because they have developed unclear models of self and others, thus rendering their attachment models unstable (Davila et al., 1997).

Therefore, the individual-difference model is a mediation model, which begins with the presence of one or more vulnerabilities. These vulnerabilities are factors that are likely to have negatively affected interpersonal development. For example, parental divorce often has negative effects on interpersonal functioning and relationship success (e.g., Amato, 2000), and parental psychopathology often affects the security and quality of parent–child and other interpersonal relationships (e.g., Eiden, Edwards, & Leonard, 2002; Hammen & Brennan, 2001; Teti, Gelfand, Messinger, & Isabella, 1995). Individual psychopathology and personality pathology also typically impair all types of interpersonal relationships. These vulnerabilities are hypothesized to impede the development of clear, stable models of the self and others. If people lack clarity in their understanding of self or others, they will be likely to report different levels or patterns of attachment security at different times, because they do not have a consistent set of models to call on. Instead, their lack of clarity results in thinking and feeling one way at one time and another way at another time.

The individual-difference model also hypothesizes that the propensity to report different attachment levels or patterns at different times may be a reflection of insecurity. The reporting of different attachment levels or patterns is thus seen as a process characteristic of insecurity, in some ways analogous to the type of incoherence in cognitive and affective processes that attachment scholars describe as characteristic of insecure individuals (e.g., Main, 1991). Therefore, the model predicts that people who change attachment patterns over time should look very much like people who are stably insecure over time in terms of vulnerabilities.

A number of studies have supported predictions of the individual-difference model. For example, in a 2-year longitudinal study of late adolescent females, individual vulnerability factors were associated with change in self-reported attachment patterns (and were better predictors than were life events; Davila et al., 1997). In addition, people who changed attachment patterns had levels of vulnerabilities comparable to stably insecure people, and they all showed significantly greater levels than stably secure people, supporting the notion that reporting different attachment patterns is a process reflective of insecurity. In a 1-year longitudinal study of late-adolescent males and females, the full mediation model was tested and supported. Personal (i.e., individual psychopathology and personality pathology) vulnerabilities were associated with lack of clarity in models of self and others, which was in turn associated with decreases in levels of security over time (Davila & Cobb, 2003).

In sum, the strength of the individual-difference model is that it identifies a group of people who are more likely than others to report fluctuating levels and patterns of security. However, numerous questions remain. For example, the exact reasons why a vulnerable person might report a different level of security at a particular time are unclear. Is it random, or is he or she responding to something in the immediate environment (e.g., priming, a life event)? In addition, the extent to which fluctuating self-reports of levels and patterns of security are representative of trait-level insecurity needs further study. If they are, then people could be more accurately classified based on self-reports measured at multiple times, which could strengthen confidence in the use of self-report measures.

Similarities and Differences among the Models

As the reader has likely noticed, the three models described herein are very different regarding the proposed source of change in attachment levels and patterns. However, they also share some important similarities. For example, the life-event and social-cognitive models both suggest that changes in security occur in response to life circumstances. The difference is that the life-event model was originally proposed as a way to understand relatively long-term adaptation to significant changes in the interpersonal world, whereas the social-cognitive model was proposed as a way to understand shorter-term changes in feelings of security in response to temporary changes in circumstances. Also, although the life-event model focuses on external events, the social-cognitive model focuses on both external and internal (e.g., how a person might be thinking or feeling) circumstances. As noted earlier, a focus on views of events, which are internal circumstances in response to external experience, brings together the social-cognitive and life-event models. The individual-difference and social-cognitive models also have an important similarity. Both suggest that change in attachment security can be a fairly transient, repetitive occurrence. However, the models focus on different sources of change. The individual-difference model focuses on a distal, dispositional source. The social-cognitive model focuses on a more proximal source with environmental origins (as does the life-event model). We believe that the fact that the different models have a number of components in common should be important to future research on change in attachment security, as well as to clinical intervention, topics that we explore in the remaining sections.

ISSUES FOR FUTURE RESEARCH

At the simplest level, research on change in adult attachment security should continue to focus on two questions that have driven research to date: Who is most likely to change? Under what circumstances do they do so? The individual-difference model speaks largely to the first question regarding who will change. The social-cognitive and life-stress models speak to the second question regarding the circumstances that lead to change. In addition to continuing to refine current models and develop new answers to the two questions, one important future direction will be to consider the similarities and differences of existing models and to develop models of change that integrate their different components.

For example, one such integration comes in the form of a *diathesis–stress model*. Generally speaking, in a diathesis–stress model, people with a vulnerability (or diathesis) are more likely than people without the vulnerability to respond in some way (e.g., change their beliefs, develop symptoms, etc.) in the face of relevant life circumstances (i.e., the "stress"). This is essentially a reactivity model in which people with certain vulnerabilities are more reactive to certain life circumstances than are other people (e.g., Bolger & Schilling, 1991; Bolger & Zuckerman, 1995).

With regard to attachment security, there are a number of possible diathesis–stress models. For example, Simpson and colleagues (2003) have suggested that preexisting deficiencies in the marital relationship (the diathesis; e.g., low perceived spousal support and high perceived spousal anger) may render spouses vulnerable to decreases in security during the transition to parenthood (the stress). Another version of a diathesis–stress model suggests that individual vulnerabilities and lack of clarity in models of self and others (the diatheses) render people more likely to experience changes in their levels or patterns of attachment security in response to relevant life circumstances (Davila et al., 1999). This diathesis–stress model combines the individual-difference model with the social-cognitive and life-event models, and it solves an important problem in the individual-difference model noted earlier: Why might a vulnerable person report a different level of security at a particular time? The two diathesis–stress models described also refine the social-cognitive and life-event models by suggesting that not everyone is equally likely to report different levels of security in response to current circumstances. Hence, a diathesis–stress model can explain how distal dispositional factors (and also preexisting contextually stable factors such as marital quality) interact with proximal contextual factors to result in changing reports of security over time. Of course, this model is speculative at present and awaits empirical verification.

In addition to the study of more integrated models of change in adult attachment security, another important issue for future research will be to examine more closely whether there are specific models of change that explain the circumstances under which people become, for example, more avoidant versus more preoccupied. That is, why would a person show one particular type of change compared with another type of change? Is it driven by specific types of events or environmental cues? Is it a product of temperamental biases or extant coping styles? There are no answers to these questions at present.

Finally, and perhaps most important, future research on change will need to consider a number of distinctions that are relevant to the conceptualization and measurement of the adult attachment construct. These include the distinction between state and trait components of security, between conscious and latent components of security, between general and specific attachment models, and between categorical and dimensional methods of describing people. Each distinction presents challenges for conceptualizing and understanding change. For example, with regard to the state–trait distinction, if there are both trait and state components of adult attachment security, then how are they related to one another? And will changes in one lead to changes in the other? For instance, if views of life events predict daily fluctuations in security (Davila & Sargent, 2003), then over time might such state fluctuations lead to a more pervasive reorganization of attachment models, especially if views disconfirm old models? The same questions apply to the distinction between conscious and latent aspects of attachment security. Do different factors lead to change at these different levels, and how is change at each level related to change at the other level, if at all?

Similarly, with regard to the general–specific attachment model distinction, how might change in general versus specific attachment models be related? Might people retain a stable general attachment model while experiencing change in their specific models? Might general models be harder to change than specific models? And with regard to the categorical–dimensional distinction, in addition to similar questions about how they change and how change in each is related, where is the "clinical significance" of changes along attachment dimensions? With classifications, it may be easy to know when someone has become predominantly more secure than insecure, but the same is not true of dimensional ratings, at least when analyzed individually and as main effects. Therefore, do our analyses of dimensional change tell us about major reorganization of attachment models? The answer is unclear.

In sum, for research on change in adult attachment security to progress, researchers must face the challenge of attending to and clarifying these important conceptual and methodological distinctions in the context of refining and extending current models of change.

IMPLICATIONS OF ATTACHMENT CHANGE MODELS FOR CLINICAL INTERVENTION

Thus far we have discussed several different models of attachment change, the existing research that speaks to each, and a number of challenges for future research. However, our analysis has been from the perspective of basic research, largely driven by social-personality and developmental psychology perspectives. An issue that is of great interest to clinical psychologists is deliberately effecting change through therapeutic intervention. Although it is important to develop and refine our models in order to understand change processes as they occur naturally, clinical psychologists are also interested in models of change because they may inform interventions. How can these models of change inform therapeutic interventions if the desired outcome is to improve an individual's mental health or interpersonal relationships through fostering increased security?

In the infant literature, there has been some limited research on how attachment security changes in response to intervention with insecurely attached infants and their caregivers. For example, Lieberman, Weston, and Pawl (1991) found that improving the quality of the interaction between mother and child over the course of 1 year significantly lowered avoidance, resistance, and anger and significantly raised partnership with mother as compared with infant–mother dyads who did not receive treatment. Although they are not specifically focused on assessing attachment change, several attachment-based interventions have been shown to successfully treat depression in adolescents (Diamond, Brendali, Diamond, Siqueland, & Isaacs, 2002) and to improve affect regulation in incarcerated adolescents (Keiley, 2002). In the literature on adult psychotherapy, there has been much theorizing about how attachment processes may be the focus of intervention with the aim of improving interpersonal relationships. Specifically, Johnson and colleagues (see Johnson, Chapter 12, this volume) have developed emotionally focused therapy for couples that has the aim of improving the quality of the relationship through a focus on attachment-relevant issues (Greenberg & Johnson, 1988; Johnson, 1996; Johnson, Hunsley, Greenberg, & Schindler, 1999; Johnson & Talitman, 1996). Although increased security is not a specific focus of the treatment, improvement in the relationship most likely has the indirect effect of increasing attachment security, if not generally then presumably at least within the context of the specific couple relationship. Although there is a lack of research documenting change in attachment over the course of treatment, Travis, Bliwise, Binder, and Horne-Moyer (2001) did find that over the course of time-limited individual psychotherapy, clients showed significant increases in attachment security, and a majority showed a change from insecure to secure attachment patterns.

For the most part, the idea of change in attachment security through therapy has been discussed as an event that alters the individual's ongoing life circumstances; in other words, such change is consistent with the life-stress model. However, therapeutic change may be accomplished through several different avenues. For example, change may occur on different levels and be attributable to different sources when it occurs naturally, as during the transition to parenthood, or when it is deliberately effected, as in an ongoing therapy relationship. Thus it is possible to interpret attachment change in therapy through the lens of each of the models presented in this chapter.

First, in the life-stress model, Bowlby (1969) proposed that therapy may be an important event that could necessitate adaptation and change in attachment models. Thus developing a new relationship with a therapist who may not react in ways consistent with insecure attachment models and who can provide support in exploring the meaning of others' and one's own interpersonal behaviors may result in the kinds of experiences that cause updating of or adaptation in attachment models.

Second, the social-cognitive model suggests that individuals have different modes of interacting depending on what attachment model is activated or is most accessible at the moment. This allows for the possibility of exploration in treatment of experiences in which the client is perhaps using more "secure" attachment models to guide behavior and interpretations as a way of strengthening or making those models more salient and thus more frequently activated. By more frequent activation of these secure models, perhaps through awareness and understanding of different patterns of behavior in different situations or in different relationships, it may be possible to induce a more lasting change by making the secure models more chronically salient.

Third, the individual-difference model presumes that changes in attachment as assessed by self-report represents an underlying insecurity that reflects unstable or unclear attachment models. Like the social-cognitive model, it implies that some attachment change is more temporary or perhaps more superficial. However, more durable changes in attachment models could be achieved through increasing the clarity and sharpness of clients' views of themselves and others. By helping clients gain a greater understanding of their own interpersonal style and the origins of their beliefs and patterns, it may be possible to begin to alter them.

In summary, just as it may be possible to integrate the three models of attachment change presented here when conceptualizing naturalistic change, it also may be possible to use an integrated approach to attachment change through treatment. Therapy involves a new experience or relationship that may be very different from the client's existing relationships (life-stress model). There may be many instances in which interactions with the therapist and others in the client's social world do not fit with the client's insecure-attachment models. Through discussion of these experiences, it may be possible to activate existing secure models (social-cognitive model). Also, understanding assumptions and interpretations of others' behaviors may facilitate a more positive adaptive view of personal relationships. This increased awareness and understanding may serve to increase the clarity of clients' views of themselves and others, and discussion of the origins of these views may be another point of change (individual-differences model).

CONCLUSIONS

In this chapter, we sought to describe recent theory and research on whether and how attachment security changes during adulthood, to identify unresolved conceptual and methodological issues and provide suggestions for future research, and to discuss implications of the models of naturalistic change for change in attachment security through clinical intervention. We hope that our review makes it possible for researchers and clinicians interested in how adult attachment security changes to better understand the relevant change processes in order to build on existing knowledge. The study of change in adult attachment security has implications for numerous aspects of social–personality, developmental, and clinical psychology with regard to basic theory and applied problems, but it is not without challenges. To the extent that we can continue to face and examine relevant conceptual and methodological issues, a more refined understanding of how and why people become more or less secure during adulthood will emerge.

REFERENCES

Ainsworth, M. D. S., Blehar, M. C., Waters, F., & Wall, S. (1978). *Patterns of attachment: A psychological study of the Strange Situation.* Hillsdale, NJ: Erlbaum.

Amato, P. R. (2000). The consequences of divorce for adults and children. *Journal of Marriage and the Family, 62,* 1269–1287.

Baldwin, M. W., & Fehr, B. (1995). On the instability of attachment style ratings. *Personal Relationships, 2,* 247–261.

Baldwin, M. W., Keelan, J. P. R., Fehr, B., Enns, V., & Koh-Rangarajoo, E. (1996). Social-cognitive conceptualization of attachment working models: Availability and accessibility effect. *Journal of Personality and Social Psychology, 71,* 94–109.

Bartholomew, K. (1998). *The Family and Peer Attachment Interview.* Unpublished manuscript, Simon Fraser University, Canada.

Bartholomew, K., & Horowitz, L. M. (1991). Attachment styles among young adults: A test of a four-category model. *Journal of Personality and Social Psychology, 61,* 226–244.

Bartholomew, K., & Shaver, P. R. (1998). Methods of assessing adult attachment: Do they converge? In J. A. Simpson & W. S. Rholes (Eds.), *Attachment theory and close relationships* (pp. 25–45). New York: Guilford Press.

Bolger, N., & Schilling, E. A. (1991). Personality and the problems of everyday life: The role of neuroticism in exposure and reactivity to daily stressors. *Journal of Personality and Social Psychology, 59,* 355–386.

Bolger, N., & Zuckerman, A. (1995). A framework for studying personality in the stress process. *Journal of Personality and Social Psychology, 69,* 890–902.

Bower, G. H. (1981). Mood and memory. *American Psychologist, 36,* 129–148.

Bowlby, J. (1969). *Attachment and loss: Vol. 1. Attachment.* New York: Basic Books.

Bowlby, J. (1973). *Attachment and loss: Vol. 2. Separation: Anxiety and anger.* New York: Basic Books.

Bridges, L., Connell, J. P., & Belsky, J. (1988). Similarities and differences in infant–mother and infant–father interaction in the Strange Situation. *Developmental Psychology, 24,* 92–100.

Caspi, A., & Roberts, B. W. (2001). Personality development across the life course: The argument for change and continuity. *Psychological Inquiry, 12,* 49–66.

Cobb, R. J., Davila, J., Rothman, A., Lawrence, E., & Bradbury, T. N. (2003). *Changes in marital satisfaction and attachment security over the transition to parenthood.* Manuscript submitted for publication.

Collins, N. L., & Read, S. J. (1994). Cognitive representations of attachment: The structure and function of working models. In K. Bartholomew & D. Perlman (Eds.), *Advances in personal relationships: Vol. 5. Attachment processes in adulthood* (pp. 53–90). London: Kingsley.

Crowell, J. A., Fraley, R. C., & Shaver, P. R. (1999). Measurement of individual differences in adolescent and adult attachment. In J. Cassidy & P. R. Shaver (Eds.), *Handbook of attachment: Theory, research, and clinical applications* (pp. 434–465). New York: Guilford Press.

Crowell, J. A., Treboux, D., & Waters, E. (2002). Stability of attachment representations: The transition to marriage. *Developmental Psychology, 38,* 467–479

Davila, J., Burge, D., & Hammen, C. (1997). Why does attachment style change? *Journal of Personality and Social Psychology, 73,* 826–838.

Davila, J., & Cobb, R. J. (2003). Predicting change in self-reported and interviewer-assessed adult attachment: Tests of the individual difference and life stress models of attachment change. *Personality and Social Psychology Bulletin, 29,* 859–870.

Davila, J., Karney, B. R., & Bradbury, T. N. (1999). Attachment change processes in the early years of marriage. *Journal of Personality and Social Psychology, 76,* 783–802.

Davila, J., & Sargent, E. (2003). The meaning of life (events) predicts change in attachment security. *Personality and Social Psychology Bulletin, 29,* 1383–1395.

Diamond, G. S., Brendali, F. R., Diamond, G. M., Siqueland, L., & Isaacs, L. (2002). Attachment-based family therapy for depressed adolescents: A treatment development study. *Journal of American Academy of Child and Adolescent Psychiatry, 41*(10), 1190–1196.

Egeland, B., & Farber, E. A. (1984). Infant–mother attachment: Factors related to its development and changes over time. *Child Development, 55,* 753–771.

Egeland, B., & Sroufe, L. A. (1981). Attachment and early maltreatment. *Child Development, 52,* 44–52.

Eiden, R. D., Edwards, E. P., & Leonard, K. E. (2002). Mother-infant and father-infant attachment among alcoholic families. *Development and Psychopathology, 14,* 253–278.

Furman, W., & Shaffer, L. (2002, April). *Conflict and conflict resolution in adolescent romantic relationships.* Poster presented at the biennial meeting of the Society for Research on Adolescence, New Orleans, LA.

George, C., Kaplan, N., & Main, M. (1985). *Attachment interview for adults.* Unpublished manuscript, University of California, Berkeley.

Greenberg, L. S., & Johnson, S. M. (1988). *Emotionally focused therapy for couples.* New York: Guilford Press.

Hamilton, C. (2000). Continuity and discontinuity of attachment from infancy through adolescence. *Child Development, 71,* 690–694.

Hammen, C., & Brennan, P. A. (2001). Depressed adolescents of depressed and nondepressed mothers: Tests of an interpersonal impairment hypothesis. *Journal of Consulting and Clinical Psychology, 69,* 284–294.

Helson, R., Kwan, V., John, O. P., & Jones, C. (2002). The growing evidence for personality change in adulthood: Findings from research with personality inventories. *Journal of Research in Personality, 36,* 287–306.

Johnson, S. M. (1996). *Creating Connection: The practice of emotionally focused marital therapy.* New York: Brunner/Mazel.

Johnson, S. M., Hunsley, J., Greenberg, L., & Schindler, D. (1999). Emotionally focused couples therapy: Status and challenges. *Clinical Psychology: Science and Practice, 6,* 67–79.

Johnson, S. M., & Talitman, E. (1996). Predictors of success in emotionally focused marital therapy. *Journal of Marital and Family Therapy, 23*(2), 135–152.

Keiley, M. K. (2002). The development and implementation of an affect regulation and attachment intervention for incarcerated adolescents and their parents. *Family Journal–Counseling and Therapy for Couples and Families, 10*(2), 177–189.

Kirkpatrick, L. A., & Hazan, C. (1994). Attachment styles and close relationships: A four-year prospective study. *Personal Relationships, 1,* 123–142.

Lamb, M. E. (1977). Father–infant and mother–infant interaction in the first year of life. *Child Development, 48,* 167–181.

Lieberman, A. F., Weston, D. R., & Pawl, J. H. (1991). Preventive intervention and outcome with anxiously attached dyads. *Child Development, 62*(1), 199–209.

Lewis, M., Feiring, C., & Rosenthal, S. (2000). Attachment over time. *Child Development, 71,* 707–720.

Main, M. (1991). Metacognitive knowledge, metacognitive monitoring, and singular (coherent) vs. multiple (incoherent) models of attachment: Findings and directions for future research. In C. M. Parkes, J. Stevenson-Hinde, & P. Marris (Eds.), *Attachment across the life cycle* (pp. 127–159). London: Tavistock/Routledge.

Main, M., & Weston, D. R. (1981). The quality of toddler's relationship to mother and father: Related to conflict behavior and the readiness to establish new relationships. *Child Development, 52,* 932–940.

McGuire, W. J., McGuire, C. V., Child, P., & Fujioka, T. (1978). Salience of ethnicity in the spontaneous self-concept as a function of one's ethnic distinctiveness in the social environment. *Journal of Personality and Social Psychology, 36,* 511–520.

Mikulincer, M., & Arad, D. (1999). Attachment working models and cognitive openness in close relationships: A test of chronic and temporary accessibility effects. *Journal of Personality and Social Psychology, 77,* 710–725.

Mikulincer, M., Gillath, O., & Shaver, P. R. (2002). Activation of the attachment system in adulthood: Threat-related primes increase the accessibility of mental representations of attachment figures. *Journal of Personality and Social Psychology, 83,* 881–895.

Morse, S., & Gergen, K. J. (1970). Social comparison, self-consistency, and the concept of self. *Journal of Personality and Social Psychology, 16,* 148–156.

Nisbett, R. E., & Wilson, T. D. (1977). Telling more than we can know: Verbal reports on mental processes. *Psychological Review, 84,* 231–259.

Scharfe, E., & Bartholomew, K. (1994). Reliability and stability of adult attachment patterns. *Personal Relationships, 1,* 23–43.

Segal, Z. V. (1988). Appraisal of the self-schema construct in cognitive models of depression. *Psychological Bulletin, 103,* 147–162.

Shaver, P. R., Belsky, J., & Brennan, K. (2000). The Adult Attachment Interview and self-reports of romantic attachment: Associations across domains and methods. *Personal Relationships, 7,* 25–43.

Simpson, J. A., Rholes, W. S., Campbell, L., & Wilson, C. L. (2003). Changes in attachment orientations across the transition to parenthood. *Journal of Experimental Social Psychology, 39,* 317–331.

Simpson, J. A., Rholes, W. S., Oriña, M. M., & Grich, J. (2002). Working models of attachment, support giving, and support seeking in a stressful situation. *Personality and Social Psychology Bulletin, 28,* 598–608.

Teti, D. M., Gelfand, D. M., Messinger, D. S., & Isabella, R. (1995). Maternal depression and the quality of early attachment: An examination of infants, preschoolers, and their mothers. *Developmental Psychology, 31,* 364–376.

Travis, L. A., Bliwise, N. G., Binder, J. L., & Horne-Moyer, H. L. (2001). Changes in clients' attachment styles over the course of time-limited dynamic psychotherapy. *Psychotherapy, 38,* 149–159.

Vaughn, B. E., Egeland, B. R., Sroufe, L. A., & Waters, E. (1979). Individual differences in infant/mother attachment at twelve and eighteen months: Stability and change in families under stress. *Child Development, 50,* 971–975.

Waters, E., Crowell, J. A., Elliott, M., Corcoran, D., & Treboux, D. (2002). Bowlby's secure base theory and the social/personality psychology of attachment style: Work(s) in progress. *Attachment and Human Development, 4,* 230–242.

Waters, E., Merrick, S. K., Treboux, D., Crowell, J., & Albersheim, L. (2000). Attachment security in infancy and early adulthood: A twenty-year longitudinal study. *Child Development, 71,* 684–689.

Wegner, D. M., & Bargh, J. A. (1998). Control and automaticity in social life. In D. T. Gilbert, S. T. Fiske, & G. Lindzey (Eds.), *The handbook of social psychology* (4th ed., Vol. 1, pp. 446–496). New York: McGraw-Hill.

Weinfeld, N. S., Sroufe, L. A., & Egeland, B. (2000). Attachment from infancy to early adulthood in a high-risk sample: Continuity, discontinuity, and their correlates. *Child Development, 71,* 695–702.

PART III

INTRAPERSONAL ASPECTS OF ATTACHMENT

Cognitive Organization, Structure, and Information Processing

CHAPTER 6

Security-Based Self-Representations in Adulthood

Contents and Processes

Mario Mikulincer
Phillip R. Shaver

According to attachment theory (Bowlby, 1969/1982, 1973, 1980), a person's self-concept (*model of self*) and ability to regulate emotions (*affect regulation*) are products of attachment relationships, beginning with those formed in infancy and continuing with new ones established throughout life. Psychoanalytic theorists have characterized the process of self-construction and acquisition of affect-regulation strategies using terms such as "identification," "introjection," and "transmuting internalization" (e.g., Blatt & Behrends, 1987; Kohut, 1971; Schafer, 1968), whereas social–personality and developmental psychologists have used such terms as "modeling," "socialization," and "reflected appraisals" (e.g., Andersen & Chen, 2002; Bandura, 1986; Deci & Ryan, 1991). In attachment theory—a conceptual framework resting on a broad foundation of clinical observation and psychoanalytic, cognitive, developmental, personality, and social psychology—repeated interactions with protective and supportive others are said to produce a relatively stable sense of attachment security (i.e., a sense that one can rely on close relationship partners for protection and support, can safely and effectively explore the environment, and can engage effectively with other people), which somehow leads to the development of a stable, positive model of self and a set of effective and largely autonomous affect-regulation strategies (Mikulincer & Shaver, 2003). This mysterious "somehow" is the focus of this chapter.

According to attachment theory (e.g., Bowlby, 1988), a sense of security contributes to self-construction and affect regulation by allowing a person to benefit from the protection, support, comfort, and relief provided by loving relationship partners (*attachment figures*) during periods of stress or distress. Bowlby (e.g., 1969/1982, 1973) wrote mainly about development during infancy and early childhood and hence emphasized the regulatory importance of *actual* proximity to an emotionally available, sensitive, and responsive attachment figure. More recently, adult attachment researchers, following a path pioneered by object relations theorists (e.g., Fairbairn, Guntrip, and Winnicott; see the anthology edited by Buckley, 1986, and the overview by Greenberg & Mitchell, 1983), have emphasized the regulatory impact of *internal, mental representations* of security-enhancing attachment figures (e.g., Baldwin & Meunier, 1999; Mikulincer, Gillath, & Shaver, 2002; Pierce & Lydon, 1998). Bowlby (1969/1982, 1980) called these representations "internal working models." According to attachment theory, the ability to rely on either external or internalized attachment figures is the most important consequence of attachment security, allowing for the gradual acquisition of personal, social, and affect-regulatory skills that together form a well-adjusted, autonomous personality (Bowlby, 1988).

Because Bowlby (1969/1982) focused on infancy in his initial theoretical writings, he was more explicit about actual reliance on "stronger and wiser" attachment figures than about the resulting personal strengths that culminate, perhaps paradoxically, in a relatively autonomous, although not "compulsively self-reliant," personality—that is, a set of skills and qualities that allow secure adults to fend for themselves without constant reliance on an external partner or particular internalized figures. This important lacuna in Bowlby's writings, and in those of his partner in theory construction, Ainsworth (e.g., 1973), has left researchers with important unanswered questions concerning relations between experiences with attachment figures, the sense of attachment security, and the acquisition of autonomous self-regulation skills.

Is it possible, we have wondered, for a secure person to build and maintain a model of self that includes procedures for self-soothing and self-care, a model based partly on qualities of interactions with attachment figures? To what extent do secure adults possess models of self that include images of themselves as cared for, valued, and supported—images based on actual experiences with attachment figures? To what extent can a secure adult cope autonomously without calling on external or internal attachment figures for support? Under what conditions does a secure person rely on attachment figures for help rather than coping autonomously?

In this chapter, we focus on ways in which the sense of attachment security contributes to self-construction and explore how internal representations of attachment figures are related to self-representations. We expand on and deepen ideas that we summarized recently in a model of the activation and dynamics of the attachment system in adulthood

(Mikulincer & Shaver, 2003; Shaver & Mikulincer, 2002) and present new data concerning attachment security and the development of an autonomous self. We evaluate the proposition that representations of security-enhancing interactions with attachment figures are integrated into a person's self-representations and can be employed in the service of self-soothing and self-regulation.

ATTACHMENT-FIGURE AVAILABILITY, THE SENSE OF ATTACHMENT SECURITY, AND AFFECT REGULATION

According to attachment theory (Bowlby, 1969/1982, 1973), human infants are born with a repertoire of behaviors aimed at attaining or maintaining proximity to attachment figures. The evolutionary function of this behavioral repertoire is to protect infants from physical and psychological threats and alleviate their distress, with the ultimate goal of increasing their chances of survival and successful reproduction. These proximity-seeking behaviors, which are organized by an innate, biologically evolved regulatory system (the *attachment behavioral system,* or *attachment system*), are automatically activated by encounters with threats. As a result, infants are driven to maintain proximity to an attachment figure who, ideally, offers an available and responsive target for proximity seeking; serves as a *safe haven,* providing support, comfort, reassurance, and relief; and constitutes a *secure base,* facilitating engagement in exploration and play. Bowlby (1988) assumed that the attachment system is active throughout life and is manifested in thoughts and behaviors related to proximity and support seeking.

Bowlby (1973) also outlined individual differences in the functioning of the attachment system, which he had apparently observed in his clinical work. He theorized that these variations derive from interactions with actual attachment figures and result in the internalization, or mental representation, of these interactions in *working models* of the self and others. On the one hand, interactions with attachment figures who are available and responsive to one's needs facilitate the optimal functioning of the attachment system and promote the formation of a sense of attachment security. This sense consists of positive expectations about others' availability in threatening situations, positive views of the self as competent and valued, and increased confidence in support seeking as a protective device. The sense of attachment security also facilitates engagement in exploration and play (Bowlby, 1988). Attachment research has confirmed that the sense of attachment security contributes to subjective well-being, self-esteem, positive perceptions of others, and adjustment-enhancing interpersonal cognitions and behaviors (for reviews, see Collins & Read, 1994; Mikulincer & Shaver, 2003).

On the other hand, interactions with significant others who are unresponsive to one's attachment needs arouse insecurity about others' goodwill and doubts about the effectiveness of proximity seeking. During these painful interactions, distress is not properly managed, a sense of attachment security is not attained, negative models of the self and others are formed, and support seeking is replaced by what Main (1990) called secondary attachment strategies. Attachment theorists, following Main's lead, have delineated two major secondary strategies: *hyperactivation* and *deactivation* of the attachment system (e.g., Cassidy & Kobak, 1988). Hyperactivation is characterized by recurrent attempts to minimize distance from attachment figures and to elicit and ensure their support through the use of clinging, angry, and controlling responses. In contrast, deactivation consists of attempts to maximize distance from attachment figures and to adopt a self-reliant attitude.

According to attachment theory, individual differences in the sense of attachment security are manifested in modes of affect regulation (Magai, 1999; Mikulincer & Shaver, 2003; Shaver & Mikulincer, 2002; Sroufe, 1996). On the one hand, repeated interactions with security-enhancing attachment figures foster what Mikulincer and Shaver (2003) called security-based strategies and a "broaden and build" cycle of attachment security (based on Fredrickson's, 2001, theory of positive emotions). In our view, this cycle consists of three stages. First, the appraisal of threats activates the attachment system, which heightens the accessibility of internalized representations of security-enhancing attachment figures and favors the seeking of proximity and support from external attachment figures. These regulatory efforts are reinforced by optimistic beliefs about the availability and responsiveness of attachment figures. Second, both external and internalized attachment figures have a soothing effect and are a source of comfort and relief that facilitate effective coping and mood repair. Third, the alleviation of distress contributes to the activation of other behavioral systems (e.g., exploration, affiliation), which broaden the individual's capacities and perspectives. On the other hand, attachment insecurities keep people from relying comfortably on external or internalized attachment figures and thus reduce the soothing, regulatory impact these figures might otherwise have (Mikulincer & Shaver, 2003).

Most empirical tests of these ideas in adult samples have focused on *attachment style*—the pattern of relational expectations and behavior that results from a particular history of interactions with significant others (Fraley & Shaver, 2000). Initially, research on attachment style was based on Ainsworth, Blehar, Waters, and Wall's (1978) typology of three infant attachment patterns—secure, anxious, and avoidant (Hazan & Shaver, 1987). However, subsequent studies (e.g., Bartholomew & Horowitz, 1991; Brennan, Clark, & Shaver, 1998; Fraley & Waller, 1998) revealed that adult attachment styles are best characterized in terms of two continuous dimensions: attachment-related *anxiety* and *avoidance*. Whereas attachment anxiety is characterized by a strong need for closeness, worries about relationships, and reliance on hyperactivating strategies, attachment avoidance is characterized by compulsive self-reliance, preference for emotional distance from others, and reliance on deactivating strategies. In this model, high scores on one or both dimensions indicate attachment insecurity, and low scores on both dimensions indicate attachment security.

Adult attachment studies have consistently shown that secure attachment, assessed with self-report measures of either styles (types) or dimensions, is positively associated with the tendency to seek support under threatening conditions (e.g., Larose, Bernier, Soucy, & Duchesne, 1999; Ognibene & Collins, 1998) and to rely on it effectively as a means of coping with both attachment-related and attachment-unrelated threats (e.g., Berant, Mikulincer, & Florian, 2001; Birnbaum, Orr, Mikulincer, & Florian, 1997; Mikulincer, Florian, & Weller, 1993). This secure–insecure difference has been documented not only in studies using self-report measures but also in observational studies of actual support-seeking behavior (e.g., Collins & Feeney, 2000; Simpson, Rholes, & Nelligan, 1992).

Recent studies have also shown that attachment-related security is associated with cognitive activation of representations of security-enhancing attachment figures in threatening contexts (Mikulincer, Birnbaum, Woddis, & Nachmias, 2000; Mikulincer, Gillath, & Shaver, 2002). In these studies, participants performed a lexical decision task, deciding whether each of a series of letter strings was or was not a word. On each trial, a threat word (e.g., "failure") or a neutral word (e.g., "hat") was subliminally primed. In Mikulincer and colleagues' (2000) study, the visible letter strings included nonwords, attachment-figure-availability words (e.g., "love"), attachment-figure-unavailability words (e.g., "rejection"), and words that had no apparent attachment connotations. In Mikulincer and colleagues' (2002) study, the letter strings consisted of nonwords, names of security-enhancing attachment figures, and names of other known or unknown persons. In these studies, secure participants exhibited greater access to thoughts about attachment-figure availability and to the names of attachment figures in threatening but not unthreatening contexts. In addition, secure individuals' reactions to threat primes were limited to words implying attachment-figure availability; unlike insecure participants, these individuals were relatively slow at accessing words connoting separation or rejection.

Attachment-style differences in the accessibility of mental representations of attachment figures during periods of stress were also evident in retrospective accounts of captivity by Israeli ex-prisoners (POWs) of the Yom Kippur War, assessed 18 years after the war (Solomon, Ginzburg,

Mikulincer, Neria, & Ohry, 1998). A content analysis of these accounts revealed that, as compared with insecure ex-POWs, securely attached ex-POWs were more likely to report having dealt with captivity by recruiting positive relationship memories or creating positive imaginary encounters with loved ones. That is, secure soldiers coped with the threat of captivity, isolation, and torture by seeking symbolic support from internalized attachment figures.

Adult attachment research has also provided important information about the positive affective consequences of attachment-figure availability. Findings show, as intuition and televised reunions might lead one to expect, that reunion with a spouse after wartime or job-related separations is often experienced as a highly exciting and exhilarating event (e.g., Gerstel & Gross, 1984). However, Medway, Davis, Cafferty, and Chappell (1995) found that securely attached people experienced more positive emotions and less conflict on reunion than anxious and avoidant people. The same pattern of attachment-style differences was found in two laboratory studies, in which women's physiological responses to stressful events were examined in either the presence or absence of their romantic partners (Carpenter & Kirkpatrick, 1996; Feeney & Kirkpatrick, 1996). Whereas the presence of a romantic partner attenuated secure women's distress-related physiological responses, partner presence actually heightened the physiological responses of insecure women. That is, the calming effect of proximity to an external attachment figure occurred only among securely attached people. For insecure people, proximity seemed to be distressing rather than calming.

A recent series of studies revealed that contextual activation of representations of attachment-figure availability also evokes positive affective reactions (Mikulincer, Gillath, et al., 2001; Mikulincer, Hirschberger, Nachmias, & Gillath, 2001; Mikulincer & Shaver, 2001). Contextual activation of representations of attachment-figure availability improved people's mood and unconsciously infused formerly neutral stimuli with positive affect. For example, Mikulincer, Hirschberger, and colleagues (2001) found that subliminal priming of the names of security-enhancing attachment figures led to higher liking ratings of unfamiliar Chinese ideographs. McGowan (2002) noted, however, that internalized representations of attachment figures have calming effects only for people who are relatively secure. In her study, participants were asked to think about a significant other or about an acquaintance while waiting to undertake a stressful task. McGowan found that thinking about a significant other but not an acquaintance led to lower levels of distress only among securely attached people. In contrast, insecure people actually reacted to these thoughts with heightened distress.

Overall, extensive evidence indicates that attachment security contributes to affect regulation in ways compatible with attachment theory.

Secure individuals tend to deal with stress and distress by seeking proximity to and support from attachment figures and relying on internalized representations of supportive attachment figures. As a result they feel comforted and soothed by either the actual presence of an attachment figure or thoughts about attachment-figure availability. These affect-regulation strategies do not work as well for insecure individuals.

ATTACHMENT-FIGURE AVAILABILITY, SECURITY-BASED STRATEGIES, AND THE AUTONOMOUS SELF

The emphasis placed by attachment theory on external or internalized attachment figures raises important questions about the dynamic interplay between the sense of attachment security, security-based strategies, and the development of autonomous self-regulation skills. At first, one might guess that the sense of attachment security, which encourages people to rely on assistance and support from an external or internalized attachment figure, interferes with self-reliance and the development of an autonomous self (e.g., Kirkpatrick, 1998). That is, attachment-figure availability might favor reliance, even overreliance, on others for coregulation of distress at the expense of autonomous self-regulation. As a result, securely attached individuals might have dependent personalities and be chronically driven to seek support to regulate distress.

The equation of secure attachment and overdependence is at odds, however, with both attachment theory (e.g., Bartholomew, 1990; Bowlby, 1969/1982) and empirical findings concerning the development of secure attachment (e.g., Sroufe, Fox, & Pancake, 1983). Recently, Mikulincer, Shaver, and Pereg (2003) proposed a developmental sequence in which attachment-figure availability not only reinforces reliance on external and internalized attachment figures but also provides a basis for the development of self-regulatory skills. In this developmental sequence, the emergence of a sense of attachment security during the first year of life allows children to become more tolerant of temporary separations from attachment figures (between 12 and 30 months of age) and to use these figures as a secure base from which to explore the environment (from early childhood). This confident exploration of the environment is a crucial step in the development of an autonomous self. Secure children distance themselves to an extent from attachment figures, learn new things about the world and the self that enrich their competency and regulatory skills, and discover that they can be in the world alone and do new things without others' help. (This early move from being supported to being relatively independent has been the focus of most attachment research in developmental psychology; for reviews, see Thompson, 1999; Weinfield, Sroufe, Egeland, & Carlson, 1999.)

In middle childhood, the sense of attachment security allows children to become more active and responsible in the coregulation of distress and to engage effectively with other people (e.g., peers; Rubin, Bukowski, & Parker, 1998; Weinfield et al., 1999; Zeifman & Hazan, 1997). This engagement in affiliative activities is an additional step in the development of an autonomous self. It provides an increased range of social options for exploring personal interests, developing skills, and broadening one's self-conception (Berlin & Cassidy, 1999). During adolescence and young adulthood, secure individuals are able to form reciprocal and equal relationships with special peers, in which they become sources of comfort for their partners and learn how to help regulate partners' distress (Allen & Land, 1999; Furman & Wehner, 1994; Zeifman & Hazan, 1997). This learning strengthens their sense of mastery and adds skills that can be used in the regulation of their own distress. In this way, secure attachment increases children and adolescents' confidence that they can rely on their own self-regulatory skills for handling distress.

The equation of attachment security and overdependence is also at odds with empirical findings concerning the characteristics of securely attached adults. First, secure adults have been found to report higher levels of self-esteem, to describe themselves in more positive terms, and to appraise themselves as having higher levels of personal resources for coping with threats than insecurely attached persons (e.g., Bartholomew & Horowitz, 1991; Mikulincer, 1995; Mikulincer & Florian, 1995, 1999). Second, self-ratings of attachment security are positively associated with reliance on instrumental problem solving and active transformational methods of coping that do not require others' assistance in dealing with stressful events (e.g., Birnbaum et al., 1997; Mikulincer & Florian, 1998, 2000). Third, people who scored low on attachment anxiety or avoidance also had the lowest scores on a dependent personality disorder scale, as well as on scales tapping emotional and instrumental dependency (Alonso-Arbiol, Shaver, & Yarnoz, 2002; Brennan & Shaver, 1998). Fourth, securely attached people, as compared with their relatively insecure counterparts, hold more positive attitudes toward work and autonomous exploration (e.g., Green & Campbell, 2000; Hazan & Shaver, 1990; Mikulincer, 1997). All of these findings fit Main, Kaplan, and Cassidy's (1985) definition of securely attached individuals as "autonomous with respect to attachment"—that is, people who value attachment relationships and regard attachment-related experiences as influential but seem relatively independent and autonomous regarding any particular experience or relationship (Hesse, 1999).

These findings imply that secure attachment is associated not only with support seeking but also with establishing the self as the mind's main executive agency. It seems that securely attached people can rely on either attachment figures or their own resources and skills when dealing with threats. That is, they can choose to deal with threats autonomously or rely on others without feeling that support seeking implies personal helplessness or vulnerability. The main question here is how secure attachment becomes related to the development and consolidation of an autonomous self. Our tentative answer is that security-enhancing interactions with attachment figures, the building blocks of attachment security, facilitate the construction of specific soothing processes within the self. In our view, these security-based self-representations and procedures become a source of comfort during threatening events, thereby reducing dependency on external or internalized attachment figures.

SECURITY-BASED SELF-REPRESENTATIONS: DEFINITION AND BASIC PROPOSITIONS

Security-based self-representations are mental constructs derived from the internalization of security-enhancing interactions with attachment figures. They are similar to, or overlap with, representations of the self and others in such interactions and are interconnected with other attachment-related representations in the mind's semantic network. As a result, the strength and centrality of security-based self-representations within a person's model of self should be positively associated with the number or quality of security-enhancing interactions he or she has experienced with attachment figures. Furthermore, these self-representations should become contextually accessible on activation of the attachment system and should provide some of the same psychological benefits as does a security-enhancing attachment figure, offering comfort and relief, fostering security, and allowing a person to engage in valuable nonattachment activities. That is, security-based self-representations should be capable of complementing or replacing reliance on security-enhancing attachment figures.

In this section we attempt to delineate the nature and functions of security-based self-representations. We assume that these representations, in the case of insecure individuals, are blocked or superseded in particular ways by insecurity-based self-representations. We focus here mainly on securely attached individuals and their use of security-based self-representations. Only occasionally do we contrast them explicitly with specific kinds of insecurity-based representations and mental processes. Our conceptualization of security-based self-representations is based on four major theoretical propositions:

Proposition 1

The first proposition is that many aspects of the self are construed in terms of internalized patterns of interaction with significant others. This proposition is based on Bowlby's (1973) statement that models of the self are derived from actual or anticipated experiences with attachment figures. According to his analysis, interactions with security-enhancing attachment figures contribute to the formation of self-representations that include or evoke the positive and soothing consequences of actual interactions with these figures. In contrast, interactions with unresponsive and rejecting figures contribute to the formation of insecurity-based self-representations that include or evoke the frustrating and painful consequences of actual interactions with these figures.

The importance of interactions with significant others for self-construction has long been recognized by psychodynamic and object relations theorists (e.g., Blatt & Behrends, 1987; Kohut, 1971, 1977; Schafer, 1968). Their theories emphasize the process of internalization, by which people adopt, as their own, features that once existed in relationships or relationship partners. According to Schafer (1968), "internalization refers to all those processes by which the subject transforms real or imagined regulatory interactions with his environment, and real or imagined characteristics of his environment, into inner regulation and characteristics" (p. 9). Similar ideas have appeared in classic theories of the self (e.g., James, 1890; Rogers, 1951; Sullivan, 1953) and in more recent social-cognitive perspectives on the self (e.g., Aron, Aron, & Norman, 2001; Baldwin, 1992; Higgins, 1987). Recently, Andersen and Chen (2002) proposed the concept of "relational self" and advanced the proposition that "given the profound importance of significant others in people's lives, the self and personality are shaped largely by experiences with significant others" (p. 621).

Proposition 2

The second proposition is that security-based self-representations coexist in a semantic network with less secure models of the self and that the relative strength of these representations (i.e., their availability in the semantic network) is a function of a person's attachment history. According to Bowlby (1973), any interaction with an attachment figure can affect working models of the self, which implies that a person can form different and even contradictory self-representations because he or she can experience contradictory interactions with attachment figures. That is, with respect to a particular relationship and across different relationships, everyone constructs both secure and insecure models of the self and can therefore sometimes think about the self in either secure or insecure terms (Baldwin, Keelan, Fehr, Enns, & Koh-Rangarajoo, 1996).

The question then becomes, Which of these models of self has the greatest likelihood of being available in the semantic network? As with other mental representations, the strength or availability of each model is determined by the amount of experience on which it is based, the number of times it has been applied in the past, and the density of its connections with other cognitive representations (e.g., Baldwin, 1992; Collins & Read, 1994; Higgins, 1987). In our opinion, the relative strength of security-based self-representations is likely to depend on a person's history of attachment interactions (the number and salience of security-enhancing interactions with attachment figures) and the consequent formation of other cognitive representations with which they are connected (i.e., the sense of attachment security, security-based strategies, positive models of others). The more frequently one experiences security-enhancing interactions with attachment figures (e.g., parents, spouse) and the stronger the consequent sense of attachment security, the better the chances of security-based self-representations constituting the most available model of self in the semantic network. As a result, securely attached people, or those with a secure attachment history, should have more available security-based self-representations than insecurely attached people or those with an insecure attachment history.

Proposition 3

The third proposition is that security-based self-representations are rendered contextually accessible by the activation of the attachment system. Social cognition research has shown that, although the entire pool of a person's self-representations is available and generally well organized in a semantic network, only a subset of this pool is rendered accessible (i.e., ready to influence information processing) in the working memory at a given time (e.g., Higgins & Bargh, 1987; Mischel & Shoda, 1995). Research has also shown that contextual cues in the immediate situation, such as social roles or relationships, contribute to the transient activation of a particular self-representation (e.g., Baldwin, 1992). Contextual cues can also include a person's current motives, which are often related to particular self-representations (e.g., Cantor, Markus, Niedenthal, & Nurius, 1986; Chartrand & Bargh, 2002). For example, mood-repair motives may activate soothing self-representations, whereas achievement motives may activate achievement-related self-knowledge. Andersen and Chen (2002) also included the activation of a specific significant-other representation, which can draw into working memory self-representations that were formed during interactions with that particular person.

We hypothesize that activation of the attachment system in securely attached individuals is automatically followed by heightened accessibility of security-based self-representations. This accessibility is the result of both associative-transferential processes and strategic maneuvers. As stated earlier, the attachment system is usually activated by the appraisal of threatening events and is followed by a search for internalized attachment figures. For secure people, activation of threat-related thoughts is accompanied by heightened accessibility of representations of security-enhancing attachment figures, which can serve as contextual cues for bringing security-based self-representations into working memory. These self-representations are presumed to have been formed originally in connection with threats that were alleviated by security-enhancing attachment figures. As a result, they became associated with threat-related and attachment-figure-related representations, and hence they can be automatically activated in new situations appraised as threatening. Beyond this associative process, attachment-system activation includes particular motives and directs a person's thoughts toward security attainment, distress alleviation, and threat removal (Bowlby, 1969/1982). Therefore, it can strategically invoke security-based self-representations, which are capable of soothing the securely attached person and restoring a sense of safety and security, as explained in the following section.

Proposition 4

The fourth proposition is that security-based self-representations accomplish a regulatory, self-soothing function during periods of stress and distress. Social-cognition research has already established that self-representations have important affective and motivational consequences (e.g., Bandura, 1986; Higgins, 1987; Markus & Nurius, 1986). For example, Bandura (1986) and his followers have shown that self-efficacy representations have a strong effect on the regulation of emotions and behavior. Markus and Nurius (1986) noted some of the affective consequences of mental representations of "possible selves" (a person's ideas about what he or she would like to become, is afraid of becoming, and could become). Higgins (1987) presented a comprehensive theory and carried out a program of research on the affective impact of discrepancies between representations of self-standards (ideal self, ought self) and actual-self representations. We propose that security-based self-representations, formed during positive interactions with security-enhancing attachment figures, become associated with the positive feelings (e.g., comfort, security, relief) arising from such interactions. As a result, contextual activation of these representations can automatically elicit positive feelings and serve as a source of comfort.

Broadening the Model

Based on these propositions, we add a complementary path to one previously included in our (Mikulincer & Shaver, 2003) model of attachment-system activation and functioning (see Figure 6.1). In addition to the path that connects attachment-system activation in times of threat or stress with search for external attachment figures or activation of internal, men-

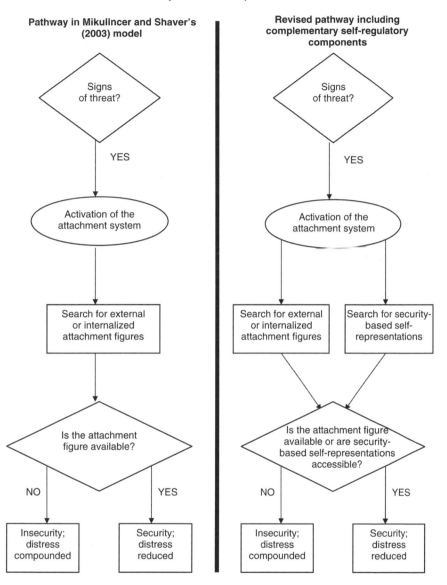

FIGURE 6.1. Extension of part of Mikulincer and Shaver's (2003) model of attachment-system activation and functioning.

tal representations of attachment figures, the possibility exists of attaining relief and an increased sense of security by activating security-based self-representations. According to this new path, activation of the attachment system during an encounter with threats leads to a search for self-representations that were originally formed during security-enhancing interactions with attachment figures. If these representations are readily available in the semantic network, they become contextually accessible and serve a soothing function, increasing a person's sense of security and contributing to the "broaden and build" cycle of security, competence, and autonomy. However, if security-based self-representations are not accessible due to lack of frequent security-enhancing interactions with attachment figures, this regulatory path is unavailable, causing the person to rely more exclusively on hyperactivating or deactivating strategies.

In the following sections we expand our discussion of this regulatory path and present preliminary data on its nature. We attempt to determine how security-enhancing interactions with attachment figures are represented in the mind as aspects of the self. Specifically, we focus on two closely related kinds of security-based self-representations: (1) representations of the self derived from the way a person sees and evaluates himself or herself during interactions with an attachment figure (self-in-relation-with-an-attachment-figure) and (2) representations of the self derived from identification with features and traits of an attachment figure.

SECURITY-BASED REPRESENTATIONS OF SELF-IN-RELATION-WITH-AN-ATTACHMENT-FIGURE

One important kind of security-based self-representation is organized around self-aspects (e.g., roles, traits, behaviors, expectations) encoded during security-enhancing interactions with attachment figures. According to attachment theory (Bowlby, 1973), these interactions are an important source of positive information about oneself. During such interactions, a person can construe himself or herself as active, strong, and competent based on having effectively coped with the threatening events that originally activated the attachment system. He or she can also feel calm, soothed, and secure because of the emotional availability of a "stronger and wiser" other (Bowlby, 1973). Moreover, one can construe oneself as valuable and special—thanks to feeling valued, loved, and accepted by the caring attachment figure—and able to form and maintain close and satisfactory relationships with others and to mobilize others' support when needed.

We suggest that these self-aspects become integrated into representations of the self-in-relation-with-an-attachment-figure, the conception a person has of himself or herself during security-enhancing interactions with such a figure. These representations are stored in semantic memory and are strongly interconnected with representations of available attachment figures and soothing feelings derived from interactions with these figures. Like other aspects of self-models (Collins & Read, 1994), these representations probably range from relationship specific (security-based models of self-in-relation-with-a-particular-attachment-figure) to abstract and general (security-based models of self-in-relation-with-attachment-figures-in-general).

This line of reasoning suggests three testable hypotheses. First, threat appraisal and consequent activation of the attachment system can increase the accessibility not only of thoughts about an available attachment figure but also of the closely associated representation of self-in-relation-with-this-attachment-figure. That is, exposure to threatening events should heighten the accessibility of this representation within a person's self-concept. Second, this accessibility should be most pronounced among securely attached people (those with relatively low scores on the attachment anxiety and avoidance dimensions). These people are presumed to have experienced more security-enhancing interactions with attachment figures than their insecure counterparts; hence they should more readily locate positive representations of the self-with-an-attachment-figure within their semantic networks. Third, whenever the representation of the self-with-an-attachment-figure becomes accessible and ready for use in affective and cognitive processing, it should bring to mind the associated soothing and comforting feelings. Therefore, heightened accessibility of this representation should be associated with distress alleviation and more effective functioning in threatening situations.

To test these hypotheses, we conducted an exploratory two-session laboratory study (Study 1) involving 64 Israeli university students (43 women and 21 men). We exposed participants differing in their attachment orientations to a threat or no-threat condition. We then measured the accessibility of the self-with-an-attachment-figure representations within participants' active self-concepts, as well as their emotional and cognitive state during the experimental session. (We refer to this active self-concept simply as "self-concept," for sake of brevity, but it is important to remember that it is conceptualized as a contextually influenced mental construction.)

The first session of Study 1 was designed to assess participants' attachment orientations and to create individually tailored lists of traits corresponding to each participant's own representation of self-with-an-attachment-figure. Specifically, participants completed (1) filler scales; (2) scales tapping attachment anxiety and avoidance (the 36-item Experiences in Close Relationships [ECR] scale; Brennan et al., 1998), and (3) Hinkley and Andersen's (1996) procedure for assessing representations of the self-in-relation-to-significant-others. The order of the scales was randomized across participants.

In the self-description task, participants were asked to describe what they are like when with (1) a security-enhancing attachment figure, (2) a person with whom they enjoy collaborative learning and working (i.e., an exploration partner), or (3) a person with whom they have fun (an affiliation partner). The description of self-with-an-attachment-figure was the main focus of the study. The other two self-descriptions were collected to control for the accessibility of self-traits that were internalized during interpersonal interactions involving the activation of other behavioral systems, such as exploration and affiliation, that do not serve protective or soothing functions. For research purposes, participants were asked to name three different people, one for each function, even though in reality one individual might serve more than one function.

For the attachment figure, we asked participants to name a significant other who serves the attachment functions of proximity and safe haven. Specifically, participants were told to name "a person from whom you seek and receive support and comfort in times of need and who helps you to be calm, solve problems, and endure difficult situations." For the exploration partner, participants were asked to name a different person "with whom you enjoy working and learning new things, and around whom you feel particularly good when undertaking new projects and tasks." For the affiliation partner, participants were asked to name another person "with whom you enjoy having fun; going to parties, movies, or restaurants; and engaging in 'small talk.'" (The actual instructions were written in Hebrew because the study was conducted in Israel.)

After identifying each of the three significant others by first name, participants were asked to visualize themselves in the presence of each of these people, one at a time, and to describe themselves as they are when they interact with that person. In performing each of the three tasks, participants completed 10 sentences beginning with, "When I am with [Name], I. . . ." The order of the three tasks was randomized across participants.

No participant had any difficulty naming the three designated partners. Of all the significant others described, 28% were family members (12% mothers, 6% fathers, and 10% others, such as sisters, brothers, cousins, or uncles) and the others were close friends (47%) or romantic partners (25%). Parents were more frequently nominated as attachment figures than as exploration or affiliation partners (14% vs. 3% and 1%, respectively). The exclusion of participants who nominated parents as attachment figures did not change the findings, implying that the observed accessibility of representations of self-with-attachment-figures cannot be attributed to the fact that these figures were the participants' parents.

In the second session, conducted 2 weeks later by a different experimenter, participants performed four cognitive tasks while an ego-relevant threat—failure feedback—was imposed on half of them. Specifically, participants were randomly divided into two groups according to the feed-back they received during the four tasks. In the threat condition ($n = 32$), participants were exposed to four unsolvable problems and told that they had failed every one. Exposure to uncontrollable failures has consistently been found to be ego relevant and distressing (see Mikulincer, 1994, for a review). In the no-threat condition ($n = 32$), participants were exposed to four solvable problems and received no feedback concerning their perfor-mance.

Afterward, we assessed the accessibility of the self-with-an-attach-ment-figure representation within a person's active self-concept. Spe-cifically, participants were given a list of 50 traits and were asked to rate "the extent to which the traits describe you as you are here and now." Rat-ings were made on a 5-point scale, ranging from 1 (*not at all*) to 5 (*very much*). For each participant, we constructed an idiosyncratic, individually tailored list of 50 traits. The list included all of the nonoverlapping traits that appeared in the three representations of the self-in-relation-with-significant-others generated in the first session. The remaining traits were taken from the traits generated by other participants in the first session that did not correspond semantically to the traits generated by the partici-pant. The order of the traits was randomized across participants.

For each participant we computed four scores by averaging ratings of (1) traits taken from his or her description of self-with-an-attachment-figure, (2) traits taken from his or her description of self-with-an-exploration-partner, (3) traits taken from his or her description of self-with-an-affiliation-partner, and (4) traits taken from other participants' self-descriptions. The higher these scores, the higher the accessibility of each trait category was judged to be in a participant's currently activated self-concept.

Following this procedure, we assessed participants' emotional and cognitive states during the experimental session. They rated their feelings during the experimental sessions (*good, bad, sad, happy*) on a 4-point scale, ranging from 1 (*not at all*) to 4 (*very much*). They also completed the 21-item Cognitive Interference Questionnaire (CIQ; Sarason, Sarason, Keefe, Hayes, & Shearin, 1986) tapping the frequency of interfering task-related worries and task-irrelevant thoughts during the experimental ses-sion. These ratings were made on a 4-point scale, ranging from 1 (*not at all*) to 4 (*very frequent*). For each participant, we computed (1) a negative-mood score by averaging the 4 emotion ratings (Cronbach's alpha = .87 after reversing the positive emotion items) and (2) a cognitive-interference score by averaging the 21 CIQ items (alpha = .93).

To examine variations in the accessibility of representations of self-with-significant-others within a participant's self-concept, we conducted three-step hierarchical regression analyses with threat induction, attach-ment anxiety, and attachment avoidance as the predictor variables. In the first step of these regressions, we entered threat induction (a dummy variable comparing the threat and the no-threat conditions), attachment anxiety, and attachment avoidance as a block in order to examine the unique main effects of these predictors. In the second step, the two-way interactions for threat induction × attachment anxiety, threat induction × attachment avoidance, and attachment anxiety × attachment avoidance were entered as additional predictors. The three-way interaction term was added in the third step of the regressions.

The regressions performed on self-with-an-exploration-partner traits, self-with-an-affiliation-partner traits, and other participants' self-traits revealed no significant effects (see Table 6.1). However, the regression performed on traits taken from the self-with-an-attachment-figure description revealed a significant main effect for threat induction. Threat induction, as compared with no-threat induction, heightened the accessibility of self-with-an-attachment-figure traits within the self-concept. The main effect for attachment anxiety closely approached statistical significance ($p = .06$): the lower the attachment anxiety, the higher the accessibility of the traits.

The regression analysis also yielded a significant interaction between attachment anxiety and threat induction (see Table 6.1). No other effects were significant. Examination of the significant interaction (using Aiken & West's [1991] procedure) revealed that the regression for accessibility of self-with-an-attachment-figure traits predicted by threat induction was significant when attachment anxiety was one standard deviation below the mean, *beta* = .53, $p < .01$, but not when attachment anxiety was one standard deviation above the mean, *beta* = .05. That is, threat induction significantly heightened the accessibility of the self-with-an-attachment-figure representation within the self-concept mainly among low-anxious persons.

TABLE 6.1. Standardized Regression Coefficients for Accessibility of Representations of the Self-with-Significant-Others as Predicted by Threat Induction and Attachment Scores

Effect	Self-with-attachment-figure	Self-with-exploration-partner	Self-with-affiliation-partner	Other participants' representations
Threat induction	0.28*	0.03	−0.10	−0.08
Attachment anxiety	−0.23[a]	0.04	−0.01	0.08
Attachment avoidance	−0.03	−0.17	−0.01	−0.13
Threat × anxiety	−0.39*	0.02	−0.01	−0.03
Threat × avoidance	−0.05	0.16	0.14	−0.01
Anxiety × avoidance	−0.06	0.01	−0.01	0.08
Three-way interaction	−0.23	0.26	0.05	0.19

*$p < .05$; [a]$p = .06$.

To examine the possible soothing function of the self-with-an-attachment-figure representation, we computed Pearson correlations between the accessibility of this representation within the self-concept and reports of negative emotion and cognitive interference. We found that the higher the accessibility of self-with-an-attachment-figure traits, the less intense the reported negative emotion, and the less frequent the occurrence of interfering thoughts (r's of $-.30$ and $-.26$, p's $< .05$). As expected, the accessibility of the self-with-an-attachment-figure representation seemed to have a soothing effect. These associations were statistically significant only in the threat condition (r's of $-.55$ and $-.46$, p's $< .01$), not in the no-threat condition (r's of $-.21$ and $-.18$). However, statistical tests revealed no significant differences between the relevant pairs of correlations with the current sample size. Pearson correlations between the accessibility of the other trait categories and reports of negative emotion and cognitive interference were not significant. This implies that the emotional and cognitive impact of self-with-an-attachment-figure traits does not generalize to other representations of the self-with-significant-others.

Hierarchical regression analyses performed on reports of negative emotion and cognitive interference indicated that threat induction heightened the intensity of negative emotions, $beta = .32$, $p < .01$, and the frequency of interfering thoughts, $beta = .41$, $p < .01$. In addition, attachment anxiety was positively associated with negative emotion, $beta = .30$, $p < .01$, and cognitive interference, $beta = .25$, $p < .05$. Attachment avoidance was not significantly associated with negative emotion or cognitive interference.

Interestingly, the significant contributions of attachment anxiety to negative emotions and cognitive interference in the threat condition (*betas* of .43 and .51) were notably weakened by the introduction of the accessibility of self-with-an-attachment-figure traits as an additional predictor (*betas* of .09 and .32, representing a 79% and a 37% reduction, respectively). After the mediator was entered into the equation, attachment anxiety was no longer significantly associated with negative emotions and cognitive interference. This finding implies that the accessibility of self-with-an-attachment-figure traits mediated the emotional and cognitive impact of attachment anxiety following a threat induction (the pattern of mediation is shown in Figure 6.2). That is, participants who scored low on attachment anxiety displayed relatively high accessibility of self-with-an-attachment-figure traits following a threat induction, which in turn led to less intense negative emotions and less frequent interfering thoughts. In contrast, introduction of the accessibility of self-with-an-attachment-figure traits as a predictor in the regression equation did not change the emotional and cognitive impact of attachment anxiety in the no-threat condition.

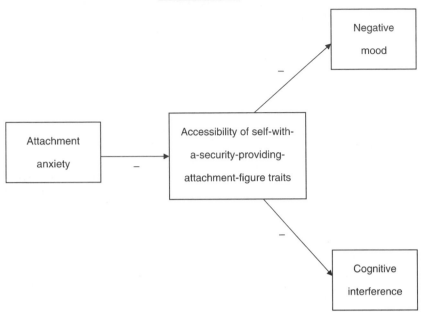

FIGURE 6.2. The mediational role of representations of self-with-a-security-enhancing-attachment-figure in the threat condition.

Overall, the findings provide encouraging preliminary evidence for the regulatory function of the representation of self-with-an-attachment-figure. As expected, exposure to an ego-relevant threat heightened the accessibility of this representation, which in turn was associated with less intense negative mood and less frequent interfering thoughts. Although we expected this regulatory path to be especially active among people who scored low on attachment anxiety and avoidance, the findings showed that it was active for low-anxious individuals regardless of their scores on the avoidance dimension (i.e., for the people Bartholomew and Horowitz [1991] called secure and dismissingly avoidant). It therefore seems that dismissing individuals possess available representations of self during security-enhancing interactions with an attachment figure and can use them in threat contexts. Avoidant deactivating strategies, which foster self-reliance and defensive construal of the self (Mikulincer & Shaver, 2003), may increase the accessibility of remembered episodes in which the self is construed as strong and competent and thus may strengthen the activation of positive representations of the self-with-an-attachment-figure. Further research is needed to explore similarities and differences between secure and dismissing individuals' formation and use of security-enhancing self-representations.

SECURITY-BASED REPRESENTATIONS OF SELF-CAREGIVING

Another important kind of security-based self-representation is one that includes internalized characteristics of particular supportive attachment figures. According to attachment theory (Bowlby, 1973), security-enhancing interactions with an attachment figure are an important source of information about the figure's intentions and responses and an important foundation of one's positive views of others. During these interactions, a person construes the attachment figure as available, sensitive, empathic, caring, and kindhearted. Moreover, the person learns about the particular supportive, comforting, and soothing qualities and behaviors of this figure. These learned features and traits of the attachment figure may then become incorporated into the self as positive, caring self-traits.

The idea that self-representations can resemble representations of significant others appears ubiquitously in psychodynamic and object relations theories (e.g., Blatt & Behrends, 1987; Greenberg & Mitchell, 1983; Sandler & Rosenblatt, 1962; Schafer, 1968). These theories emphasize the processes of incorporation, introjection, and identification, which allow the transformation of regulatory functions provided by others into inner regulatory mechanisms. In infancy, this transformation is thought to take the form of incorporation, which involves little or no self–other differentiation (Meissner, 1981). With higher levels of self–other differentiation, children can introject features or traits identified as being outside the self, but they seem to continue to experience these features as part of an internalized other (Schafer, 1968). In its most mature form, this process is one of identification, in which features of a well-differentiated other are transformed into self-representations and identified as integral parts of the self (Schafer, 1968). We hypothesize that this identification process results in the formation of security-based self-representations that resemble features and traits of security-enhancing attachment figures.

The process of identification with a significant other is one of the core developmental processes in Kohut's (1971, 1977) self psychology. Kohut (1971) labeled this process "transmuting internalization"—the internalization of regulatory functions that were originally performed by a significant other, with the individual gradually acquiring the capacity to perform these functions autonomously. Kohut (1971, 1977) claimed that caregivers' empathic responses to children's needs foster the development of an inner state of stability, security, and self-cohesion, which in turn makes external regulation less necessary. In Kohut's view, the self incorporates the features and traits of the external figure and thereby gradually acquires self-soothing, self-approving, and self-regulatory capacities. Specifically, the person can internally regulate self-esteem and ambitions instead of requiring admiration from others. The person can develop his or her own system of ideals and maintain a sense of direction in life instead of needing to rely on external guides. In this way, he or she becomes less dependent on external sources of regulation and can relate to others in a more autonomous and reciprocal fashion.

A related process is what Aron and colleagues (2001) called "expansion of the self." These authors claimed that one important cognitive consequence of close relationships is the inclusion of a partner's resources and features in one's self-concept. We believe this process of self-expansion can be set in motion during security-enhancing interactions with an attachment figure. During these positive interactions, a partner's responses are smoothly synchronized with a person's needs (Tronick, 1989), and the partner can easily be experienced as part of the self. As a result, the person can incorporate the partner's features and traits into the self, which in turn facilitates the development of a belief that the self has caregiving and soothing capacities that were originally experienced as qualities of the attachment figure.

We wish to advance what may be a novel proposition: that the process of identification with attachment figures leads to the internalization of their features and traits in a specific component or subroutine of the self—a component that characterizes one's relation to and treatment of oneself. That is, the features and behaviors of one's key attachment figures are integrated into the self and come to characterize the way one relates to and treats oneself. Thus a person's relation to and treatment of the self during periods of stress and distress tend to resemble the treatment the person has received from attachment figures. Specifically, a person whose attachment figures have been compassionate, sensitive, caring, punishing, rejecting, or forgiving will exhibit a similar approach to comforting or punishing himself or herself and will harbor self-representations of being comforted, punished, and so on. We tentatively call these mental processes *representations of self-caregiving.* These self-representations are more or less direct internalizations of attachment figures' characteristics and behaviors, and they allow a person to provide much of his or her own caregiving and emotion regulation.

Our conceptualization of self-caregiving representations resembles Bollas's (1987) psychoanalytic concept of the "self as object." Following Winnicott's (1965) idea that adults relate to and treat themselves as a mother or father treats a child, Bollas claimed that "in the course of a person's object relations he re-presents various positions in the historical theatre of lived experiences between elements of mother, father, and his infant-child self. One idiom of representation is the person's relation to the self as an object, an object relation where the individual may objectify, imagine, analyze, and manage the self through identification with primary others who have been involved in that very task" (p. 41).

In the case of security-enhancing attachment figures, the process of identification fosters the formation of security-based representations of self-caregiving—representations based on features and traits of security-enhancing attachment figures. These self-representations include strategies for being available, sensitive, compassionate, caring, and comforting toward oneself in times of need, and they resemble the way a person was previously treated by security-enhancing attachment figures. These security-based self-representations become stored in the semantic network, together with other representations of self-caregiving, and are especially associated with representations of available attachment figures. This idea is very compatible with Kohut's (1971) aforementioned notion of transmuting internalization, a process by which the self takes over functions that were originally accomplished by a comforting and soothing significant other (e.g., a parent or lover). It is also compatible with Moretti and Higgins's (1999) ideas and evidence that some aspects of our self-guides (ideal self, ought self) are derived from identification with parental guides.

Based on this line of reasoning, we derived three testable hypotheses. First, threat appraisal and the consequent activation of internalized representations of available attachment figures will automatically heighten the accessibility of these figures' traits within a person's representations of self-caregiving. That is, exposure to threatening events will heighten the accessibility of security-based representations of self-caregiving; hence a person's description of the way he or she currently relates to and treats the self will resemble the traits of security-inducing attachment figures. Second, this heightened accessibility will be most pronounced among secure individuals. They presumably have experienced more security-enhancing interactions with attachment figures than have insecurely attached people, so there should be more security-based representations of self-caregiving available within their semantic networks. Third, whenever security-based representations of self-caregiving become accessible and ready for use in affective and cognitive processing, they should soothe and comfort a person in the same way helpful attachment figures have done.

These hypotheses were assessed in another two-session laboratory study (Study 2) with 60 different Israeli university students (39 women and 21 men). In Study 2, we exposed participants differing in their attachment orientations to a threat or no-threat condition and assessed the accessibility of the representation of a particular attachment figure within their own self-caregiving representations. In addition, we assessed participants' emotional and cognitive state during the experimental session.

In the first session, participants completed the ECR scale and provided descriptions of three significant others: a security-enhancing attachment figure, an exploration partner, and an affiliation partner (see Study 1 for methodological details). Participants received instructions identical to those of Study 1, and then, after identifying each of the three significant others by first name, were asked to describe each of these people by completing 10 sentences beginning with "Generally, [Name]. . . ." The order of the three tasks was randomized across participants. The identities of the different people resembled those of Study 1.

In the second session, conducted 2 weeks later by a different experimenter, participants were randomly divided into the two conditions described in Study 1: (1) threat condition ($n = 30$), which involved failing at four unsolvable cognitive tasks; (2) no-threat condition ($n = 30$), which involved no feedback following four solvable cognitive tasks. The procedure and materials were identical to those used in Study 1. Afterward, we measured the accessibility of traits of participants' attachment figures within their own self-caregiving representations. Specifically, participants were given a list of 50 traits and were asked to rate the extent to which each of these traits described the ways they felt and related to themselves during the experimental session (self-caregiving representations). Ratings were made on a 5-point scale, ranging from 1 (*not at all*) to 5 (*very much*).

For each participant, we constructed an idiosyncratic, individually tailored list of 50 traits. This list included all of the nonoverlapping traits that appeared in the descriptions of the three significant others generated by a participant in the first session. The remaining traits were taken from those generated by other participants in the first session that did not correspond semantically to traits generated by the participant. The order of the traits was randomized across participants. For each participant, we computed four scores by averaging ratings of (1) traits taken from his or her description of an attachment figure, (2) traits taken from his or her description of an exploration partner, (3) traits taken from his or her description of an affiliation partner, and (4) traits taken from other participants' descriptions of significant others. The higher these scores, the higher the accessibility of each trait category in a participant's self-caregiving representations.

Following this procedure, we assessed participants' emotional and cognitive states during the experimental session using the same scales employed in Study 1. Specifically, participants rated their feelings during the experimental session (*good, bad, sad, happy*) and completed the CIQ. As in Study 1, we computed a negative-mood score (alpha = .85) and a total cognitive-interference score (alpha = .94).

Hierarchical regression analyses performed on the accessibility of exploration-partner traits, affiliation-partner traits, and other participants' traits revealed no significant main or interactive effects of threat induction, attachment anxiety, or attachment avoidance. However, the regression performed on attachment-figure traits revealed that the main effect of attachment avoidance approached statistical significance (p = .07; see Table 6.2), with higher avoidance scores being associated with less accessibility of these traits within a participant's self-caregiving representation. That is, people who scored high on the avoidance dimension, as compared with those who scored low, were less likely to rate traits of their attachment figure as describing how they felt and related to themselves during the experimental situation.

This regression analysis also revealed significant two-way interactions for threat × anxiety and anxiety × avoidance as well as a significant three-way interaction for threat × anxiety × avoidance (see Table 6.2). Further regression analyses (using Aiken & West's [1991] procedure) indicated that threat induction significantly heightened the accessibility of attachment-figure traits only among secure persons (one standard deviation below the mean on both attachment anxiety and avoidance), $beta$ = .52, p < .01, but not among the three groups (quadrants) that Bartholomew and Horowitz (1991) labeled "preoccupied," "dismissingly avoidant," and "fearfully avoidant" (one standard deviation above the mean on anxiety and/or avoidance), $betas$ < .23, p's > .15. That is, only secure participants reacted to threatening events by relating to themselves the same way their attachment figure treated them.

Pearson correlations between the accessibility of attachment-figure traits and reports of negative emotion and cognitive interference revealed significant associations (r's of –.28 and –.39, p's < .05). Supporting our hypotheses, the more accessible attachment-figure traits were within a participant's self-caregiving representation, the less intense was the reported

TABLE 6.2. Standardized Regression Coefficients Predicting Accessibility of Significant-Others' Traits within Self-Caregiving Representations by Threat Induction and Attachment Scores

Effect	Attachment-figure traits	Exploration-partner traits	Affiliation-partner traits	Other participants' representations
Threat induction	0.18	–0.14	–0.01	–0.15
Attachment anxiety	–0.13	0.15	0.12	–0.01
Attachment avoidance	–0.24[a]	0.19	0.08	0.18
Threat × anxiety	–0.33*	0.03	–0.04	0.17
Threat × avoidance	0.01	–0.15	0.12	0.19
Anxiety × avoidance	0.29*	–0.12	0.12	–0.01
Three-way interaction	0.34*	0.16	–0.18	–0.05

*p < .05; [a]p = .07.

negative emotion, and the less frequent was the occurrence of interfering thoughts. These associations were statistically significant only in the threat condition (r's of $-.44$ and $-.53$, p's $< .01$), not in the no-threat condition (r's of $-.08$ and $-.28$). However, statistical tests revealed no significant differences between the relevant pairs of correlations with the current sample size. Pearson correlations also indicated that none of the other trait categories were significantly associated with negative emotion or cognitive interference.

As in Study 1, additional hierarchical regressions indicated that threat induction heightened the intensity of negative emotions, $beta = .25$, $p < .05$, and the frequency of interfering thoughts, $beta = .27$, $p < .05$. In addition, attachment anxiety was positively related to negative emotion, $beta = .29$, $p < .05$, and cognitive interference, $beta = .36$, $p < .01$. Furthermore, the significant association between attachment anxiety and reports of negative emotions and cognitive interference in the threat condition (*betas* of .35 and .43) were notably weakened by the introduction of the accessibility of attachment-figure traits as an additional predictor (*betas* of .14 and .17, reductions of 60% in both cases). After the accessibility mediator was introduced into the equation, attachment anxiety was no longer significantly associated with reports of negative emotions and cognitive interference. This finding supports the following sequence of mediational events: Participants scoring low on attachment anxiety exhibited relatively high accessibility of attachment-figure traits within their self-caregiving representations, which in turn led to less intense negative emotions and less frequent interfering thoughts during the experimental session (this pattern of mediation is displayed in Figure 6.3).

Overall, the findings of Study 2 support our ideas about the regulatory function of security-based representations of self-caregiving. First, exposure to an ego-relevant threat heightened the accessibility of traits of a security-enhancing attachment figure within participants' representations of self-caregiving. Second, heightened accessibility of security-based representations of self-caregiving was associated with less intense negative mood and less frequent interfering thoughts during the encounter with a threat. Third, this regulatory sequence was most pronounced among persons who scored low on attachment anxiety and avoidance. That is, reliance on security-based representations of self-caregiving as a regulatory device for coping with threats seems to be especially characteristic of secure people.

CONCLUSIONS AND CHALLENGES

In this chapter we have attempted to explain how security-enhancing interactions with attachment figures increase a person's capacity for inner reg-

Threat Condition

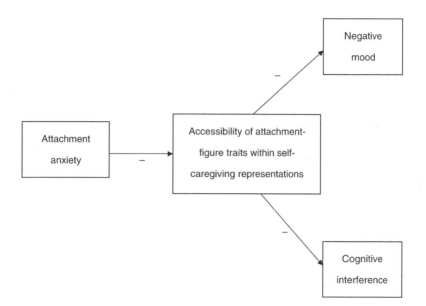

FIGURE 6.3. The mediational role of security-based self-caregiving representations in the threat condition.

ulation and make dependence on others for affect regulation less necessary. We developed and tested the idea that attachment-figure availability is related to the development of specific soothing subroutines within the self: security-based self-representations, which are made accessible during periods of stress and distress and become an inner source of comfort and relief. Specifically, we proposed that the prototypical security-enhancing interaction with an attachment figure is reproduced within a person's self-representations and that securely attached people tend to react to threats with the activation of these self-representations.

Figure 6.4 summarizes the hypothesized mediational processes by which the prototypical security-enhancing interaction with an attachment figure is integrated into self-representations that accomplish self-regulatory functions during encounters with threats. The first step involves the internalization of soothing interactions with an actual attachment figure into representations of the security-enhancing attachment figure and the self-with-this-figure. The second step involves storage of these representations in the semantic network and their integration into a person's model of self. Specifically, the attachment figure is integrated into representations of self-caregiving, and the self-with-an-attachment-figure is integrat-

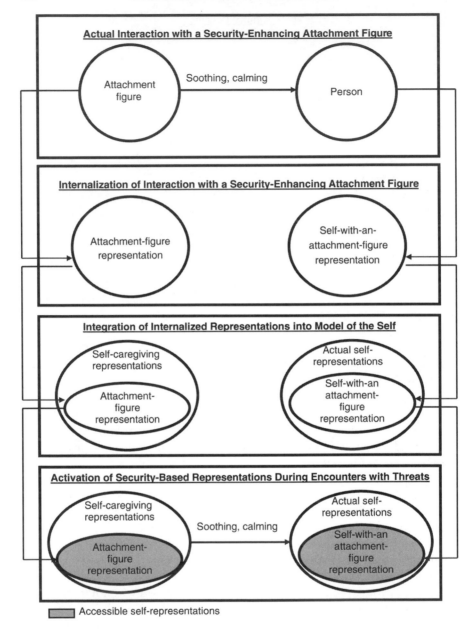

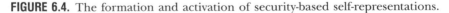
Accessible self-representations

FIGURE 6.4. The formation and activation of security-based self-representations.

ed into the actual self. The third step involves reactivation of these representations during periods of stress as part of the process of searching for attachment-related sources of comfort. As a result of this reactivation, caregiving and soothing processes are reproduced internally and no longer require external support. In other words, some parts of the self are represented as sensitive and caring toward other parts, and the latter parts are represented as secure, calm, and able to deal with threats.

All of the mental processes described in Figure 6.4 seem to characterize people who have generally and repeatedly experienced security-enhancing interactions with attachment figures. These people possess highly available security-based self-representations in their semantic networks and can rely on these self-representations during encounters with threats. Activation of these representations in response to threatening events can be viewed as an important security-based strategy and an integral part of the "broaden and build" cycle of attachment security. People who can count on such self-representations should find it easier to develop themselves along the lines of exploration, affiliation, and self-actualization.

Our findings revealed that attachment insecurities of the anxious and avoidant kinds have differential effects on the accessibility of security-based self-representations. Whereas attachment anxiety inhibited, or was associated with the relative absence of, activation of positive self-with-an-attachment-figure representations and security-based representations of self-caregiving, attachment avoidance inhibited, or was associated with the relative absence of, only the activation of self-caregiving representations. It therefore appears that both avoidant and anxious people lack available representations of security-enhancing attachment figures who could serve as models of caregiving and hence also lack representations of parts of themselves as sensitive, caring, and kind toward other parts. However, only the anxiety dimension was associated with a relative absence of positive representations of self-with-an-attachment-figure, which seemed to reduce individuals' ability to feel secure, calm, and effective in coping with threats. In contrast, avoidant individuals seemed to be able to call on positive representations of self-with-an-attachment-figure when reporting on their models of their actual selves. Whether this ability reflects actual experiences with attachment figures or a defensive means of increasing self-reliance and maintaining a sense of self-worth remains to be seen. Further research will be needed to distinguish between the contents and developmental foundations of secure and avoidant individuals' representations of self-with-an-attachment-figure.

Although our preliminary studies generated what we believe are new and exciting findings concerning the internalization of security-enhancing interactions with attachment figures into self-representations, we view the studies as only initial steps in examining the regulatory function of these representations. First, the accessibility of security-based self-representations was assessed in a trait-cued self-rating task, a task in which participants received specific traits they had named in an earlier session and were asked to indicate the extent to which those same traits described themselves at the moment. Further studies should include open-ended descriptions of participants' current selves and computation of semantic similarity scores between the generated traits and the traits appearing in representations of the attachment figure and the self-with-an-attachment-figure. Second, although the associations between security-based self-representations and both negative emotions and cognitive interference were higher in the threat than in the no-threat condition, the differences were not statistically significant. To be sure of those differences, we would need to increase the sample sizes. Third, we provided only these correlational data on the association between accessibility of security-based self-representations and a participant's emotional and cognitive state. In future studies, we plan to manipulate the contextual accessibility of security-based self-representations and examine the emotional and cognitive impact of this manipulation. Fourth, in each study we focused on only one of each participant's attachment figures; security in threatening situations is probably a function of mental representations of interactions with more than one attachment figure.

Beyond these methodological issues, several conceptual issues have yet to be fully worked out. First, we assumed that the attachment figure is integrated into representations of self-caregiving. However, the attachment figure might also be integrated into representations of the actual self. Specifically, people might perceive themselves in relation to others in the same way they earlier perceived their attachment figures in relation to themselves. For example, a person who perceived an attachment figure as sensitive and caring might also view himself or herself as sensitive and caring toward other people in need. This identification process and the integration of the attachment-figure representation into the actual self may be crucial for understanding securely attached persons' sensitive, empathic, and altruistic attitudes toward others' needs (e.g., Collins & Feeney, 2000; Kunce & Shaver, 1994; Mikulincer, Gillath, et al., 2001). These mental processes may also underlie securely attached people's sensitive parenting, their ability to provide a secure base for their offspring, and the intergenerational transmission of attachment security (see De Wolff & van IJzendoorn, 1997, for a review). Future studies should examine the incorporation of attachment-figure representations into the actual self and its impact on a person's reactions to others' needs.

Second, we assumed that attachment-figure availability is the crucial factor underlying the formation of security-based self-representations. However, other features or components of security-enhancing interactions with attachment figures might also contribute to the formation of these self-representations. For example, recall Kohut's (1971) ideas about the idealization and mirroring functions that a good parental caregiver provides to promote the development of healthy self-representations in a child. Children need a caregiver who admires them, celebrates their progress, and applauds their accomplishments. According to Kohut, children also need to possess an image of idealized caregivers toward whom they can feel admiration and with whom they can identify to the point of feeling that they share those people's admirable qualities. In our view, an attachment figure who fulfills idealization needs and serves as an ideal model for identification facilitates the transfer of desirable caregiving traits into representations of self-caregiving. Moreover, we think it likely that an attachment figure who provides mirroring experiences (e.g., describing and celebrating the child's desirable, admirable traits and achievements) facilitates the integration of the self-with-an-attachment-figure into the actual self.

Third, the main goal of this chapter was to understand how secure attachment promotes autonomy and self-regulation. However, our ideas also have important implications for attachment insecurities and for insecure individuals' self-representations. For example, our findings show that insecurity is associated with relative inaccessibility of security-based self-representations during encounters with threats. In addition, our studies imply that anxious and avoidant people, who, we assume, have experienced insecure interactions with unreliable or rejecting attachment figures, may integrate negative representations of attachment figures into their representations of self-caregiving. The results also imply that anxious people may possess negative representations of self-with-an-attachment-figure, representations that become highly accessible during threatening experiences, thereby adding to the anxious person's tension and distress. In future studies, we plan to assess these self-representations and examine their accessibility and effects during encounters with threats.

Fourth, we added a new regulatory path through the "broaden and build" cycle of attachment security outlined in our previous research (Mikulincer & Shaver, 2003). Several questions remain, however, about how this path of autonomy is integrated with other security-based strategies. For example, how do the various paths—seeking actual proximity to attachment figures, heightening the accessibility of attachment-figure representations in working memory, and heightening the accessibility of security-based self-representations—complement each other or interact during stressful experiences? To what extent can a secure adult do without external support from actual attachment figures, and under what circumstances does such a person need, and actively seek, a safe haven and a secure base in the form of an actual, physically present attachment figure? To what extent can a secure adult rely on symbolic figures, such as God or guardian angels or the spirits of deceased attachment figures, as "mentally actual" safe havens and secure bases? Further studies are needed to explore the interplay and integration of the various security-based strategies.

ACKNOWLEDGMENTS

Preparation of this chapter was facilitated by a grant from the Fetzer Institute.

REFERENCES

Aiken, L. S., & West, S. G. (1991). *Multiple regression: Testing and interpreting interactions.* Newbury Park, CA: Sage.

Ainsworth, M. D. S. (1973). The development of infant–mother attachment. In B. M. Caldwell & H. N. Ricciuti (Eds.), *Review of child development research* (Vol. 3, pp. 1–94). Chicago: University of Chicago Press.

Ainsworth, M. D. S., Blehar, M. C., Waters, E., & Wall, S. (1978). *Patterns of attachment: A psychological study of the Strange Situation.* Hillsdale, NJ: Erlbaum.

Allen, J. P., & Land, D. (1999). Attachment in adolescence. In J. Cassidy & P. R. Shaver (Eds.), *Handbook of attachment: Theory, research, and clinical applications* (pp. 319–335). New York: Guilford Press.

Alonso-Arbiol, I., Shaver, P. R., & Yarnoz, S. (2002). Insecure attachment, gender roles, and interpersonal dependency in the Basque Country. *Personal Relationships, 9,* 479–490.

Andersen, S. M., & Chen, S. (2002). The relational self: An interpersonal social-cognitive theory. *Psychological Review, 109,* 619–645.

Aron, A., Aron, E. N., & Norman, C. (2001). Self-expansion model of motivation and cognition in close relationships and beyond. In G. J. O. Fletcher & M. S. Clark (Eds.), *Blackwell handbook of social psychology: Interpersonal processes* (pp. 478–501). Malden, MA: Blackwell.

Baldwin, M. W. (1992). Relational schemas and the processing of social information. *Psychological Bulletin, 112,* 461–484.

Baldwin, M. W., Keelan, J. P. R., Fehr, B., Enns, V., & Koh-Rangarajoo, E. (1996). Social-cognitive conceptualization of attachment working models: Availability and accessibility effects. *Journal of Personality and Social Psychology, 71,* 94–109.

Baldwin, M. W., & Meunier, J. (1999). The cued activation of attachment relational schemas. *Social Cognition, 17,* 209–227.

Bandura, A. (1986). *Social foundations of thought and action: A social cognitive theory.* Englewood Cliffs, NJ: Prentice Hall.

Bartholomew, K. (1990). Avoidance of intimacy: An attachment perspective. *Journal of Social and Personal Relationships, 7,* 147–178.

Bartholomew, K., & Horowitz, L. M. (1991). Attachment styles among young adults: A test of a four-category model. *Journal of Personality and Social Psychology, 61,* 226–244.

Berant, E., Mikulincer, M., & Florian, V. (2001). The association of mothers' attachment style and their psychological reactions to the diagnosis of infant's congenital heart disease. *Journal of Social and Clinical Psychology, 20,* 208–232.

Berlin, L. J., & Cassidy, J. (1999). Relations among relationships: Contributions from attachment theory and research. In J. Cassidy & P. R. Shaver (Eds.), *Handbook of attachment: Theory, research, and clinical applications* (pp. 688–712). New York: Guilford Press.

Birnbaum, G. E., Orr, I., Mikulincer, M., & Florian, V. (1997). When marriage breaks up: Does attachment style contribute to coping and mental health? *Journal of Social and Personal Relationships, 14,* 643–654.

Blatt, S. J., & Behrends, R. S. (1987). Internalization, separation–individuation, and the nature of therapeutic action. *International Journal of Psychoanalysis, 68,* 279–297.

Bollas, C. (1987). *The shadow of the object.* New York: Columbia University Press.

Bowlby, J. (1973). *Attachment and loss: Vol. 2. Separation: Anxiety and anger.* New York: Basic Books.

Bowlby, J. (1980). *Attachment and loss: Vol. 3. Sadness and depression.* New York: Basic Books.

Bowlby, J. (1982). *Attachment and loss: Vol. 1. Attachment* (2nd ed.). New York: Basic Books. (Original work published 1969)

Bowlby, J. (1988). *A secure base: Clinical applications of attachment theory.* London: Routledge.

Brennan, K. A., Clark, C. L., & Shaver, P. R. (1998). Self-report measurement of adult attachment: An integrative overview. In J. A. Simpson & W. S. Rholes (Eds.), *Attachment theory and close relationships* (pp. 46–76). New York: Guilford Press.

Brennan, K. A., & Shaver, P. R. (1998). Attachment styles and personality disorders: Their connections to each other and to parental divorce, parental death, and perceptions of parental caregiving. *Journal of Personality, 66,* 835–878.

Buckley, P. (Ed.). (1986). *Essential papers on object relations.* New York: New York University Press.

Cantor, N., Markus, H., Niedenthal, P., & Nurius, P. (1986). On motivation and the self-concept. In R. M. Sorrentino & E. T. Higgins (Eds.), *Handbook of motivation and cognition: Foundations of social behavior* (pp. 96–121). New York: Guilford Press.

Carpenter, E. M., & Kirkpatrick, L. A. (1996). Attachment style and presence of a romantic partner as moderators of psychophysiological responses to a stressful laboratory situation. *Personal Relationships, 3,* 351–367.

Cassidy, J., & Kobak, R. R. (1988). Avoidance and its relationship with other defensive processes. In J. Belsky & T. Nezworski (Eds.), *Clinical implications of attachment* (pp. 300–323). Hillsdale, NJ: Erlbaum.

Chartrand, T. L., & Bargh, J. A. (2002). Nonconscious motivations: Their activation, operation, and consequences. In A. Tesser & D. A. Stapel (Eds.), *Self and motivation: Emerging psychological perspectives* (pp. 13–41). Washington, DC: American Psychological Association.

Collins, N. L., & Feeney, B. C. (2000). A safe haven: An attachment theory perspective on support seeking and caregiving in intimate relationships. *Journal of Personality and Social Psychology, 78,* 1053–1073.

Collins, N. L., & Read, S. J. (1994). Cognitive representations of attachment: The structure and function of working models. In K. Bartholomew & D. Perlman

(Eds.), *Advances in personal relationships: Vol. 5. Attachment processes in adulthood* (pp. 53–90). London: Kingsley.

Deci, E. L., & Ryan, R. M. (1991). A motivational approach to self: Integration in personality. In R. Dienstbier (Ed.), *Nebraska Symposium on Motivation: Vol. 38. Perspectives on motivation* (pp. 237–288). Lincoln: University of Nebraska Press.

De Wolff, M. S., & van IJzendoorn, M. H. (1997). Sensitivity and attachment: A meta-analysis on parental antecedents of infant attachment. *Child Development, 68,* 571–591.

Feeney, B. C., & Kirkpatrick, L. A. (1996). Effects of adult attachment and presence of romantic partners on physiological responses to stress. *Journal of Personality and Social Psychology, 70,* 255–270.

Fraley, R. C., & Shaver, P. R. (2000). Adult romantic attachment: Theoretical developments, emerging controversies, and unanswered questions. *Review of General Psychology, 4,* 132–154.

Fraley, R. C., & Waller, N. G. (1998). Adult attachment patterns: A test of the typological model. In J. A. Simpson & W. S. Rholes (Eds.), *Attachment theory and close relationships* (pp. 77–114). New York: Guilford Press.

Fredrickson, B. L. (2001). The role of positive emotions in positive psychology: The broaden-and-build theory of positive emotions. *American Psychologist, 56,* 218–226.

Furman, W. W., & Wehner, E. A. (1994). Romantic views: Toward a theory of adolescent romantic relationships. In R. Montemayor, G. R. Adams, & T. P. Gullotta (Eds.), *Personal relationships during adolescence* (pp. 168–195). Thousand Oaks, CA: Sage.

Gerstel, N., & Gross, H. (1984). *Commuter marriage: A study of work and family.* New York: Guilford Press.

Green, J. D., & Campbell, W. K. (2000). Attachment and exploration in adults: Chronic and contextual accessibility. *Personality and Social Psychology Bulletin, 26,* 452–461.

Greenberg, J. R., & Mitchell, S. A. (1983). *Object relations in psychoanalytic theory.* Cambridge, MA: Harvard University Press.

Hazan, C., & Shaver, P. R. (1987). Romantic love conceptualized as an attachment process. *Journal of Personality and Social Psychology, 52,* 511–524.

Hazan, C., & Shaver, P. R. (1990). Love and work: An attachment-theoretical perspective. *Journal of Personality and Social Psychology, 59,* 270–280.

Hesse, E. (1999). The Adult Attachment Interview: Historical and current perspectives. In J. Cassidy & P. R. Shaver (Eds.), *Handbook of attachment: Theory, research, and clinical applications* (pp. 395–433). New York: Guilford Press.

Higgins, E. T. (1987). Self-discrepancy theory: A theory relating self and affect. *Psychological Review, 94,* 319–340.

Higgins, E. T., & Bargh, J. A. (1987). Social cognition and social perception. In M. R. Rosenzweig & L. W. Porter (Eds.), *Annual review of psychology* (Vol. 38, pp. 369–425). Palo Alto, CA: Annual Reviews.

Hinkley, K., & Andersen, S. M. (1996). The working self-concept in transference: Significant-other activation and self-change. *Journal of Personality and Social Psychology, 71,* 1279–1295.

James, W. (1890). *The principles of psychology* (Vol. 1). Cambridge, MA: Harvard University Press.

Kirkpatrick, L. A. (1998). Evolution, pair-bonding, and reproductive strategies: A reconceptualization of adult attachment. In J. A. Simpson & W. S. Rholes (Eds.), *Attachment theory and close relationships* (pp. 353–393). New York: Guilford Press.

Kohut, H. (1971). *The analysis of the self.* New York: International Universities Press.

Kohut, H. (1977). *The restoration of the self.* New York: International Universities Press.

Kunce, L. J., & Shaver, P. R. (1994). An attachment-theoretical approach to caregiving in romantic relationships. In K. Bartholomew & D. Perlman (Eds.), *Advances in personal relationships: Vol. 5. Attachment processes in adulthood* (pp. 205–237). London: Kingsley.

Larose, S., Bernier, A., Soucy, N., & Duchesne, S. (1999). Attachment style dimensions, network orientation, and the process of seeking help from college teachers. *Journal of Social and Personal Relationships, 16,* 225–247.

Magai, C. (1999). Affect, imagery, and attachment: Working models of interpersonal affect and the socialization of emotion. In J. Cassidy & P. R. Shaver (Eds.), *Handbook of attachment: Theory, research, and clinical applications* (pp. 787–802). New York: Guilford Press.

Main, M. (1990). Cross-cultural studies of attachment organization: Recent studies, changing methodologies, and the concept of conditional strategies. *Human Development, 33,* 48–61.

Main, M., Kaplan, N., & Cassidy, J. (1985). Security in infancy, childhood, and adulthood: A move to the level of representation. *Monographs of the Society for Research in Child Development, 50*(1 & 2, Serial No. 209), 66–104.

Markus, H., & Nurius, P. (1986). Possible selves. *American Psychologist, 41,* 954–969.

McGowan, S. (2002). Mental representations in stressful situations: The calming and distressing effects of significant others. *Journal of Experimental Social Psychology, 38,* 152–161.

Medway, F. J., Davis, K. E., Cafferty, T. P., & Chappell, K. D. (1995). Family disruption and adult attachment correlates of spouse and child reactions to separation and reunion due to Operation Desert Storm. *Journal of Social and Clinical Psychology, 14,* 97–118.

Meissner, W.W. (1981). *Internalization in psychoanalysis.* New York: International Universities Press.

Mikulincer, M. (1994). *Human learned helplessness: A coping perspective.* New York: Plenum Press.

Mikulincer, M. (1995). Attachment style and the mental representation of the self. *Journal of Personality and Social Psychology, 69,* 1203–1215.

Mikulincer, M. (1997). Adult attachment style and information processing: Individual differences in curiosity and cognitive closure. *Journal of Personality and Social Psychology, 72,* 1217–1230.

Mikulincer, M., Birnbaum, G., Woddis, D., & Nachmias, O. (2000). Stress and accessibility of proximity-related thoughts: Exploring the normative and intraindividual components of attachment theory. *Journal of Personality and Social Psychology, 78,* 509–523.

Mikulincer, M., & Florian, V. (1995). Appraisal of and coping with a real-life stressful situation: The contribution of attachment styles. *Personality and Social Psychology Bulletin, 21,* 406–414.

Mikulincer, M., & Florian, V. (1998). The relationship between adult attachment styles and emotional and cognitive reactions to stressful events. In J. A. Simpson & W. S. Rholes (Eds.), *Attachment theory and close relationships* (pp. 143–165). New York: Guilford Press.

Mikulincer, M., & Florian, V. (1999). Maternal–fetal bonding, coping strategies, and mental health during pregnancy: The contribution of attachment style. *Journal of Social and Clinical Psychology, 18,* 255–276.

Mikulincer, M., & Florian, V. (2000). Exploring individual differences in reactions to mortality salience: Does attachment style regulate terror management mechanisms? *Journal of Personality and Social Psychology, 79,* 260–273.

Mikulincer, M., Florian, V., & Weller, A. (1993). Attachment styles, coping strategies, and posttraumatic psychological distress: The impact of the Gulf War in Israel. *Journal of Personality and Social Psychology, 64,* 817–826.

Mikulincer, M., Gillath, O., Halevy, V., Avihou, N., Avidan, S., & Eshkoli, N. (2001). Attachment theory and reactions to others' needs: Evidence that activation of the sense of attachment security promotes empathic responses. *Journal of Personality and Social Psychology, 81,* 1205–1224.

Mikulincer, M., Gillath, O., & Shaver, P. R. (2002). Activation of the attachment system in adulthood: Threat-related primes increase the accessibility of mental representations of attachment figures. *Journal of Personality and Social Psychology, 83,* 881–895.

Mikulincer, M., Hirschberger, G., Nachmias, O., & Gillath, O. (2001). The affective component of the secure base schema: Affective priming with representations of attachment security. *Journal of Personality and Social Psychology, 81,* 305–321.

Mikulincer, M., & Shaver, P. R. (2001). Attachment theory and intergroup bias: Evidence that priming the secure base schema attenuates negative reactions to out-groups. *Journal of Personality and Social Psychology, 81,* 97–115.

Mikulincer, M., & Shaver, P. R. (2003). The attachment behavioral system in adulthood: Activation, psychodynamics, and interpersonal processes. In M. P. Zanna (Ed.), *Advances in experimental social psychology* (Vol. 35, pp. 53–152). San Diego, CA: Academic Press.

Mikulincer, M., Shaver, P. R., & Pereg, D. (2003). Attachment theory and affect regulation: The dynamics, development, and cognitive consequences of attachment-related strategies. *Motivation and Emotion, 27,* 77–102.

Mischel, W., & Shoda, Y. (1995). A cognitive–affective system theory of personality: Reconceptualizing situations, dispositions, dynamics, and invariance in personality structure. *Psychological Review, 102,* 246–268.

Moretti, M. M., & Higgins, E. T. (1999). Internal representations of others in self-regulation: A new look at a classic issue. *Social Cognition, 17,* 186–208.

Ognibene, T. C., & Collins, N. L. (1998). Adult attachment styles, perceived social support, and coping strategies. *Journal of Social and Personal Relationships, 15,* 323–345.

Pierce, T., & Lydon, J. (1998). Priming relational schemas: Effects of contextually activated and chronically accessible interpersonal expectations on responses to a stressful event. *Journal of Personality and Social Psychology, 75,* 1441–1448.

Rogers, C. (1951). *Client-centered therapy.* Boston: Houghton Mifflin.

Rubin, K. H., Bukowski, W., & Parker, J. G. (1998). Peer interactions, relationships, and groups. In W. Damon (Series Ed.) & N. Eisenberg (Vol. Ed.), *Handbook of child psychology: Vol. 3. Social, emotional, and personality development* (5th ed., pp. 619–700). New York: Wiley.

Sandler, J., & Rosenblatt, B. (1962). The concept of the representational world. *Psychoanalytic Study of the Child, 27,* 128–145.

Sarason, I. G., Sarason, B. R., Keefe, D. E., Hayes, B. E., & Shearin, E. N. (1986). Cognitive interference: Situational determinants and traitlike characteristics. *Journal of Personality and Social Psychology, 51,* 215–226.

Schafer, R. (1968). *Aspects of internalization.* New York: International Universities Press.

Shaver, P. R., & Mikulincer, M. (2002). Attachment-related psychodynamics. *Attachment and Human Development, 4,* 133–161.

Simpson, J. A., Rholes, W. S., & Nelligan, J. S. (1992). Support seeking and support giving within couples in an anxiety-provoking situation: The role of attachment styles. *Journal of Personality and Social Psychology, 62,* 434–446.

Solomon, Z., Ginzburg, K., Mikulincer, M., Neria, Y., & Ohry, A. (1998). Coping with war captivity: The role of attachment style. *European Journal of Personality, 12,* 271–285.

Sroufe, L. A. (1996). *Emotional development: The organization of emotional life in the early years.* New York: Cambridge University Press.

Sroufe, L. A., Fox, N., & Pancake, V. (1983). Attachment and dependency in developmental perspective. *Child Development, 54,* 1615–1627.

Sullivan, H. S. (1953). *The interpersonal theory of psychiatry* (H. S. Perry & M. L. Gawel, Eds.). New York: Norton.

Thompson, R. A. (1999). Early attachment and later development. In J. Cassidy & P. R. Shaver (Eds.), *Handbook of attachment: Theory, research, and clinical applications* (pp. 265–286). New York: Guilford Press.

Tronick, E. Z. (1989). Emotions and emotional communication in infants. *American Psychologist, 44,* 112–119.

Weinfield, N. S., Sroufe, L. A., Egeland, B., & Carlson, E. A. (1999). The nature of individual differences in infant–caregiver attachment. In J. Cassidy & P. R. Shaver (Eds.), *Handbook of attachment: Theory, research, and clinical applications* (pp. 68–88). New York: Guilford Press.

Winnicott, D. W. (1965). *The maturational process and the facilitating environment.* London: Hogarth.

Zeifman, D., & Hazan, C. (1997). A process model of adult attachment formation. In S. Duck (Ed.), *Handbook of personal relationships* (2nd ed., pp. 179–195). Chichester, UK: Wiley.

CHAPTER 7

Working Models of Attachment
New Developments and Emerging Themes

NANCY L. COLLINS
ANAMARIE C. GUICHARD
MAIRE B. FORD
BROOKE C. FEENEY

> Every situation we meet with in life is constructed in terms of the
> representational models we have of the world about us and of ourselves.
> Information reaching us through our sense organs is selected and
> interpreted in terms of those models, its significance for us and for those
> we care for is evaluated in terms of them, and plans of action conceived
> and executed with those models in mind. On how we interpret and
> evaluate each situation, moreover, turns also how we feel.
> —BOWLBY (1980, p. 229)

A fundamental assumption of attachment theory is that adults do not enter relationships as tabula rasas, or blank slates. Instead, they bring with them a history of social experiences and a unique set of memories, expectations, goals, and action tendencies that guide how they interact with others and how they construe their social world. Although these mental representations continue to evolve as individuals develop new relationships throughout their lives, attachment theory assumes that representational models that begin their development early in one's personal history are likely to remain influential. Internal *working models* of attachment are thought to be core features of personality that shape the manner in which the attachment system is expressed by directing cognitive, affective, and behavioral response patterns in attachment-relevant contexts. Furthermore, individual differences in *attachment style* observed between children and adults are attributed to systematic differences in underlying models of self and others, and whatever continuities exist in these styles across the lifespan are proposed to be largely a function of the enduring quality of these models (Bowlby, 1973; Bretherton, 1985; Collins & Read, 1994; Main, Kaplan, & Cassidy, 1985).

The working-models concept is thus a cornerstone of attachment theory; working models are presumed to organize attachment behavior, mediate individual differences in attachment style, and explain stability in attachment functioning across the lifespan. Because of its central theoretical relevance, researchers have devoted considerable attention in recent years to understanding the nature of working models in adulthood. These efforts have resulted in a growing body of work that includes increasingly detailed theories about the content and functioning of working models and increasingly sophisticated methodologies for studying them. Nevertheless, although significant gains have been made, there are still many unanswered questions and many topics in need of theoretical and empirical clarification. Our goal in this chapter is to provide an in-depth review of theory and empirical work on working models of attachment in adulthood and to identify untested assumptions, gaps in our knowledge, and contemporary trends in the field (see also Pietromonaco & Feldman Barrett, 2000). In our prior work on attachment representations, we proposed a framework for understanding the content, structure, and function of working models by integrating attachment theory with research and theory in the social-cognitive literature on the nature of mental representation and its role in social experience (Collins & Allard, 2001; Collins & Read, 1994; Shaver, Collins, & Clark, 1996). Because this approach has proven useful to attachment scholars, we continue to utilize it as a framework for organizing this discussion.

We begin by briefly reviewing the major propositions outlined by Bowlby and others on the early development and nature of working models. Next, we specify the components of working models and discuss how these components are useful for mapping out differences in adult attachment styles. We then discuss how working models are likely to be structured in memory, focusing on the complex and multidimensional nature of attachment representations and the distinction between general and relationship-specific working models. Finally, we consider how working models function and the processes through which they shape cognitive, affective, and behavioral response patterns in adulthood.

WORKING MODELS FROM CHILDHOOD TO ADULTHOOD

Bowlby (1973) used the term "working models" to describe the internal mental representations that children develop of the world and of significant people within it, including the self (Bretherton, 1985). These representations evolve out of experiences with attachment figures and center around the regulation and fulfillment of attachment needs—namely, the maintenance of proximity to a nurturing caregiver and the regulation of felt security (Bretherton, 1985; Sroufe & Waters, 1977). Of course, not all infants will have access to caretakers who respond to their needs in a consistent and loving manner. Thus the quality of the infant–caretaker relationship and hence the nature of one's working models are expected to be largely determined by the caregiver's emotional availability and responsiveness to the child's needs. Working models are hypothesized to include two complementary components, one referring to the attachment figure and the other referring to the self. The former characterizes whether the caregiver will be available, sensitive, and responsive when needed, and the latter characterizes the self as either worthy or unworthy of love and care.

Early working models are thus composed of schemata that reflect a child's attempts to gain comfort and security, along with the typical outcome of those attempts (Main, Kaplan, & Cassidy, 1985), and they are expected to be fairly accurate reflections of social reality as experienced by the developing child (Bowlby, 1973). One central aspect of working models adopted by Bowlby is the idea that working models are used to predict the behavior of others and to plan one's own behavior in social interaction. Working models shape how the attachment behavioral system is expressed, and are dynamic and functional. For this reason, individual differences in infant *behavioral* patterns, as displayed in diagnostic situations, are used to infer underlying differences in internal working models (Main et al., 1985) and serve as the basis for categorizing infants into secure and various forms of insecure attachment styles (Ainsworth, Blehar, Waters, & Wall, 1978).

In early childhood, attachment models appear to be relatively open to change if the quality of caregiving changes (see Bretherton & Munholland, 1999, for an overview). However, given a fairly consistent pattern of caregiving throughout childhood and adolescence, working models are expected to become solidified through repeated experience and increasingly generalized over time. Thus what begins as a schema of a specific child–caretaker relationship results in the formation of more abstract representations of oneself and the social world (Shaver, Collins, & Clark, 1996). Once formed, these representations are likely to operate automatically and unconsciously, thereby making them resistant (but certainly not impervious) to dramatic change (Bowlby, 1979). Thus working models of self and others that take root in childhood and adolescence become core features of personality that are carried forward into adulthood, where they continue to shape social perception and behavior in close relationships.

On the basis of this assumption, attachment theory has become a widely used model for understanding interpersonal behavior and romantic experience in adult close relationships (see Feeney, 1999a, for a review). Inspired by Hazan and Shaver's (1987) seminal paper on romantic love as an attachment process, much of the empirical work has focused on individual differences in adult *attachment styles.* These styles reflect chronic differences in the way individuals think, feel, and behave in close relationships, and they are believed to be rooted in systematic differences in working models of self and others.

Adult attachment researchers typically define four prototypic attachment styles derived from two underlying dimensions (Bartholomew & Horowitz, 1991; Brennan, Clark, & Shaver, 1998). The first dimension, labeled *anxiety,* reflects the degree to which individuals worry about being rejected, abandoned, or unloved by significant others. The second dimension, labeled *avoidance,* reflects the degree to which individuals limit intimacy and interdependence with others. *Secure* individuals are low in both anxiety and avoidance. They feel valued by others and worthy of affection, and they perceive attachment figures as generally responsive, caring, and reliable. They are comfortable developing close relationships and depending on others when needed. *Preoccupied* individuals (also called *anxious–ambivalent*) are high in anxiety but low in avoidance. They have an exaggerated desire for closeness but lack confidence in others' availability and likely responsiveness to their needs. They depend greatly on the approval of others for a sense of personal well-being but have heightened concerns about being rejected or abandoned. *Fearful–avoidant* individuals are high in both anxiety and avoidance. They experience a strong sense of distrust in others coupled with heightened expectations of rejection, which result in discomfort with intimacy and avoidance of close relationships. Finally, *dismissing–avoidant* individuals are low in anxiety but high in avoidance. They perceive attachment figures as generally unreliable and unresponsive but view themselves as confident and invulnerable to negative feelings. They attempt to maintain a positive self-image in the face of potential rejection by minimizing attachment needs, distancing themselves from others, and restricting expressions of emotionality.

These attachment styles represent theoretical prototypes that individuals can approximate to varying degrees (Griffin & Bartholomew, 1994), and there is growing consensus that individual differences are best measured in terms of the two continuous dimensions (anxiety and avoidance) that underlie the prototypes (Brennan, Clark, & Shaver, 1998; Crowell, Fraley, & Shaver, 1999; Fraley & Waller, 1998). However, because researchers in the past have used a variety of methods for conceptualizing and measuring attachment style, our review of the literature will necessarily involve some inconsistencies in terminology.

Despite differences in the conceptualization and measurement of attachment style, adult attachment researchers agree that individual differences in attachment patterns are rooted in the nature and content of working models. We begin our discussion of working models in adulthood by identifying their components and exploring how they may differ for adults with different attachment styles.

THE CONTENT OF WORKING MODELS

What are working models? Working models of attachment are similar in many ways to other cognitive structures studied by social psychologists, including schemas, scripts, and prototypes. Like all such constructs, working models are hypothetical cognitive–affective structures that are presumed to be stored in long-term memory and activated in response to attachment-relevant cues. They organize past experience and provide a framework for understanding new experiences and guiding social interaction (Bretherton & Munholland, 1999; Collins & Allard, 2001; Shaver, Collins, & Clark, 1996). However, unlike traditional approaches to schemas, which tend to focus on semantic knowledge and verbal propositions, attachment theory places greater emphasis on the representation of motivation and action tendencies. In addition, because working models are formed in the context of emotional experiences with significant others and center around the fulfillment of emotional needs, they are more heavily affect laden and more explicitly interpersonal than other knowledge structures typically studied by social psychologists. Despite these differences, the working-models construct is highly compatible with a number of contemporary theories in social and personality psychology that emphasize the importance of cognitive–motivational representations of the self in relation to others (e.g., Andersen & Chen, 2002; Baldwin, 1992; Mischel & Shoda, 1995). Indeed, attachment theory provides an important point of contact between the close-relationships literature, which is increasingly interested in the cognitive processes that shape interpersonal experience (e.g., Berscheid, 1994; Holmes, 2002), and the social-cognition literature, which is increasingly interested in mental processes in the context of significant relationships (e.g., Fitzsimons & Bargh, 2003; Moretti & Higgins, 1999; Shah, 2003).

Building Blocks of Working Models

Because working models are built within the context of the attachment behavioral system, Collins and Read (1994) proposed that they should include four interrelated components: (1) memories of attachment-related experience, (2) beliefs, attitudes, and expectations about self and others in relation to attachment processes, (3) attachment-related goals and needs, and (4) strategies and plans associated with achieving attachment goals.

Attachment-Related Memories

Memories and accounts of attachment-related experiences are important components of working models. These should include not only representations of specific interactions and concrete episodes but also constructions placed on those episodes, such as appraisals of experience and explanations for one's own and others' behavior. Because these memories should be based, in part, on actual experience, we would expect that secure adults would be more likely than insecure adults to report positive relationship experiences with key attachment figures. Evidence for this assumption has been obtained in a number of studies involving retrospective reports of relationships with parents (Collins & Read, 1990; Feeney & Noller, 1990, Hazan & Shaver, 1987; Rothbard & Shaver, 1994). For example, Hazan and Shaver (1987) found that secure adults remembered their relationships with their parents as more affectionate and warm than did avoidant or anxious adults. In a more recent study of community women, Shaver, Belsky, and Brennan (2000) examined memory for attachment experiences as coded from the Adult Attachment Interview (AAI; George, Kaplan, & Main, 1984). Overall, insecure women had more negative attachment memories than secure women. For example, avoidant women (those uncomfortable with closeness and with depending on others) described their mothers as less loving and more neglecting, their fathers as neglecting and rejecting, and a mother–daughter relationship that involved role reversal (in which the mother relied on the daughter for care).

In addition to differing in the *content* of their attachment memories, secure and insecure adults also differ in the degree to which they effectively process information about their past attachment experiences. Relative to secure individuals, anxious and avoidant individuals appear to have less integrated and organized attachment memories, which makes it difficult for them to provide a coherent account of their early attachment experiences (Shaver et al., 2000). Secure and insecure adults also differ in the cognitive *accessibility* of their attachment-related memories. Avoidant adults have greater difficulty retrieving attachment memories (Mikulincer & Orbach, 1995; Shaver et al., 2000), and preoccupied adults have more ready access to negative than positive memories (Mikulincer, 1998b, Study 1; Mikulincer & Orbach, 1995). For example, Mikulincer and Orbach (1995) asked young adults to recall childhood experiences in which they felt a particular emotion (anger, sadness, anxiety, and happiness), and the time taken to retrieve each episode was then recorded. Anxious–ambivalent individuals showed the fastest responding (highest accessibility) to sadness and anxiety memories, whereas avoidant individuals showed the slowest responding (lowest accessibility). In addition, anxious–ambivalent individuals were faster to retrieve negative than positive memories, whereas secure individuals showed the opposite pattern.

Attachment-Related Beliefs, Attitudes, and Expectations

A person's knowledge about self, others, and relationships is likely to be extremely complex in adulthood. It will include not only static *beliefs* (e.g., "relationships require a lot of work") but also *attitudes* (e.g., "relationships are not worth the effort") and *expectations* (e.g., "I am unlikely to find someone who will love me completely"). This knowledge is abstracted, in part, from concrete experiences with key attachment figures and can vary in level of abstraction. Some will be associated with particular attachment figures (e.g., "my mother is emotionally distant"); others will be broader generalizations about relationships (e.g., "friends can be counted on for support") or about people (e.g., "people are trustworthy").

Although empirical work is still in its early stages, important links have been found between self-reported attachment style and general beliefs about the self and the social world. Overall, relative to avoidant and anxious adults, secure adults have more positive beliefs about the self in relation to others (Collins & Read, 1990; Hazan & Shaver, 1987; Mikulincer, 1995, Studies 1 & 2). For example, Collins and Read (1990) found that secure adults were higher in global self-worth, saw themselves as more confident in social situations, were more interpersonally oriented, and were more assertive as compared with anxious individuals. Avoidant individuals did not differ from the secure group in their global self-worth or assertiveness, but they did view themselves as less confident in social situations and less interpersonally oriented. Subsequent studies that have differentiated dismissing from fearful avoidance consistently find that dismissing individuals report high levels of self-worth, similar to secure individuals, but fearful individuals report very low levels of self-worth (Bartholomew & Horowitz, 1991; Brennan & Bosson, 1998; Brennan & Morris, 1997; Griffin & Bartholomew, 1994). However, although secure and dismissing adults report similar *levels* of global self-esteem, they differ in the relative importance they place on different *sources* of self-worth (Brennan & Bosson, 1998; Brennan & Morris, 1997). Dismissing adults place greater weight on competence-based sources of esteem (e.g., autonomy, environmental mastery), whereas secure adults place greater weight on interpersonal sources (e.g., positive relations with others). In future work, it would be interesting to study attachment differences in other contingencies of self-worth (Crocker & Wolf, 2001), as well as the degree to which self-worth is stable or unstable (Kernis & Waschull, 1995).

In addition to identifying the content of self-knowledge, secure and insecure adults also differ in the way their self-knowledge is organized. For example, secure individuals have more balanced, complex, and coherent self-structures than anxious and avoidant individuals (Mikulincer, 1995, Studies 3 & 4); they also report fewer discrepancies between their *actual* self and their *ideal* self and between their actual self and their *ought* self (Mikulincer, 1995, Studies 5 & 6). In addition, although the self-concepts of secure individuals include both positive and negative features, their positive features are more central than their negative features, whereas fearful individuals show the opposite pattern (Clark, Shaver, & Calverley, cited in Shaver & Clark, 1996).

Relatively fewer studies have investigated attachment differences in beliefs about others and the social world, but these studies consistently reveal that secure adults have more optimistic expectations about relationships and about the general benevolence of others (Collins & Read, 1990; Hazan & Shaver, 1987; Mikulincer, 1995, Studies 1 & 2). For example, Collins and Read (1990) found that secure adults viewed people in general as trustworthy, dependable, and altruistic; whereas avoidant adults were suspicious of human motives, viewed others as not trustworthy and not dependable, and doubted the honesty and integrity of social role agents such as parents. Anxious adults thought others were complex and difficult to understand and that people have little control over the outcomes in their lives. Baldwin, Fehr, Keedian, Seidel, and Thomson (1993) have shown that attachment-related beliefs about relationships may be stored as "if–then" propositions that reflect one's expectations about their social interactions with others. In one study, they asked participants to consider a number of hypothetical, attachment-relevant behaviors (e.g., "If I depend on my partner . . .") and then to rate the likelihood that their partner would respond in various positive and negative ways (e.g., "then my partner will leave me" or "then my partner will support me"). Results indicated that secure participants held more positive if–then expectancies than did avoidant or anxious–ambivalent (preoccupied) participants. In a second study, reaction time data provided further evidence that insecure adults hold more pessimistic interpersonal expectations than secure adults. For example, when avoidant participants were given a prime that involved trusting a romantic partner, they showed particularly quick reactions to the negative outcome word "hurt."

Finally, one study has examined attachment differences in the complexity of one's relationship knowledge. Fishtein, Pietromonaco, and Feldman Barrett (1999) found that preoccupied individuals who were involved in high-conflict relationships had more complex knowledge structures than those in low-conflict relationships; these differences were primarily due to their use of distinct, positive attributes. These authors suggest that this pattern may result from preoccupied individuals' tendency to encode high-conflict interactions in both positive and negative terms because conflict provides an opportunity for increased closeness and intimacy (Pietromonaco & Feldman Barrett, 1997). In future research, it will be important to investigate other structural features of relationship knowledge (e.g., coherence, integration, differentiation, elaboration, compartmentalization) and to study their implications for information processing and relationship resilience (e.g., Murray & Holmes, 1999; Showers & Kevlyn, 1999). Holmes (2002) offers some valuable insights concerning the nature of relationship expectations and some suggestions about the ways in which secure and insecure adults may differ in the structure of their mental models of others.

Attachment-Related Goals and Needs

Although the attachment behavioral system serves the broad goal of maintaining felt security, a person's history of achieving or failing to achieve this goal is expected to result in a characteristic hierarchy of attachment-related social and emotional needs. For example, people differ in the extent to which they are motivated to develop intimate relationships, avoid rejection, maintain privacy, seek approval from others, and so on. As such, the goal structures of secure and insecure individuals should differ considerably. For example, secure adults are likely to desire intimate relationships with others and to seek a balance of closeness and autonomy within relationships. Preoccupied (anxious–ambivalent) adults also desire close relationships, but their additional need for approval and fear of rejection may lead them to seek extreme intimacy and lower levels of autonomy. Avoidant adults are guided by a need to maintain distance; dismissing avoidants seek to limit intimacy in the service of satisfying their desire for autonomy and independence, but fearful avoidants do so to avoid rejection (Bartholomew & Horowitz, 1991).

Although there is little empirical work that directly addresses these hypotheses, several studies have explored the goal structures of adults with different attachment styles (Collins, Ford, Guichard, & Allard, 2003; Feeney, 1999b; Mikulincer, 1998b). For example, Collins and colleagues (2003) asked participants to rate the importance of their romantic partner fulfilling specific attachment-related needs for comfort, support, and proximity (e.g., "How important is it that your partner comforts you when you are feeling down?"). Preoccupied and fearful individuals (those high in attachment-related anxiety) rated these needs as very important, whereas dismissing individuals rated them as relatively unimportant; secure individuals fell in between these two extremes. Along similar lines, Feeney (1999b) found that when dating partners were asked to describe their relationships, dismissing men were more likely to spontaneously mention goal conflicts centering on their need to remain self-reliant, to maintain distance, and to control the emotional climate of their relationship, whereas anxious women were more likely to mention goal conflicts centering on their need for greater closeness. Relative to secure and preoccupied adults, avoidant adults also place greater weight on non-attachment-related goals and needs, such as achievement in school or career

(Brennan & Bosson, 1998; Brennan & Morris, 1997; Hazan & Shaver, 1990), which may be one method of minimizing attachment concerns and managing their need for social distance.

Finally, two recent studies point to the importance of studying broader motivational systems. Based on models that postulate the existence of distinct appetitive (approach) and aversive (avoidance) motivational systems (e.g., Gray, 1987), Feeney and Collins (2003) explored the specific motives that promote or inhibit caregiving behavior in couples. Overall, secure and anxious individuals were more likely than avoidant individuals to endorse approach motives, although their specific approach goals differed. Secure individuals (those lower in anxiety and avoidance) provided care to their partners for relatively altruistic reasons—because they wanted to increase their partners' well-being and because they enjoyed helping their partners. Anxious individuals provided care for relatively egoistic reasons—because they wanted to create closeness, to make their partners dependent on them, and to feel in control. In contrast, avoidant individuals tended to endorse aversive (avoidance) motives. Specifically, they often *failed* to provide care to their partners because they were uncomfortable with their partners' distress, perceived that helping would lead to negative consequences (e.g., that their partners would be difficult to interact with or would lack appreciation), and because their partners were too dependent on them. In another study, Elliot and Reis (2003) investigated the links between approach and avoidance motives in the domain of achievement. In a series of studies, they found that secure participants had higher achievement motivation and lower fear of failure and that they adopted more approach versus avoidance goals (e.g., seeking to master course content versus seeking to avoid doing poorly) and appraised specific achievement tasks (e.g., an upcoming exam) as a positive challenge rather than a threat. In contrast, anxious individuals adopted more avoidance goals and tended to appraise tasks as threatening. These authors speculate that secure attachment will facilitate approach-oriented motivational processes in *all* spheres of functioning because it enables individuals to pursue their goals with confidence that support and acceptance are readily available if needed. In contrast, insecure attachment is likely to facilitate avoidance-oriented motivational processes because it orients individuals toward the prevention of negative outcomes that could place them at risk for rejection or abandonment. These processes are worth studying in future research.

Plans, Strategies, and Action Tendencies

Individuals are expected to have encoded as part of their working models a set of plans and strategies for regulating their attachment-related needs, and these strategies should be contingent, at least in part, on a person's history of experiences with key attachment figures (Main, 1981). Thus attachment-style differences are expected in one's plans and strategies for dealing with socioemotional needs and goals, including strategies for regulating emotional distress (Kobak & Sceery, 1988), obtaining comfort when needed, maintaining autonomy, developing intimacy with others, giving comfort to others, and so on.

Identifying individual differences in plans and action tendencies poses some difficulties because such representations are likely to be stored as procedural knowledge that is difficult to articulate and that may operate largely outside awareness. One way to identify plans and strategies is to examine how different individuals respond to the same controlled social stimulus. For example, in a series of studies, Collins and colleagues (Collins, 1996; Collins et al., 2003) asked respondents to imagine a variety of attachment-relevant events (e.g., "imagine that your partner didn't comfort you when you were feeling down") and then to describe how they would respond in each situation. Content coding of these descriptions revealed important differences in behavioral strategies. Overall, relative to insecure adults, secure adults tended to choose behavioral strategies that were less punishing toward their partners and less likely to lead to conflict. In another study, Ognibene and Collins (1998) asked young adults to describe how they would cope with a series of hypothetical stressful life events. Results revealed systematic differences in the coping strategies of adults with different attachment styles. For example, secure and preoccupied adults were more likely than avoidant adults to say that they would seek social support. Finally, Pierce and Lydon (1998) found that both chronic and temporarily primed attachment schemas were linked to coping behavior. Participants with different attachment styles were asked to imagine a stressful situation and to report their likely coping responses after being subliminally primed with accepting or rejecting interpersonal expectancies. Women who were chronically secure, as well as those primed with accepting interpersonal expectancies, were more likely to seek social support and less likely to engage in self-denigrating coping.

Another useful research strategy is to employ response-latency paradigms to uncover unconscious action tendencies that may be linked to particular interpersonal contexts. For example, Mikulincer (1998b, Study 5) used a lexical decision task to study attachment style differences in the way people cope with trust violations. Secure and anxious–ambivalent adults responded quicker to the word "talk," whereas avoidant adults responded quicker to the word "escape." Finally, action tendencies can, of course, be illuminated by observing actual behavior in attachment-relevant contexts. A growing number of studies reveal differences in a variety of attachment-relevant behaviors, including support seeking and caregiving (Collins & Feeney, 2000; Feeney & Collins, 2001; Simpson, Rholes, &

Nelligan, 1992), conflict and problem solving (Feeney, Noller, & Callan, 1994; Simpson, Rholes, & Phillips, 1996), self-disclosure (Mikulincer & Nachshon, 1991), and responses to separation from one's partner (Fraley & Shaver, 1998).

Emerging Themes Concerning the Content of Working Models

The existing literature provides strong evidence that adults with different attachment styles differ in the content of their working models. Nevertheless, a number of topics need further investigation. Here we highlight two that we believe are especially important.

Implicit and Explicit Working Models

One important issue in need of further study concerns the distinction between *implicit* and *explicit* aspects of working models. Until recently, most of the work on the content of working models has relied on explicit, self-report measures. Although such measures can be extremely useful for identifying conscious features of working models that individuals can introspect and articulate, many aspects of working models are presumed to lie outside conscious awareness and are therefore not available for reflection and report. Moreover, even when individuals *are* capable of providing accurate reports of their working models, they may sometimes be motivated to mask their true thoughts and feelings in the service of self-regulation and self-presentation. There are also important theoretical reasons to measure both implicit and explicit features of working models. Bowlby (1973) suggested that, for some individuals, conscious and unconscious elements of working models will be inconsistent and that such inconsistencies can have important consequences for attachment experience (see also Crittenden, 1990; Main, 1991). Hence, in future work, it will be important for researchers to develop valid and reliable assessments of implicit attachment-related representations and methods for identifying individuals who hold compatible versus incompatible explicit and implicit models.

At present, few empirical studies directly assess implicit features of working models, and none systematically compare explicit and implicit content. Fortunately, adult attachment researchers are beginning to utilize tools from cognitive social psychology to explore unconscious aspects of working models. For example, the response-latency paradigms used by Baldwin and colleagues (1993) and Mikulincer (1998b) are especially useful. Another tool that holds promise is the Implicit Association Test (IAT; e.g., Greenwald, McGhee, & Schwartz, 1998), which measures the strength of automatic associations between a target concept (e.g., *self*) and an attribute (e.g., *good*). In a recent study, Zayas (2003) used the IAT to explore attachment style differences in automatic affective associations to three targets—self, mother, and romantic partner. Secure and preoccupied individuals showed stronger positive associations toward their romantic partners and their mothers than did fearful and dismissing individuals. In addition, dismissing individuals had relatively stronger automatic positive associations toward self than toward their romantic partners, whereas all other groups showed the opposite pattern. This finding suggests that dismissing individuals hold a higher automatic regard for the self than for others.

In addition to social-cognitive paradigms such as these, implicit features of working models may also be revealed in physiological responses (see Diamond & Hicks, Chapter 8, this volume), in nonverbal behavior, and in unstructured or projective tasks that can be used to infer unconscious thoughts and feelings. And, of course, interview assessments of adult attachment patterns, such as the Adult Attachment Interview (AAI; George et al., 1984) and the Current Relationship Interview (CRI; Crowell & Owens, 1996) offer valuable tools for identifying both implicit and explicit features of working models. Although the AAI and CRI depend on verbal reports, the critical coding dimensions (e.g., coherence of transcript, coherence of mind) used to distinguish secure and insecure models are not based on the explicit content of respondents' attachment memories (e.g., whether they report good or bad relationships with attachment figures) but on their ability to talk coherently about attachment issues and to effectively access memories of attachment experiences. Another promising new tool is the secure-base script assessment, which measures the degree to which individuals have knowledge of effective secure-base script dynamics (see Waters, 2003). A secure-base script is defined as a general interpersonal script that involves an attachment figure (mother or romantic partner) being responsive to the needs of an attached person in a distressing situation (Waters & Rodrigues-Doolabh, 2001). To measure *scriptedness,* participants are presented with a set of prompt words and asked to construct a story. These narratives are then rated for the degree to which they reveal knowledge of prototypical secure-base dynamics. This measure can be adapted to correspond to different types of attachment relationships or to a specific relationship (Wais, Treboux, & Waters, 2003), and there is accumulating evidence for its construct and predictive validity (Waters & Rodrigues-Doolabh, 2001).

One final note concerning implicit measures: Because implicit measures lie outside conscious control and are not easily distorted by forces that might motivate false responding, it is tempting to assume that they are more valid than explicit measures—that is, more reflective of an individual's *true* thoughts or feelings. We caution against such reasoning. There is ample evidence that people process social information at both an explicit and an implicit level and that implicit and explicit mental processes have unique influences on social judgment and behavior (see Bargh, 1997; Greenwald & Banaji, 1995). For example, Spalding and Hardin (1999) found that *explicit* self-esteem predicted conscious (self-reported) experiences of anxiety during a laboratory interview, whereas *implicit* self-esteem predicted nonverbal expressions of anxiety (rated by observers), a form of behavior that is typically outside of conscious awareness and control. Based on findings such as these, it is reasonable to assume that implicit and explicit attachment models will shape attachment behavior through different but *equally valid* streams of influence. Thus the important question for attachment scholars is not which feature of working models is more valid but how explicit and implicit features jointly contribute to attachment experience.

Accessibility of Working Models

In addition to investigating the content of attachment models, another important topic for future research concerns the accessibility of attachment-related representations. Construct accessibility refers to the degree to which a psychological construct is easily activated or brought to mind. The accessibility of a construct can be increased either by recent activation (a *temporarily accessible* construct) or frequent activation over time (a *chronically accessible* construct). Prior studies on mental constructs such as stereotypes and attitudes have shown that both temporary activation and chronic activation increase the likelihood that a construct will influence social judgment (e.g., Fincham, Garnier, Gano-Phillips, & Osborne, 1995; Higgins, King, & Mavin, 1982) and behavior (e.g., Bargh, Chen, & Burrows, 1996; Fazio & Williams, 1986).

Construct accessibility is important to study for at least two reasons. First, individual differences in attachment style may be more strongly linked to construct accessibility than to content per se. That is, secure and insecure individuals may share similar knowledge or goals but may differ in the degree to which those constructs are easily accessible. For example, although most individuals are assumed to have a need for acceptance, this goal should be most chronically activated for preoccupied adults. In this way, differences in attachment style can be conceptualized in terms of differences in *chronically accessible* mental representations. Second, individuals with the same attachment style may differ in the degree to which their models are currently accessible, and knowledge accessibility may moderate the degree to which attachment models shape social perception and behavior. Specifically, the link between attachment style and important personal and interpersonal outcomes should be stronger when attachment models are more accessible (either chronically or temporarily). Consistent with this idea, Whitaker, Beach, Etherton, Wakefield, and Anderson (1999) found that attachment style differences in expectations for future satisfaction and problem-solving efficacy in long-term relationships was moderated by the accessibility of internal models. For example, individuals who were high in attachment-related anxiety expected to be less satisfied in their marriages and less effective at solving marital problems, but this effect was considerably stronger for those whose attachment constructs were highly accessible.

THE STRUCTURE OF WORKING MODELS: A COMPLEX REPRESENTATIONAL NETWORK

Until recently, there has been a strong tendency to discuss working models and attachment style in the singular, as if an individual can have only one. However, most attachment scholars now agree that representational models of attachment are complex and multifaceted (Baldwin et al., 1996; Bretherton, Biringen, Ridgeway, Maslin, & Sherman, 1989; Crittenden, 1990; George & Solomon, 1999; Pierce & Lydon, 2001; Trinke & Bartholomew, 1997). Collins and Read (1994) suggest that working models may be best conceptualized as a network of interconnected models that may be loosely organized as a *default hierarchy*. At the top of the hierarchy is the default model that corresponds to the most general representations about self and others, abstracted from a history of experiences with key attachment figures. Further down in the hierarchy are *domain-specific* models that correspond to particular kinds of relationships (parent–child relationships, romantic relationships), and lowest in the hierarchy are *relationship-specific* models that correspond to particular relationships. Although models within the network are conceptually distinct, they are presumed to be linked through a rich set of associations.

Consistent with these ideas, a growing number of studies provide evidence for the multidimensional nature of attachment representations in adulthood. Several studies find that adults have different working models of attachment in different relationship *domains*. For example, representations of attachment with respect to parents are only moderately or weakly correlated with representations of attachment with respect to peers (Bartholomew & Horowitz, 1991) or romantic partners (Shaver, Belsky, & Brennan, 2000; Simpson, Rholes, Orina, & Grich, 2002). Other studies find that *general* (or domain-specific) working models and *relationship-specific* working models are correlated but not redundant constructs (Baldwin et al., 1996; Cozzarelli, Hoekstra, & Bylsma, 2000; Crowell & Owens, 1996; Pierce & Lydon, 2001). Moreover, several studies find that different working models predict unique variance in interpersonal behavior and relationship outcomes. For example, in a longitudinal study of young couples who were about to marry (summarized in Crowell, Fraley, & Shaver, 1999), security of attachment to one's fiancé (measured with the CRI) uniquely predicted feelings of commitment, intimacy, and aggression 18 months later, whereas security of attachment to parents (measured with the AAI) uniquely predicted intimacy, threats to abandon the partner, and partner's physical aggression (see also Bartholomew & Horowitz, 1991; Cozzarelli et al., 2000; Pierce & Lydon, 2001; Simpson et al., 2002). Taken together, these studies are consistent with the idea that individuals possess a complex associative network of working models that contains abstract representations (a general model or style), as well as specific exemplars (relationship-specific models).

Other researchers have explored the multidimensional nature of attachment representations by using sophisticated statistical models to examine between- and within-person variability in attachment security (Cook, 2000; La Guardia, Ryan, Couchman, & Deci, 2000; Pierce & Lydon, 2001). These studies suggest that the degree to which an individual feels secure in a specific relationship is partly due to that person's general propensity to feel secure or insecure (a general attachment style) and partly due to features of the specific relationship. However, these studies consistently find that the majority of the variance in attachment security lies at the relationship (within-person) level. For example, La Guardia and colleagues (2000) asked young adults to complete measures of attachment security with respect to a variety of specific relationships (e.g., mother, father, romantic partner, best friend). Across three samples, hierarchical linear modeling analyses revealed that 21–44% of the variability in felt security occurred at the between-person level (reflecting individual differences in general attachment models) and that the remaining variability occurred at the within-person level (reflecting relationship-specific models). As we discuss in more detail later, studies such as these highlight the importance of understanding attachment dynamics within specific relationships.

The studies cited previously provide evidence that adults possess multiple attachment representations, but they do not speak directly to the structural relations underlying these various representational models. More direct evidence for the hierarchical nature of attachment representations was provided in a recent study by Overall, Fletcher, and Friesen (2003). In this study, respondents completed measures of attachment style in three domains—close family relationships, close friendships, and romantic relationships. Within each domain, they also completed attachment measures for their three most important relationships. Confirmatory factor analyses revealed that the structural model that best fit the data was one consistent with the default hierarchy originally proposed by Collins and Read (1994), indicating that relationship-specific models are nested under domain-specific representations (family, friends, romantic partners), which are nested under an overarching global working model.

Emerging Themes Concerning the Structure of Working Models

As the previous discussion makes clear, there is now a good deal of evidence that adults possess a rich network of attachment representations that vary in their level of specificity. However, we still know relatively little about the relationship between general and relationship-specific models and the ways in which these models work together to shape social perception and behavior in close relationships. Given the growing interest in relationship-specific working models, we highlight two issues in need of consideration.

How Do Relationship-Specific Models Develop, and How Are They Related to More General Models?

In order to be functional, relationship-specific models should be rooted in interpersonal transactions and features of one's relationship as experienced by the individual. Just as parent–child relationships differ in their attachment quality, adult intimate relationships will differ in the degree to which they provide partners with a safe haven of comfort and security and a secure base from which to explore interests outside of the relationship. Felt security within a specific relationship should therefore depend in large part on whether one's partner is perceived to be both willing and able to be responsive to one's needs in attachment-relevant contexts (Collins & Feeney, 2000).

It is important to clarify what we mean by *felt security* in adulthood. Collins and Feeney (2004) distinguish between two different but compatible uses of the term. First, *situation-specific* felt security reflects the degree to which an individual feels free from physical and emotional threat. When felt security is threatened (by either a threat to the self or a threat to the attachment relationship), the attachment system will be activated, and individuals will take steps to restore feelings of security (through real or imagined contact with attachment figures or through other means of coping). Thus acute threats to felt security trigger the attachment system and motivate attachment behavior (Mikulincer, Gillath, & Shaver, 2002). This form of felt security is distinct from *relationship-specific* felt security, which refers to an individual's overall sense of confidence in a partner's love and commitment and expectations concerning the partner's responsiveness to need. Individuals will feel more secure in their relationships to the extent that they feel valued and cared for by partners who are emotionally available and responsive to their needs. Consistent with this perspective, Murray, Holmes, Griffin, Bellavia, and Rose (2001) argue that felt security requires two conjunctive beliefs: (1) that one's partner loves oneself and is thus *willing* to be available and caring and (2) that the partner is a good, responsive person who is *capable* of fulfilling one's needs.

Thus a secure relationship-specific working model simultaneously evaluates the self as loved and the partner as trustworthy and reliable.

If relationship-specific felt security requires individuals to believe that their partners are responsive to their needs and uniquely committed to them, such inferences should be based on past experience in diagnostic situations that enable individuals to draw inferences about their partner's motives and attitudes toward them (Holmes & Rempel, 1989; Weiselquist, Rusbult, Foster, & Agnew, 1999). Collins and Feeney (2004) suggest that intimate interactions, in which partners reveal private aspects of themselves, provide a critical testing ground for drawing such inferences. After all, in order for individuals to feel secure in their partners' love, they must perceive that their partners know, understand, and value them for their true selves. A sense of felt security also requires evidence that one's partner is willing and able to be responsive to one's needs. Therefore, care-seeking and caregiving interactions, which are a special form of intimate interaction, should be especially informative. Through such interactions, individuals learn whether they can count on their partners to understand their needs, accept responsibility for their well-being, follow communal norms, and make themselves emotionally (and physically) available to them. Furthermore, it is precisely because care-seeking interactions involve vulnerability (e.g., expressions of fear, weakness, sadness, hurt) that they offer such a critical testing ground for felt security; they provide evidence of a partner's willingness to care for us when we are at our weakest (e.g., when we are emotionally vulnerable, socially isolated, physically ill, down on our luck) and perhaps least able to reciprocate. Under these circumstances, a partner's continued acceptance and nurturance provides diagnostic evidence of his or her deep investment in our well-being (Tooby & Cosmides, 1996).

Although these hypotheses have not been directly addressed in the literature, several studies demonstrate that relationship-specific security is rooted in evidence of partner responsiveness. For example, La Guardia and colleagues (2000) examined the association between relationship-specific security and need satisfaction across a variety of specific relationships (e.g., mother, father, romantic partner, best friend). Results revealed that feelings of security varied substantially across different relationships and, more important, that individuals felt more secure in relationships that did a better job of meeting their needs for relatedness (feeling accepted and cared for by the partner), competence (feeling that the partner supports their sense of confidence and self-efficacy), and autonomy (feeling that their partner supports their desire to engage in independent activities).

Other studies have shown that relationship-specific security is associated with partner sensitivity and responsiveness in laboratory interactions. For example, Kobak and Hazan (1991) used a Q-sort procedure to measure relationship-specific working models and then observed couples during a conflict discussion and a confiding/support discussion. Husbands who had more secure working models of their marriages (who felt their partners were psychologically available to them) had wives who expressed more support validation and less rejection in the problem-solving task. In addition, wives who had more secure working models (who felt they could rely on their husbands and perceived their husbands to be psychologically available) had husbands who expressed more acceptance during the confiding task. Along similar lines, Collins and Feeney (2000) found that couples who perceived their relationships as more secure engaged in more effective support and caregiving interactions when one member of the couple was discussing a personal stressor. To the extent that behavior in these laboratory interactions is representative of behavior outside the lab, these studies are consistent with the idea that relationship-specific security is rooted in diagnostic situations that enable individuals to draw inferences about their partners' acceptance of them and concern for their well-being (see also Wais, Treboux, & Waters, 2003).

Although relationship-specific models show evidence of being tied to the raw data of relationship experience, they are nevertheless subjective construals that should be influenced by more general attachment models. Indeed, attachment theory explicitly assumes that new experiences will, at least to some extent, be assimilated into existing expectations. Consistent with this assumption, in studies that have measured both general and relationship-specific models, the two constructs were found to be moderately correlated (Baldwin et al., 1996; Cozzarelli et al., 2000; Pierce & Lydon, 2001, Study 1). However, because general and relationship-specific models were assessed concurrently in these studies, it is not clear whether general models shaped specific ones or whether specific models contributed to the general ones. Of course, it is likely that both processes are at work, and several longitudinal studies support this assumption (Murray, Holmes, & Griffin, 1996; Pierce & Lydon, 2001, Study 2; Simpson, Rholes, Campbell, & Wilson, 2003; Wais et al., 2003).

Before concluding our discussion, we note one final measurement issue. At present, there are no agreed-on measures of relationship-specific working models. Researchers typically measure relationship-specific models by simply modifying scales that were originally developed to assess general attachment styles and by asking respondents to complete these scales with a specific partner in mind (e.g. LaGuardia et al., 2000; Pierce & Lydon, 2001). Although this procedure has been fruitful, researchers may want to consider additional means of assessing relationship-specific attachment representations that focus more precisely on the interpersonal expectancies, goals, and action tendencies that are relevant to attachment dynamics in couples. For example, it would be useful to assess the degree to which individuals feel that they can rely on their partners as a safe haven of comfort and support and a secure base for exploration. In addition, it remains to be seen whether the two dimensions of attachment (anxiety and avoidance) that have been useful for conceptualizing individual differences in general attachment style are equally relevant at the relationship-specific level or whether the particular patterns of insecurity will be tied to particular patterns of partner responsiveness in ways that parallel the parent–child patterns. For example, when a partner's affections and responsiveness are inconsistent but not necessarily neglecting or rejecting, we might expect that an individual would develop a relationship-specific pattern that is relatively preoccupied (high anxiety and low avoidance). In this way, relationship-specific attachment styles may reflect functional adaptations to expectations about a partner's responsiveness in attachment-relevant contexts, in much the same way that infant attachment styles are presumed to be adaptations to various caregiving environments.

How Do General and Relationship-Specific Models Work Together to Shape Interpersonal Experience?

If individuals possess both general and relationship-specific working models, how do they work together to shape thought and behavior in specific relationships? At present, researchers have not yet articulated a clear model or set of models for explaining the unique and shared roles of different attachment representations. If we assume that general and relationship-specific models are correlated but not redundant constructs (as the existing data suggest), there are a number of alternative causal models that might explain their joint influence on attachment behavior. Figure 7.1 presents three simplified models. Model 1, the independence model, proposes that general and relationship-specific models influence attachment outcomes through independent channels. According to this model, general and relationship-specific models would have additive effects on behavior, and these effects need not be convergent. For example, the degree to which an individual seeks support may be shaped independently by the degree to which the individual is generally avoidant and the degree to which he or she believes that this particular partner will be emotionally available and responsive. Thus Model 1 predicts that aspects of one's general working model will continue to be activated and used to guide behavior even in the presence of a more specific relational model. It is reasonable to assume, for example, that well-learned behavioral routines that are linked to general models and that lie outside conscious awareness may be automatically activated and therefore difficult to modify even when they may not be optimally suited to the current relationship. Consistent with Model 1, Cozzarelli and colleagues (2000) and Pierce and Lydon (2001)

1. Independence model

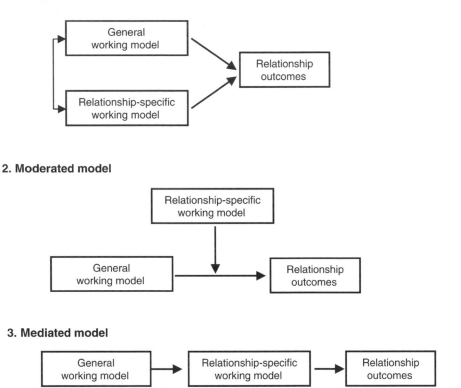

2. Moderated model

3. Mediated model

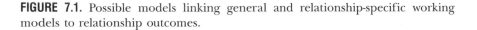

FIGURE 7.1. Possible models linking general and relationship-specific working models to relationship outcomes.

found that global and specific attachment representations independently predicted outcomes such as life satisfaction and the quality of social interactions.

A second possibility is that general and relationship-specific models have interactive effects. Model 2, the moderated model, proposes that the effects of general working models are moderated by relationship-specific models. In other words, this model assumes that the impact of general attachment representations will depend on current relationship circumstances. For example, individuals who are generally insecure may function relatively well if they are involved with a partner who is highly responsive to their needs and is perceived to be deeply committed to them. Thus insecure chronic models may represent a vulnerability factor that may or may not be expressed, depending on current circumstances (Collins et al.,

2003). Consistent with Model 2, Pierce and Lydon (2001, Study 2) found that global and relationship-specific models interacted to predict daily social experience. Specifically, chronically anxious individuals functioned well if they were interacting with a partner whom they perceived as responsive; but, when their partner was less responsive, their social interactions were lower in quality and less intimate than those of secure individuals. A similar pattern was obtained in two longitudinal studies conducted by Simpson, Rholes, and colleagues (Rholes, Simpson, Campbell, & Grich, 2001; Simpson, Rholes, Campbell, Tran, & Wilson, 2003), who investigated attachment processes during the transition to parenthood. In these studies, women who were high in chronic anxiety and who perceived that their husbands were unsupportive and angry during their pregnancies experienced increases in depressive symptoms (Simpson et al., 2003) and decreases in marital satisfaction (Rholes et al., 2001) 6 months postpartum. However, when spousal support was perceived to be high, anxious women were functioning as well as nonanxious women. Model 2 is compatible with contemporary theories of personality (Andersen & Chen, 2002; Mischel & Shoda, 1995) and relationship interdependence (e.g., Holmes, 2002) that emphasize the importance of studying stable person × situation interactions, in which long-term romantic partners (and one's expectations concerning those partners) represent a stable feature of one's interpersonal environment.

Models 1 and 2 assume that general and relationship-specific models are either uncorrelated or modestly correlated. However, if we assume that they are moderately or strongly related and that general models shape the development of relationship-specific models, then their joint effects may be best represented as a mediated model. Model 3 proposes a mediated model in which the effects of general attachment models on behavior are fully mediated by relationship-specific models. For example, this model might predict that individuals who are chronically high in attachment-related anxiety will be more likely to doubt the love of their current partners, which will in turn lead them to engage in high levels of reassurance-seeking behavior. Thus this model assumes that general models exert their influence on current functioning by shaping the development of relationship-specific models. At present, we are not aware of any studies that directly or indirectly test a mediated model.

These models are, of course, a simplification of what are surely more complex processes, and they are not intended to provide an exhaustive list of the possible causal models that might underlie the links between general and relationship-specific working models. Our goal was simply to encourage attachment scholars to be more explicit about their assumptions when investigating the joint effects of general and relationship-specific models and to stimulate thoughtful research on the topic.

THE FUNCTIONS OF WORKING MODELS IN ADULTHOOD

Working models are a central component of the attachment behavioral system that are expected to play a critical role in shaping how individuals operate in their relationships and how they construe their social world. However, the specific mechanisms through which this occurs are not fully understood. One way to understand these mechanisms is to consider working models of attachment as part of a broader system of cognitive–motivational processes that enable individuals to make sense of their experiences and to function in ways that meet their personal needs (Collins & Read, 1994). We assume that working models of attachment are highly accessible cognitive–affective constructs that will be automatically activated whenever attachment-relevant events occur. Once activated, they should play an important role in shaping cognitive, affective, and behavioral response patterns. Moreover, we need not assume that people are consciously directing these processes or even that they are aware of them. It is likely that that much of this system will operate automatically; that is, spontaneously, with little effort, and outside of awareness (Bargh, 1997). In the following sections, we specify these processes in greater detail and review relevant empirical work.

Cognitive Response Patterns

Working models of attachment contain a rich network of memories, beliefs, and goals that should have a critical role in shaping how individuals think about themselves and their relationships. This assumption is consistent with a large body of research in social psychology on the role of prior knowledge in information processing and social judgment. This research demonstrates that social perception is heavily influenced by top-down, theory-driven processes in which existing goals, schemas, and expectations shape the way individuals view new information. Here we consider four cognitive processes that should be strongly influenced by working models and should have important implications for personal and interpersonal functioning.

Selective Attention

Empirical, as well as anecdotal, evidence indicates that two people experiencing the same event rarely agree about what took place. Indeed, Bargh (1984) concludes that social perception involves "an interaction between the environmental stimuli that are currently present and the individual's readiness to perceive some over others" (p. 15). But what determines a person's readiness to attend to particular features of the environment and to disregard others? Evidence suggests that individuals are apt to attend to information that is relevant to their currently active goals and consistent with their existing attitudes and expectations (Bargh, 1984; Roskos-Ewoldsen & Fazio, 1992; Srull & Wyer, 1986).

If goals and expectations predispose individuals to attend to particular features of their environment, then working models of attachment should play an important role in directing mental resources in attachment-relevant situations. And, as a result, information available for further processing may tend to be biased in a goal-relevant and expectation-consistent manner. For example, anxious–ambivalent (preoccupied) adults are expected to have "seeking approval" and "avoiding rejection" as chronically active goals. As a result, they are likely to have a threat-oriented focus that keeps them vigilant for signs of disapproval by others. In addition, because they expect the worst, they may easily notice evidence that confirms their fears. Avoidant adults should be characterized by a very different pattern. Their motivation to maintain autonomy should make them highly sensitive to signs of intrusion or control by others, and their desire to minimize attachment concerns will tend to direct their attention away from features of the environment that make attachment needs salient (Fraley, Davis, & Shaver, 1998).

Although these specific hypotheses have not been directly tested, several studies indicate that individuals with different attachment styles differ in their ability to regulate their attention to threatening stimuli. Fraley and Shaver (1997) used a thought-suppression paradigm to examine whether individuals with different attachment styles differed in their ability to suppress unwanted attachment-related thoughts. After being asked to suppress thoughts about losing their partners, dismissing individuals were successful at reducing the subsequent intrusion of unwanted thoughts, and they also evidenced lower physiological arousal. In contrast, preoccupied adults experienced a rebound in thoughts of losing their partners and became more physiologically aroused. These data suggest that dismissing adults have well-developed defense systems that enable them to regulate negative affect by deactivating their attachment systems and reducing the accessibility of attachment-related thoughts. In contrast, preoccupied adults have difficulty turning their attention away from such thoughts, even when explicitly attempting to do so, which may result in hyperactivation of the attachment system and increased negative affect. Consistent with these findings, Baldwin and colleagues have shown that anxious individuals have difficulty inhibiting the activation of rejection cues (Baldwin & Kay, 2003; Baldwin & Meunier, 1999). In one study, Baldwin and Kay (2003) exposed participants to tones paired with symbols of interpersonal rejection (frowning faces) and acceptance (smiling faces). In a subsequent lexical decision task, secure and, especially, dismissing individuals were slower to respond to rejection target words in the presence of either the rejection or the acceptance tones (relative to a neutral tone). In contrast, fearful and preoccupied individuals (those high in anxiety) were quick to respond to rejection words, even when primed with a tone that was previously linked to acceptance. To the extent that slow responding reflects the inhibition of rejection thoughts, these findings indicate that secure and dismissing individuals are able to direct their attention away from threatening stimuli, whereas anxious individuals are hypervigilent to such cues and have a low threshold for detecting potential threats to acceptance.

Other studies show that attachment-related goals can influence how people allocate their attention to social and nonsocial tasks (Mikulincer, 1997; Miller & Noroit, 1999). For example, Mikulincer (1997, Study 2), asked participants to select how much information they wanted to hear about a new product. They were told that time spent on this task would affect how much time they had left for a second task (either a social interaction or a sensory test). Avoidant adults selected more information during the first task when the second task was social rather than nonsocial; anxious–ambivalent adults showed the opposite pattern. These data suggest that insecure participants allocated their attention in ways that served their personal goals. Anxious–ambivalent adults—who value social connection and social approval—limited their attention to a competing task when it interfered with a social task. In contrast, avoidant adults—who value social distance—increased their attention to a nonsocial task, thereby decreasing their available attention for a social task. Finally, independent of individual differences, adults normatively turn their attention to attachment figures in response to threatening cues. In a series of studies, Mikulincer, Gillath, and Shaver (2002) found that when individuals were primed with threatening words, mental representations of attachment figures became more accessible in memory (and this was true regardless of the individual's chronic attachment style).

Cognitive Openness

One of the hallmarks of effective personality functioning is a flexible cognitive system that is open to new information. Individuals with different working models of attachment may differ in their willingness and ability to update their mental representations of self and others and to incorporate new information in ways that enable them to cope with and adapt to changing circumstances (Kobak & Hazan, 1991). To the extent that cognitive openness reflects, at least to some extent, a willingness to take risks and explore novel stimuli, then secure individuals are likely to have a more open and flexible cognitive style than insecure individuals, who are likely to be more risk averse. Consistent with this idea, several studies indicate that secure individuals have a less rigid cognitive style and are more likely to integrate new information into their existing expectations about others (Green-Hennessy & Reis, 1998; Mikulincer, 1997; Mikulincer & Arad, 1999). Secure individuals are also more open and more positively responsive to information about themselves (Brennan & Bosson, 1998). For example, relative to secure individuals, fearful and dismissing adults are less likely to desire honest feedback about themselves from their partners, and fearful adults are more likely to prefer positive feedback even if it is false. In addition, relative to secure individuals, preoccupied and fearful individuals feel more distressed in response to partner feedback, whereas dismissing individuals feel more indifferent.

Memory

One of the most robust findings in the social-cognitive literature is that existing knowledge structures shape what gets stored in memory and what is later recalled or reconstructed (Srull & Wyer, 1989). In general, aspects of experience that can be interpreted in terms of easily accessible concepts are more likely to be encoded into memory. As a result, well-established schemas bias memory toward schema-relevant, and often schema-consistent, information. In addition, once information is stored in memory, further processing gives consistent material an advantage over inconsistent material. Existing representations may also lead individuals to recall or reconstruct features of experiences that never took place. One reason for this effect is that, as episodic memory for an event fades over time, people may rely more on their generic schemas and less on the particular encounter (Graesser & Nakamura, 1982).

Evidence for these processes within the attachment domain is beginning to emerge. Consistent with a schema-driven memory model, both chronically and temporarily activated attachment models appear to shape memory for new information (Rowe & Carnelley, 2003) and to lead to false-positive memory intrusions (Mikulincer & Horesh, 1999). There is also evidence that schema-driven memory effects are likely to emerge over time. Feeney and Cassidy (2003) assessed high school students' perceptions of laboratory interactions with their parents immediately after each interaction and again 6 weeks later. Over time, adolescents *reconstructed* their memories of specific interactions in ways that confirmed their working models. Those who held positive models of their parents recalled having had more positive and less negative interactions than they had reported immediately following the interaction. These findings illustrate how memory for a specific interpersonal exchange can be revised in ways that support relationship-specific expectations (see also Collins & Feeney, in press). In another study, Pietromonaco and Feldman Barrett (1997) asked participants to provide global reports of their typical social and emotional experiences (which reflect their long-term semantic memory) and then to complete interaction records for 1 week in which they recorded their experiences immediately following each social interaction (which reflects their shorter term episodic memory). Results indicated that semantic-based reports and episodic-based reports diverged in important ways. Although preoccupied individuals reported experiencing more affect intensity than other individuals on their global reports, they did not report more extreme emotional responses immediately following their daily interactions. Likewise, although dismissing adults reported experiencing relatively low levels of affect intensity on their global reports, they reported negative emotions that were at least as intense as those of other insecure people immediately following their daily interactions. These findings provide indirect evidence that memory for interpersonal experiences may become more consistent with attachment models over time and that insecure individuals may fail to accommodate new information into their generalized representations despite evidence that disconfirms these general impressions. This study also points to the importance of investigating the processes through which episodic memories come to be generalized into more abstract, semantic memories and the impact of working models on different memory systems (Klein, Babey, & Sherman, 1997).

In addition to schema-driven processes, several studies provide evidence for motivated memory processes (Fraley, Garner, & Shaver, 2000; Miller, 2001; Miller & Noroit, 1999). For example, Fraley and colleagues (2000) investigated the role of differential attention as an explanation for differences in memory for attachment experiences. Recall that avoidant individuals have greater difficulty recalling emotional experiences from their pasts (Mikulincer & Orbach, 1995; Shaver et al., 2000). Fraley and colleagues reasoned that this pattern may occur either because avoidant individuals (1) limit their attention to emotional information and hence their encoding of it (labeled a "preemptive defense") or (2) limit their elaboration, rehearsal, and processing of emotional information they have encoded (labeled a "postemptive defense"). To test these alternatives participants were asked to listen to an interview in which a woman discussed emotionally sensitive attachment experiences and then measured recall immediately following the task and at various delayed intervals. Avoidant individuals had worse recall immediately following the task but did not differ in how much they forgot over time, suggesting that they differed in their initial encoding of the story events but not in the degree to which they subsequently processed the information. Thus avoidant individuals appear to be less attentive to emotional events while they are occurring (a preemptive defense), thereby encoding less of the information that is available to them. Consistent with these findings, Miller (2001) found that avoidant individuals (especially those who matched the dismissing profile) had poor overall recall of observed conversations, especially when those conversations involved an opposite-sex peer.

Social Construal

A large body of research in social psychology indicates that people's existing concepts and expectations play an active role in shaping the way they perceive others and interpret their social experiences. Social information is filtered through existing schemas and stereotypes, which then guide social inference processes. Like other knowledge structures, working models of attachment should play an important role in guiding how people construe their interpersonal experiences and make sense of their relationships.

One process that is especially important for relationship functioning and that is expected to be strongly influenced by working models is the construction of explanations and attributions. Consistent with this idea, several studies indicate that adults with different attachment styles are predisposed to explain relationship events in ways that are consistent with their expectations concerning themselves and others (Collins, 1996; Collins et al., 2003; Gallo & Smith, 2001). Overall, relative to their insecure counterparts, secure adults tend to make more benign attributions for their partners' transgressions. For example, Collins (1996) asked participants to provide explanations for a series of potentially negative partner behaviors. Secure participants explained their partners' behavior in ways that reflected confidence in their partners' love and responsiveness, whereas anxious–ambivalent participants explained events in ways that revealed low self-worth and self-reliance, a lack of confidence in their partners' love and trustworthiness, and a belief that their partners were purposely rejecting closeness. Biases in attributions are not limited to partner transgressions. Collins and colleagues (2003, Study 2) found that adults with different attachment styles also differed in their explanations for their partners' supportive and caring behavior. Overall, insecure adults tended to make attributions that undermined their partners' good intentions. This was especially true for avoidant individuals, who tended to attribute their partners' caring behavior to selfish rather than altruistic motivation.

By presenting participants with a controlled set of social stimuli, these studies provide strong evidence that social construal processes are colored by existing expectations about oneself and others. However, because participants were asked to explain hypothetical events on the basis of very little information, the results from these studies may not generalize to more natural settings. To address this limitation, we conducted several studies to examine attachment style differences in perceptions of actual social interactions between romantic partners. In one study (Collins & Feeney, 2000), we videotaped couples while one member of the couple disclosed a personal problem or worry to his or her partner. Although attachment models did not predict the discloser's perceptions, they did predict their partners' perceptions. Specifically, partners who were higher in attachment-related anxiety and avoidance perceived their interactions more negatively, even after controlling for the discloser's perceptions *and* ratings made by outside observers. Next, to provide a more stringent test of biased construal, we *experimentally manipulated* the supportiveness of the partner's behavior to determine whether secure and insecure perceivers would differ in their construal of the *same* social support message (Collins & Feeney, in press, Study 1). For this study, we created a stressful experience for one member of the couple by asking him or her to give a videotaped speech. After couple members interacted spontaneously for 5 minutes, we then manipulated social support by having the partner copy either two *supportive* or two relatively *unsupportive* notes. The dependent variable was the speech givers' ratings of these notes and ratings of their partners' behavior during the spontaneous interaction. Results provided clear evidence that working models of attachment colored perceptions, but only in response to the unsupportive notes. When participants received the relatively unsupportive notes, insecure adults perceived them as less supportive and were more likely to infer that their partners purposely intended to hurt them. What was even more striking is that they also rated their earlier interactions as less supportive, even though these interactions occurred *prior* to the support manipulation and were unrelated to the note condition (which was randomly assigned). Thus insecure perceivers demonstrated a *retrospective contamination;* they either misremembered or reconstrued their partner's prior behavior after receiving an unsupportive note in the intervening period. We found further evidence for biased construal in a conceptual replication in which we used a similar paradigm but allowed partners to write genuine notes that were then rated by three independent observers (Collins & Feeney, in press, Study 2). Relative to secure participants, insecure support-recipients rated their partners' notes as less supportive, and they inferred more negative motivation, even after controlling for the objective content of the notes as judged by independent coders. Moreover, this effect became more pronounced as the notes became less objectively supportive and more ambiguous. Taken together, these studies provide compelling evidence that insecure working models predispose individuals to construe their social experiences in pessimistic ways, but primarily in the context of ambiguous or potentially negative interactions, perhaps because these interactions have greater latitude for construal or because they are more likely to activate the latent doubts and fears of insecure individuals. These data also point to the importance of studying person × situation interactions.

In addition to schema-driven processes such as those illustrated earlier, it is also important to explore *motivated* construal processes. Evidence for attachment style differences in strategic social construal is beginning to accumulate. For example, after receiving failure feedback, avoidant adults tend to inflate their self-views, whereas anxious–ambivalent adults tend to emphasize their negative self-aspects (Mikulincer, 1998a). Along similar lines, under conditions of threat, anxious–ambivalent individuals increase their perceptions of self–other similarity, whereas avoidant individuals decrease self–other similarity (Mikulincer, Orbach, & Iavnieli, 1998). Mikulincer suggests that these strategic patterns reflect chronic emotion-regulation strategies in which avoidant adults manage threat by avoiding recognition of personal weaknesses and by distancing self from others, whereas anxious–ambivalent adults manage threat by becoming overly attentive to inner sources of distress and by seeking closeness and connection to others. Further evidence for motivated construal was provided by Simpson, Ickes, and Grich (1999), who examined attachment style differences in empathic accuracy. Empathy accuracy refers to the degree to which individuals correctly infer their partner's thoughts and feelings. Prior research indicates that empathic accuracy is neither all good nor all bad; it can have positive consequences when it leads to greater understanding and increased intimacy, but it can also have negative consequences when it poses a threat to oneself or to one's relationship. Simpson and colleagues hypothesized that insecure individuals may be less able than secure individuals to strategically decrease their accuracy in situations that would pose a threat to their relationships. To test this idea, couples were asked to rate the attractiveness and sexual appeal of opposite-sex targets in the presence of their partners. Results indicated that individuals who were high in attachment-related anxiety had greater empathic accuracy. That is, they were more accurate in perceiving their partners' thoughts and feelings during the rating process. However, among anxious women, greater accuracy was associated with declines in feelings of closeness to the partner, and among anxious men, greater accuracy was associated with increased likelihood of breakup 4 months later. Thus, although anxious individuals were more successful at perceiving their partners' true thoughts and feelings, their greater insight had negative consequences for them. In contrast, low-anxious individuals were able to protect themselves by being less accurate in circumstances that might pose a threat to their relationships.

Finally, there is some evidence for attachment style differences in motivated person perception. For example, avoidant individuals are more conservative (more risk averse) when drawing inferences about others' personalities, whereas anxious individuals have more labile perceptions and are quick to draw both positive and negative inferences (Zhang & Hazan, 2002). Specifically, when asked to form impressions of a potential romantic partner or classmate, avoidant individuals required more evidence to confirm that someone possessed positive traits or did not possess negative ones. In other words, avoidant individuals needed more evidence to conclude that someone was good. In contrast, anxious individuals required less information to confirm positive or negative traits but also less information to overturn these impressions. In another study, Niedenthal, Brauer, Robin, and Innes-Ker (2002) found that secure and insecure adults differed in their perceptions of facial expressions in ways that may reflect attachment-related interpersonal goals. For example, under conditions of stress, insecure individuals (especially fearful individuals) tended to see the offset of negative facial expressions later than did secure people. This finding suggests that, under distress, insecure individuals may be vigilant to emotional cues that signal potential acceptance or rejection.

Affective Response Patterns

The second general function of working models is to guide affective response patterns. Emotional response patterns are of central interest to attachment theory, and individual differences in attachment style are associated with variations in emotional regulation and emotional expression (e.g., Kobak & Sceery, 1988; Shaver, Collins, & Clark, 1996). Working models of attachment may shape emotional response patterns through two general pathways: a direct path, labeled primary appraisal, and an indirect path, labeled secondary appraisal (Collins & Read, 1994).

Primary Appraisal

The primary appraisal process occurs when attachment-related events occur and working models initiate an immediate, largely automatic emotional response. Two primary mechanisms are proposed to operate here. First, attachment representations are heavily affect laden, and this affect should be automatically evoked whenever working models are activated in memory, a process referred to as "schema-triggered affect" (Andersen & Baum, 1994; Fiske & Pavelchak, 1986). Consistent with this idea, Mikulincer, Hirschberger, Nachmias, and Gillath (2001) have shown that activation of secure-base expectations (outside of awareness) automatically activates positive affect (measured implicitly). Along similar lines, Rowe and Carnelley (2003) found that individuals who were temporarily primed with a secure relationship-specific working model reported more positive affect and less negative affect than those who were primed with anxious or avoidant working models.

The second mechanism linking working models and primary emotional appraisal involves goals. In general, individuals respond with positive affect when a goal is achieved or facilitated and with negative affect when a goal is blocked (Berscheid, 1983). Because adults with different attachment styles have different personal and interpersonal goals, they are apt to have different emotional responses to the same event (Collins &

Read, 1994). Consistent with this idea, Collins and colleagues (2003, Study 1) asked young adults to imagine a series of potentially negative partner behaviors (e.g., "your partner left you standing alone at a party"). Results indicated that secure and insecure individuals differed in their emotional responses to these events and that these differences were mediated by the importance of the needs being violated in each event. Specifically, highly anxious individuals rated the attachment needs as more important and therefore experienced more emotional distress when their partners failed to meet these needs.

The outcome of the primary appraisal process is especially important because of its impact on further information processing. Affect has been shown to influence all aspects of information processing, including attention, memory, and social inference processes (Gilligan & Bower, 1984). Mood makes mood-congruent material more easily noticed and more easily encoded in memory (Forgas, Bower, & Krantz, 1984). Mood may also serve as information in subsequent social inference processes (Clore & Tamir, 2002), such that negative arousal may lead individuals to infer that a threat must be present. Finally, high levels of arousal may have a general effect on information processing by restricting cognitive resources (Kihlstrom, 1981; Kim & Baron, 1988; Sarason, 1975). As a result, intense affective reactions may lead individuals to rely on overlearned schemas at the expense of conducting more controlled and effortful processing of information. Although these processes have not been directly investigated in the domain of attachment, two studies suggest that attachment-related anxiety may interfere with information processing. Miller and Noirot (1999) found that, when participants were asked to write about a rejecting (versus a supportive) friendship experience, fearful avoidance was associated with impaired performance on a subsequent cognitive task. In a second study, Miller (1996) found that a rejection prime interfered with anxious adults' ability to effectively solve social problems. These studies provide preliminary evidence that the activation of chronic worries about rejection (for fearful and anxious–ambivalent adults) can interfere with subsequent information processing in both social and nonsocial domains.

Secondary Appraisal

A person's initial emotional response to an event can be either maintained, amplified, or altered depending on how the experience is subsequently interpreted (Lazarus & Folkman, 1984; Weiner, 1986). Collins and Read (1994) suggest that people respond to attachment experiences not just on the basis of whether or not they like the outcome but also of what the outcome means, at a symbolic level, for themselves and their relationship (Kelley, 1984). And, because adults with different attachment styles will tend to differ in the way they interpret events, they should also differ in the way they feel in response to the same events. Consistent with this idea, Collins and her colleagues (Collins, 1996; Collins et al., 2003, Study 1) have shown that attachment-style differences in emotional responses to relationship events are mediated in part by differences in attributions. For example, anxious participants are more likely to attribute their partners' transgressions to selfish motivation and a lack of responsiveness and are therefore more likely to experience anger and emotional distress. Findings such as these suggest that anxious individuals will tend to experience greater distress in their relationships, at least in part, because they are apt to interpret their partners' behavior in more threatening ways.

Behavioral Response Patterns

Just as working models can have direct and indirect effects on affective responses, they should also have direct and indirect effects on behavior. First, working models contain a rich source of plans and action tendencies that should be automatically evoked whenever working models are activated in memory. In these circumstances, working models may guide behavior by providing ready-made plans and behavioral strategies for the attainment of attachment-related goals. These action tendencies are likely to be stored in terms of "if–then" rules (Baldwin et al., 1993; Mischel & Shoda, 1995) that specify particular behavioral strategies to be used in response to particular appraisals or environmental contingencies (e.g., *if* stressed, *then* seek support; *if* hurt, *then* seek emotional distance). As a result, once a social situation is appraised, a person's behavioral response may be overdetermined. This response may be especially likely to occur under conditions of high stress and arousal, when processing capacity is limited. Evidence suggests that under such conditions, individuals may rely on readily accessible, overlearned strategies and behavioral scripts (Clark & Isen, 1982; Ellis, Thomas, & Rodriguez, 1984; Kihlstrom, 1981).

The idea that behavioral strategies can be automatically evoked by particular appraisals raises the possibility that the mere activation of an attachment model is sufficient for eliciting a behavioral response, without having to posit an intervening cognitive and emotional mediator. To be sure, some situations are so familiar, and some behaviors so overlearned, that behavioral responses can be elicited by particular features of the environment alone (Bargh, Chen, & Burrows, 1996; Bowlby, 1980). This may be especially likely to occur in long-term relationships for which people have highly elaborate and strongly held relational schemas. Although this idea has not been tested in the attachment domain, research in the broader social-cognition literature provides evidence that the activation of relational schemas can automatically elicit interpersonal goals and goal-directed behavioral responses. In a series of studies, Shah (2003) explored how activation of relationship-specific schemas (significant-other representations) may automatically direct individuals toward some goals and away from others. After being subliminally primed with the name of a significant other (e.g., mother, father, best friend), participants were more committed to the goals linked to that significant other, persisted at a goal-relevant task longer, performed better at the task, and were better able to inhibit competing goals. Along similar lines, Fitzsimons and Bargh (2003) showed that activation of significant-other representations automatically activated goal-directed behavior. For example, after imagining a close friend—which was normatively shown to be linked to prosocial goals—participants were more willing to help a stranger than when they imagined a coworker. These studies offer compelling evidence that the activation of relationship-specific schemas can automatically evoke goals and action tendencies and that these processes occur outside of awareness. It seems reasonable to assume that working models of attachment will operate in a similar fashion such that, under some conditions, goal-directed behavior may be automatically evoked when working models are activated in memory. This remains an important topic for future research.

In addition to these direct effects, working models should also have indirect effects on behavior by shaping cognitive and emotional responses. Consistent with this idea, Collins and her colleagues (Collins, 1996; Collins et al., 2003) have shown that secure and insecure adults behave differently in their relationships *because* they tend to think and feel differently in response to relationship events. In three studies, the relationship between attachment style and behavioral responses to partner transgressions was mediated by attributions and emotions. For example, highly anxious individuals endorsed more relationship-threatening attributions for their partners' behavior and responded to these transgressions with greater emotional distress; these attributions and emotional responses then strongly predicted their tendency to engage in more hostile and punishing behavior.

Emerging Themes Concerning the Function of Working Models

The existing literature provides initial evidence that working models of attachment play an important role in guiding cognitive, affective, and behavioral response patterns in attachment-relevant contexts. Nevertheless, as the preceding review indicates, there are a number of untested assumptions concerning the fundamental role of working models in shaping the manner in which the attachment system is expressed in adulthood, and there are many gaps in our knowledge of specific mechanisms. We need not reiterate these missing links. Instead, we conclude by highlighting several trends in the literature that are especially noteworthy. First, attachment scholars are beginning to investigate the joint role of cognitive and motivational processes (e.g., Collins et al., 2003; Fraley et al., 2000), which should lie at the heart of attachment dynamics. Second, in line with contemporary models of personality (e.g., Mischel & Shoda, 1995), there is increased awareness of the need to study individual differences in terms of stable person × situation interactions (e.g., Collins & Feeney, in press; Mikulincer et al., 1998). Third, the use of priming techniques and other methods of manipulating attachment representations in the lab provide critical opportunities for testing the causal role of working models in shaping important personal and interpersonal outcomes (e.g., Rowe & Carnelley, 2003). Finally, there is growing interest in normative processes, as well as in individual differences in attachment style (e.g., Mikulincer et al., 2001, 2002).

CONCLUDING COMMENTS

As we have highlighted throughout this chapter, individuals enter their relationships with a rich network of representations that shape how they construct their lives and find meaning in their personal and interpersonal experiences. Attachment theory provides an ideal framework for understanding how close relationships in adulthood may be shaped by a long history of social and emotional experiences that precede such relationships. Attachment scholars have made tremendous progress in uncovering the content and function of working models, but much remains to be discovered about the precise mechanisms through which they shape personal and interpersonal experiences across the lifespan. Our goal in this chapter was to contribute to this effort by encouraging attachment researchers to think about working models in a more precise and systematic way, by highlighting emerging themes and trends in the literature, and by stimulating thoughtful research on the topic and continued theoretical refinement.

ACKNOWLEDGMENTS

Preparation of this chapter was supported by National Science Foundation Grant No. SBR–0096506 to Nancy Collins, by National Institute of Mental Health Grant No. MH–066119 to Brooke Feeney, and by National Science Foundation Predoctoral Fellowship to Maire Ford.

REFERENCES

Ainsworth, M. D. S., Blehar, M. C., Waters, E., & Wall, S. (1978). *Patterns of attachment: A psychological study of the Strange Situation.* Hillsdale, NJ: Erlbaum.
Andersen, S. M., & Baum, A. (1994). Transference in interpersonal relations: In-

ferences and affect based on significant-other representations. *Journal of Personality, 62,* 459–497.

Andersen, S. M., & Chen, S. (2002). The relational self: An interpersonal social-cognitive theory. *Psychological Review, 109,* 619–645.

Baldwin, M. W. (1992). Relational schemas and the processing of social information. *Psychological Bulletin, 112,* 461–484.

Baldwin, M. W., Fehr, B., Keedian, E., Seidel, M., & Thomson, D. W. (1993). An exploration of the relational schemata underlying attachment styles: Self-report and lexical decision approaches. *Personality and Social Psychology Bulletin, 19,* 746–754.

Baldwin, M. W., & Kay, A. C. (2003). Adult attachment and the inhibition of rejection. *Journal of Social and Clinical Psychology, 22,* 275–293.

Baldwin, M. W., Keelan, J. P. R., Fehr, B., Enns, V., & Koh-Rangarajoo, E. (1996). Social-cognitive conceptualization of attachment working models: Availability and accessibility effects. *Journal of Personality and Social Psychology, 71,* 94–109.

Baldwin, M. W., & Meunier, J. (1999). The cued activation of attachment relational schemas. *Social Cognition, 17,* 209–227.

Bargh, J. A. (1984). Automatic and conscious processing of social information. In R. S. Wyer & T. K. Srull (Eds.), *Handbook of social cognition* (Vol. 3, pp. 1–44). Hillsdale, NJ: Erlbaum.

Bargh, J. A. (1997). The automaticity of everyday life. In R. S. Wyer, Jr. (Ed.), *Advances in social cognition* (Vol. 10, pp. 1–61). Mahwah, NJ: Erlbaum.

Bargh, J. A., Chen, M., & Burrows, L. (1996). Automaticity of social behavior: Direct effects of trait construct and stereotype activation on action. *Journal of Personality and Social Psychology, 71,* 230–244.

Bartholomew, K., & Horowitz, L. M. (1991). Attachment styles among young adults: A test of a four-category model. *Journal of Personality and Social Psychology, 61,* 226–244.

Berscheid, E. (1983). Emotion. In H. H. Kelley, E. Berscheid, A. Christensen, J. Harvey, T. Huston, G. Levinger, E. McClintock, L. A. Peplau, & D. Peterson (Eds.), *Close relationships* (pp. 110–168). San Francisco: Freeman.

Berscheid, E. (1994). Interpersonal relationships. *Annual Review of Psychology, 45,* 79–129.

Bowlby, J. (1973). *Attachment and loss: Vol. 2. Separation: Anxiety and anger.* New York: Basic Books.

Bowlby, J. (1979). *The making and breaking of affectional bonds.* London: Tavistock.

Bowlby, J. (1980). *Attachment and loss: Vol. 3. Loss: Sadness and depression.* New York: Basic Books.

Brennan, K. A., & Bosson, J. K. (1998). Attachment-style differences in attitudes toward and reactions to feedback from romantic partners: An exploration of the relational bases of self-esteem. *Personality and Social Psychology Bulletin, 24,* 699–714.

Brennan, K. A., Clark, C. L., & Shaver, P. R. (1998). Self-report measurement of adult attachment: An integrative overview. In J. A. Simpson & W. S. Rholes (Eds.), *Attachment theory and close relationships* (pp. 46–76). New York: Guilford Press.

Brennan, K. A., & Morris, K. A. (1997). Attachment styles, self-esteem, and patterns of seeking feedback from romantic partners. *Personality and Social Psychology Bulletin, 23,* 23–31.

Bretherton, I. (1985). Attachment theory: Retrospect and prospect. *Monographs of the Society for Research in Child Development, 50,* 3–35.

Bretherton, I., Biringen, Z., Ridgeway, D., Maslin, C., & Sherman, M. (1989). Attachment: The parental perspective. *Infant Mental Health Journal, 10,* 203–221.

Bretherton, I., & Munholland, K. A. (1999). Internal working models in attachment relationships: A construct revisited. In J. Cassidy & P. R. Shaver (Eds.), *Handbook of attachment: Theory, research, and clinical applications* (pp. 89–111). New York: Guilford Press.

Clark, M. S., & Isen, A. M. (1982). Toward understanding the relationship between feeling states and social behavior. In A. Hastorf & A. Isen (Eds.), *Cognitive social psychology* (pp. 73–108). New York: Elsevier North-Holland.

Clore, G. L., & Tamir, M. (2002). Affect as embodied information. *Psychological Inquiry, 13,* 37–45.

Collins, N. L. (1996). Working models of attachment: Implications for explanation, emotion, and behavior. *Journal of Personality and Social Psychology, 71,* 810–832.

Collins, N. L., & Allard, L. M. (2001). Cognitive representations of attachment: The content and function of working models. In G. J. O. Fletcher & M. S. Clark (Eds.), *Blackwell handbook of social psychology: Vol. 2. Interpersonal processes* (pp. 60–85). Oxford, UK: Blackwell.

Collins, N. L., & Feeney, B. C. (2000). A safe haven: An attachment theory perspective on support seeking and caregiving in intimate relationships. *Journal of Personality and Social Psychology, 78,* 1053–1073.

Collins, N. L., & Feeney, B. C. (2004). An attachment theory perspective on closeness and intimacy. In D. Mashek & A. Aron (Eds.), *Handbook of closeness and intimacy* (pp. 163–187). Mahwah, NJ: Erlbaum.

Collins, N. L., & Feeney, B. C. (in press). Working models of attachment shape perceptions of social support: Evidence from experimental and observational studies. *Journal of Personality and Social Psychology.*

Collins, N. L., Ford, M. B., Guichard, A., & Allard, L. M. (2003). *Working models of attachment and social construal processes in romantic relationships.* Manuscript submitted for publication, University of California at Santa Barbara.

Collins, N. L., & Read, S. J. (1990). Adult attachment, working models, and relationship quality in dating couples. *Journal of Personality and Social Psychology, 58,* 644–663.

Collins, N. L., & Read, S. J. (1994). Cognitive representations of attachment: The structure and function of working models. In K. Bartholomew & D. Perlman (Eds.), *Advances in personal relationships: Vol. 5. Attachment processes in adulthood* (pp. 53–90). London: Kingsley.

Cook, W. L. (2000). Understanding attachment security in family context. *Journal of Personality and Social Psychology, 78,* 285–294.

Cozzarelli, C., Hoekstra, S. J., & Bylsma, W. H. (2000). Gerneral versus specific mental models of attachment: Are they associated with different outcomes? *Personality and Social Psychology Bulletin, 26,* 605–618.

Crittenden, P. M. (1990). Internal representational models of attachment relationships. *Infant Mental Health Journal, 11,* 259–277.

Crocker, J., & Wolfe, C. T. (2001). Contingencies of self-worth. *Psychological Review, 108,* 593–623.

Crowell, J. A, Fraley, R. C., & Shaver, P. R. (1999). Measurement of individual differences in adolescent and adult attachment. In J. Cassidy & P. R. Shaver (Eds.), *Handbook of attachment: Theory, research, and clinical applications* (pp. 434–465). New York: Guilford Press.

Crowell, J. A., & Owens, G. (1996). *Current Relationship Interview and scoring system.* Unpublished manuscript, State University of New York at Stony Brook.

Elliot, A. J., & Reis, H. T. (2003). Attachment and exploration in adulthood. *Journal of Personality and Social Psychology, 85,* 317–331.

Ellis, H. C., Thomas, R. L., & Rodriguez, I. A. (1984). Emotional mood states and memory: Elaborative encoding, semantic processing, and cognitive effort. *Journal of Experimental Psychology: Learning, Memory, and Cognition, 10,* 470–482.

Fazio, R. H., & Williams, C. J. (1986). Attitude accessibility as a moderator of the attitude-perception and attitude-behavior relations: An investigation of the 1984 presidential election. *Journal of Personality and Social Psychology, 51,* 505–514.

Feeney, B. C., & Cassidy, J. (2003). Reconstructive memory related to adolescent–parent conflict interactions: The influence of attachment-related representations on immediate perceptions and changes in perceptions over time. *Journal of Personality and Social Psychology, 85,* 945–955.

Feeney, B. C., & Collins, N. L. (2001). Predictors of caregiving in adult intimate relationships: An attachment theoretical perspective. *Journal of Personality and Social Psychology, 80,* 972–994.

Feeney, B. C., & Collins, N. L. (2003). Motivations for caregiving in adult intimate relationships: Influences on caregiving behavior and relationship functioning. *Personality and Social Psychology Bulletin, 29,* 950–968.

Feeney, J. A. (1999a). Adult romantic attachment and couple relationships. In J. Cassidy & P. R. Shaver (Eds.), *Handbook of attachment: Theory, research, and clinical applications* (pp. 355–377). New York: Guilford Press.

Feeney, J. A. (1999b). Issues of closeness and distance in dating relationships: Effects of sex and attachment style. *Journal of Social and Personal Relationships, 16,* 571–590.

Feeney, J. A., & Noller, P. (1990). Attachment style as a predictor of adult romantic relationships. *Journal of Personality and Social Psychology, 58,* 281–291.

Feeney, J. A., Noller, P., & Callan, V. J. (1994). Attachment style, communication and satisfaction in the early years of marriage. In K. Bartholomew & D. Perlman (Eds.), *Advances in personal relationships: Vol. 5. Attachment processes in adulthood* (pp. 269–308). London: Kingsley.

Fincham, F. D., Garnier, P. C., Gano-Phillips, S., & Osborne, L. N. (1995). Preinteraction expectations, marital satisfaction, and accessibility: A new look at sentiment override. *Journal of Family Psychology, 9,* 3–14.

Fishtein, J., Pietromonaco, P. R., & Feldman Barrett, L. (1999). The contribution of attachment style and relationship conflict to the complexity of relationship knowledge. *Social Cognition, 17,* 228–244.

Fiske, S. T., & Pavelchak, M. A. (1986). Category-based versus piecemeal-based affective responses: Developments in schema-triggered affect. In R. M.

Sorrentino & E. T. Higgins (Eds.), *Handbook of motivation and cognition: Foundations of social behavior* (pp. 167–203). New York: Guilford Press.

Fitzsimons, G. M., & Bargh, J. A. (2003). Thinking of you: Nonconscious pursuit of interpersonal goals associated with relationship partners. *Journal of Personality and Social Psychology, 84,* 148–163.

Forgas, J. P., Bower, G. H., & Krantz, S. E. (1984). The influence of mood on perceptions of social interactions. *Journal of Experimental Social Psychology, 20,* 497–513.

Fraley, R. C., Davis, K. E., & Shaver, P. R. (1998). Dismissing-avoidance and the defensive organization of emotion, cognition, and behavior. In J. A. Simpson & W. S. Rholes (Eds.), *Attachment theory and close relationships* (pp. 249–279). New York: Guilford Press.

Fraley, R. C., Garner, J. P., & Shaver, P. R. (2000). Adult attachment and the defensive regulation of attention and memory: Examining the role of preemptive and postemptive defensive processes. *Journal of Personality and Social Psychology, 79,* 816–826.

Fraley, R. C., & Shaver, P. R. (1997). Adult attachment and the suppression of unwanted thoughts. *Journal of Personality and Social Psychology, 73,* 1080–1091.

Fraley, R. C., & Shaver, P. R. (1998). Airport separations: A naturalistic study of adult attachment dynamics in separating couples. *Journal of Personality and Social Psychology, 75,* 1198–1212.

Fraley, R. C., & Waller, N. G. (1998). Adult attachment patterns: A test of the typological model. In J. A. Simpson & W. S. Rholes (Eds.), *Attachment theory and close relationships* (pp. 77–114). New York: Guilford Press.

Gallo, L. C., & Smith, T. W. (2001). Attachment style in marriage: Adjustment and responses to interaction. *Journal of Social and Personal Relationships, 18*(2), 263–289.

George, C., Kaplan, N., & Main, M. (1984). *Attachment Interview for Adults.* Unpublished manuscript, University of California, Berkeley.

George, C., & Solomon, J. (1999). Attachment and caregiving: The caregiving behavioral system. In J. Cassidy & P. R. Shaver (Eds.), *Handbook of attachment: Theory, research, and clinical applications* (pp. 649–670). New York: Guilford Press.

Gilligan, S. G., & Bower, G. H. (1984). Cognitive consequences of emotional arousal. In C. E. Izard, J. Kagan, & R. B. Zajonc (Eds.), *Emotions, cognition, and behavior* (pp. 547–588). Cambridge, UK: Cambridge University Press.

Graesser, A. C., & Nakamura, G. V. (1982). The impact of a schema on comprehension and memory. In G. H. Bower (Ed.), *The psychology of learning and motivation* (Vol. 16, pp. 60–109). New York: Academic Press.

Gray, J. A. (1987). *The psychology of fear and stress* (2nd ed.). New York: Cambridge University Press.

Green-Hennessy, S., & Reis, H. T. (1998). Openness in processing social information among attachment types. *Personal Relationships, 5,* 449–466.

Greenwald, A. G., & Banaji, M. R. (1995). Implicit social cognition: Attitudes, self-esteem, and stereotypes. *Psychological Review, 102,* 4–27.

Greenwald, A. G., McGhee, D. E., & Schwartz, J. L. K. (1998). Measuring individual differences in implicit cognition: The implicit association test. *Journal of Personality and Social Psychology, 74,* 1464–1480.

Griffin, D. W., & Bartholomew, K. (1994). Models of the self and other: Fundamental dimensions underlying measures of adult attachment. *Journal of Personality and Social Psychology, 67,* 430–445.

Hazan, C., & Shaver, P. (1987). Romantic love conceptualized as an attachment process. *Journal of Personality and Social Psychology, 52,* 511–524.

Hazan, C., & Shaver, P. (1990). Love and work: An attachment-theoretical perspective. *Journal of Personality and Social Psychology, 59,* 270–280.

Higgins, E. T., King, G. A., & Mavin, G. H. (1982). Individual construct accessibility and subjective impressions and recall. *Journal of Personality and Social Psychology, 43,* 35–47.

Holmes, J. G. (2002). Interpersonal expectations as the building blocks of social cognition: An interdependence theory perspective. *Personal Relationships, 9,* 1–26.

Holmes, J. G., & Rempel, J. K. (1989). Trust in close relationships. In C. Hendrick (Ed.), *Review of personality and social psychology: Vol. 10. Close relationships* (pp. 187–220). London: Sage.

Kelley, H. II. (1984). Affect in interpersonal relations. In. P. Shaver (Ed.), *Review of personality and social psychology* (Vol. 5, pp. 89–115). Beverly Hills, CA: Sage.

Kernis, M. H., & Waschull, S. B. (1995). The interactive roles of stability and level of self-esteem: Research and theory. In M. P. Zanna (Ed.), *Advances in experimental social psychology* (Vol. 27, pp. 93–141). San Diego, CA: Academic Press.

Kihlstrom, J. F. (1981). On personality and memory. In N. Cantor & J. Kihlstrom (Eds.), *Personality, cognition, and social interaction* (pp. 123–149). Hillsdale, NJ: Erlbaum.

Kim, H., & Baron, R. S. (1988). Exercise and the illusory correlation: Does arousal heighten stereotypic processing? *Journal of Experimental Social Psychology, 24,* 366–380.

Klein, S. B., Babey, S. H., & Sherman, J. W. (1997). The functional independence of trait and behavioral self-knowledge: Methodological considerations and new empirical findings. *Social Cognition, 15,* 183–203.

Kobak, R. R., & Hazan, C. (1991). Attachment in marriage: The effects of security and accuracy of working models. *Journal of Personality and Social Psychology, 60,* 861–869.

Kobak, R. R., & Sceery, A. (1988). Attachment in late adolescence: Working models, affect regulation, and representations of self and others. *Child Development, 59,* 135–146.

La Guardia, J. G., Ryan, R. M., Couchman, C. E, & Deci, E. L. (2000). Within-person variation in security of attachment: A self-determination theory perspective on attachment, need fulfillment, and well-being. *Journal of Personality and Social Psychology, 79,* 367–384.

Lazarus, R. S., & Folkman, S. (1984). *Stress, appraisal, and coping.* New York: Springer.

Main, M. (1981). Avoidance in the service of attachment: A working paper. In K. Immelmann, G. Barlow, L. Petrinovich, & M. Main (Eds.), *Behavioral development: The Bielefeld interdisciplinary project* (pp. 651–693). New York: Cambridge University Press.

Main, M. (1991). Metacognitive knowledge, metacognitive monitoring, and singular (coherent) vs. multiple (incoherent) model of attachment: Findings and directions for future research. In C. M. Parkes, J. Stevenson-Hinde, & P. Marris (Eds.), *Attachment across the life cycle* (pp. 127–159). London: Tavistock/Routledge.

Main, M., Kaplan, N., & Cassidy, J. (1985). Security in infancy, childhood, and adulthood: A move to the level of representation. *Monographs of the Society for Research in Child Development, 50*(1 & 2, Serial No. 209), 66–104.

Mikulincer, M. (1995). Attachment style and the mental representation of the self. *Journal of Personality and Social Psychology, 69,* 1203–1215.

Mikulincer, M. (1997). Adult attachment style and information processing: Individual differences in curiosity and cognitive closure. *Journal of Personality and Social Psychology, 72,* 1217–1230.

Mikulincer, M. (1998a). Adult attachment style and affect regulation: Strategic variations in self-appraisals. *Journal of Personality and Social Psychology, 75,* 420–435.

Mikulincer, M. (1998b). Attachment working models and the sense of trust: An exploration of interaction goals and affect regulation. *Journal of Personality and Social Psychology, 74,* 1209–1224.

Mikulincer, M., & Arad, D. (1999). Attachment working models and cognitive openness in close relationships: A test of chronic and temporary accessibility effects. *Journal of Personality and Social Psychology, 77,* 710–725.

Mikulincer, M., Gillath, O., & Shaver, P. R. (2002). Activation of the attachment system in adulthood: Threat-related primes increase the accessibility of mental representations of attachment figures. *Journal of Personality and Social Psychology, 83,* 881–895.

Mikulincer, M., Hirschberger, G., Nachmias, O., & Gillath, O. (2001). The affective component of the secure base schema: Affective priming with representations of attachment security. *Journal of Personality and Social Psychology, 81,* 305–321.

Mikulincer, M., & Horesh, N. (1999). Adult attachment style and the perception of others: The role of projective mechanisms. *Journal of Personality and Social Psychology, 76,* 1022–1034.

Mikulincer, M., & Nachshon, O. (1991). Attachment styles and patterns of self-disclosure. *Journal of Personality and Social Psychology, 61,* 321–331.

Mikulincer, M., & Orbach, I. (1995). Attachment styles and repressive defensiveness: The accessibility and architecture of affective memories. *Journal of Personality and Social Psychology, 68,* 917–925.

Mikulincer, M., Orbach, I., & Iavnieli, D. (1998). Adult attachment style and affect regulation: Strategic variations in subjective self–other similarity. *Journal of Personality and Social Psychology, 75,* 436–448.

Miller, J. B. (1996). Social flexibility and anxious attachment. *Personal Relationships, 3,* 241–256.

Miller, J. B. (2001). Attachment models and memory for conversation. *Journal of Social and Personal Relationships, 18,* 404–422.

Miller, J. B., & Noirot, M. (1999). Attachment memories, models and information processing. *Journal of Social and Personal Relationships, 16,* 147–173.

Mischel, W., & Shoda, Y. (1995). A cognitive-affective system theory of personality: Reconceptualizing situations, dispositions, dynamics, and invariance in personality structure. *Psychological Review, 102,* 246–268.

Moretti, M. M., & Higgins, E. T. (1999). Own versus other standpoints in self-regulation: Developmental antecedents and functional consequences. *Review of General Psychology, 3,* 188–223.

Murray, S. L., & Holmes, J. G. (1999). The (mental) ties that bind: Cognitive structures that predict relationship resilience. *Journal of Personality and Social Psychology, 77,* 1228–1244.

Murray, S. L., Holmes, J. G., & Griffin, D. W. (1996). The self-fulfilling nature of positive illusions in romantic relationships: Love is not blind, but prescient. *Journal of Personality and Social Psychology, 71,* 1155–1180.

Murray, S. L., Holmes, J. G., Griffin, D. W., Bellavia, G., & Rose, P. (2001). The mismeasure of love: How self-doubt contaminates relationship beliefs. *Personality and Social Psychology Bulletin, 27,* 423–436.

Niedenthal, P. M., Brauer, M., Robin, L., & Innes-Ker, A.H. (2002). Adult attachment and the perception of facial expression of emotion. *Journal of Personality and Social Psychology, 82,* 419–433.

Ognibene, T. C., & Collins, N. L. (1998). Adult attachment styles, perceived social support, and coping strategies. *Journal of Social and Personal Relationships, 15,* 323–345.

Overall, N. C., Fletcher, G. J. O., & Friesen, M. D. (2003). Mapping the intimate relationship mind: Comparisons between three models of attachment representations. *Personality and Social Psychology Bulletin, 29,* 1479–1493.

Pierce, T., & Lydon, J. (1998). Priming relational schemas: Effects of contextually activated and chronically accessible interpersonal expectations on responses to a stressful event. *Journal of Personality and Social Psychology, 75,* 1441–1448.

Pierce, T., & Lydon, J. E. (2001). Global and specific relational models in the experience of social interactions. *Journal of Personality and Social Psychology, 80,* 613–631.

Pietromonaco, P. R., & Feldman Barrett, L. (1997). Working models of attachment and daily social interactions. *Journal of Personality and Social Psychology, 73,* 1409–1423.

Pietromonaco, P. R., & Feldman Barrett, L. (2000). The internal working models concept: What do we really know about the self in relation to others? *Review of General Psychology, 4,* 155–175.

Rholes, W. S., Simpson, J. A., Campbell, L., & Grich, J. (2001). Adult attachment and the transition to parenthood. *Journal of Personality and Social Psychology, 81,* 421–435.

Roskos-Ewoldsen, D. R., & Fazio, R. H. (1992). On the orienting value of attitudes: Attitude accessibility as a determinant of an object's attraction to visual attention. *Journal of Personality and Social Psychology, 63,* 198–211.

Rothbard, J. C., & Shaver, P. R. (1994). Continuity of attachment across the life span. In M. B. Sperling and W. H. Berman (Eds.), *Attachment in adults: Clinical and developmental perspectives* (pp. 31–71). New York: Guilford Press.

Rowe, A., & Carnelley, K. B. (2003). Attachment style differences in the processing of attachment-relevant information: Primed-style effects on recall, interpersonal expectations, and affect. *Personal Relationships, 10,* 59–75.

Sarason, I. G. (1975). Anxiety and self-preoccupation. In I. G. Sarason & C. D. Spielberger (Eds.), *Stress and anxiety* (Vol. 2, pp. 27–44). New York: Wiley.

Shah, J. (2003). Automatic for the people: How representations of significant others implicitly affect goal pursuit. *Journal of Personality and Social Psychology, 84,* 661–681.

Shaver, P. R., Belsky, J., & Brennan, K. A. (2000). The Adult Attachment Interview and self-reports of romantic attachment: Associations across domains and methods. *Personal Relationships, 7,* 25–43.

Shaver, P. R., & Clark, C. L. (1996). Forms of adult romantic attachment and their cognitive and emotional underpinnings. In G. G. Noam & K. W. Fischer (Eds.), *Development and vulnerability in close relationships* (pp. 29–58). Mahwah, NJ: Erlbaum.

Shaver, P. R., Collins, N. L., & Clark, C. L. (1996). Attachment styles and internal working models of self and relationship partners. In G. J. O. Fletcher & J. Fitness (Eds.), *Knowledge structures in close relationships: A social psychological approach* (pp. 25–61). Mahwah, NJ: Erlbaum.

Showers, C. J., & Kevlyn, S. B. (1999). Organization of knowledge about a relationship partner: Implications for liking and loving. *Journal of Personality and Social Psychology, 76,* 958–971.

Simpson, J. A., Ickes, W., & Grich, J. (1999). When accuracy hurts: Reactions of anxious–ambivalent dating partners to a relationship-threatening situation. *Journal of Personality and Social Psychology, 76,* 754–769.

Simpson, J. A., Rholes, W. S., Campbell, L., Tran, S., & Wilson, C. L. (2003). Adult attachment, the transition to parenthood, and depressive symptoms. *Journal of Personality and Social Psychology, 84,* 1172–1187.

Simpson, J. A., Rholes, W. S., Campbell, L., & Wilson, C. L. (2003). Changes in attachment orientations across the transitions to parenthood. *Journal of Experimental Social Psychology, 39,* 317–331.

Simpson, J. A., Rholes, W. S., & Nelligan, J. S. (1992). Support seeking and support giving within couples in an anxiety-provoking situation: The role of attachment styles. *Journal of Personality and Social Psychology, 62,* 434–446.

Simpson, J. A., Rholes, W. S., Orina, M. M., & Grich, J. (2002). Working models of attachment, support giving, and support seeking in a stressful situation. *Personality and Social Psychology Bulletin, 28,* 598–608.

Simpson, J. A., Rholes, W. S., & Phillips, D. (1996). Conflict in close relationships: An attachment perspective. *Journal of Personality and Social Psychology, 71,* 899–914 .

Spalding, L. R., & Hardin, C. D. (1999). Unconscious unease and self-handicapping: Behavioral consequences of individual differences in implicit and explicit self-esteem. *Psychological Science, 10,* 535–539.

Sroufe, L. A., & Waters, E. (1977). Attachment as an organizational construct. *Child Development, 48,* 1184–1199.

Srull, T. K., & Wyer, R. S., Jr. (1986). The role of chronic and temporary goals in social information processing. In R. M. Sorrentino & E. T. Higgins (Eds.), *Handbook of motivation and cognition: Foundations of social behavior* (pp. 503–549). New York: Guilford Press.

Tooby, J., & Cosmides, L. (1996). Friendship and the banker's paradox: Other pathways to the evolution of adaptations for altruism. *Proceedings of the British Academy, 88,* 119–143.

Trinke, S. J., & Bartholomew, K. (1997). Hierarchies of attachment relationships in young adulthood. *Journal of Social and Personal Relationships, 14,* 603–625.

Wais, D., Treboux, D., & Waters, H. S. (2003, April). *Current relationships attachment scripts: Correlates and partner-specific contributions.* Paper presented at the conference of the Society for Research in Child Development, Tampa, FL. Retrieved November 10, 2003, from *http://www.psychology.sunysb.edu/attachment/srcd2003/srcd2003.htm*

Waters, E. (2003, April). *Script-like representations of secure base experience: Evidence of cross-age, cross-cultural, and behavioral links.* Paper presented at the conference of the Society for Research in Child Development, Tampa, FL. Retrieved November 10, 2003, from *http://www.psychology.sunysb.edu/attachment/srcd2003/srcd2003.htm*

Waters, H. S., & Rodrigues-Doolabh, L.M. (2001, April). *Are attachment scripts the building blocks of attachment representations? Narrative assessment of representations and the AAI.* Paper presented at the meeting of the Society for Research in Child Development, Minneapolis, MN. Retrieved November 10, 2003, from *http://www.psychology.sunysb.edu/attachment/ srcd2001/HSWScripts/index.htm*

Weiner, B. (1986). Attribution, emotion, and action. In R. M. Sorrentino & E. T. Higgins (Eds.), *Handbook of motivation and cognition: Foundations of social behavior* (pp. 281–312). New York: Guilford Press.

Whitaker, D. J., Beach, S. R. H., Etherton, J., Wakefield, R., & Anderson, P. L. (1999). Attachment and expectations about future relationships: Moderation by accessibility. *Personal Relationships, 6,* 41–56.

Wieselquist, J., Rusbult, C. E., Foster, C. A., & Agnew, C. R. (1999). Commitment, pro-relationship behavior, and trust in close relationships. *Journal of Personality and Social Psychology, 77,* 942–966.

Zayas, V. (2003). *Personality in context: An interpersonal systems perspective.* Unpublished doctoral dissertation, University of Washington.

Zhang, F., & Hazan, C. (2002). Working models of attachment and person perception processes. *Personal Relationships, 9,* 225–235.

CHAPTER 8

Psychobiological Perspectives on Attachment

Implications for Health over the Lifespan

LISA M. DIAMOND
ANGELA M. HICKS

One of the most robust findings to emerge from health psychology over the past 30 years is that individuals in enduring, committed romantic relationships have longer, healthier, and happier lives than unmarried individuals (Kitigawa & Hauser, 1973; Ryff, Singer, Wing, & Love, 2001; Stack & Eshleman, 1998). This effect cannot be attributed to overall social integration, given that individuals' *most intimate* relationships appear to promote health and well-being above and beyond generalized social support (Ryff et al., 2001). Rather, the key variable appears to be the existence of an enduring, emotionally intimate affectional bond (Ross, 1995).

According to attachment theory, feelings of security derived from such bonds play critical roles in regulating our positive and negative emotional responses to internal and external stimuli (Porges, Doussard-Roosevelt, & Maiti, 1994). Because such emotional experiences are directly linked to multiple physiological processes underlying health and disease (Kiecolt Glaser, McGuire, Robles, & Glaser, 2002; Repetti, Taylor, & Seeman, 2002; Ryff et al., 2001), this suggests that attachment relationships—at all stages of life—critically influence physical, as well as psychological, functioning. In this chapter, we review research linking attachment phenomena to specific biological systems and processes that have direct implications for health and well-being over the lifespan.

BOWLBY AND THE PSYCHOBIOLOGY OF ATTACHMENT

Bowlby conceptualized attachment as a fundamentally psychobiological system, especially with regard to its emotion-regulating functions. Specifically, he posited two different "rings" of homeostasis that assist the individual in responding to major and minor stressors (Bowlby, 1973). The inner ring comprises life-maintaining biological systems that govern ongoing physiological adaptation to external demands. The outer ring comprises behavioral (and particularly, interpersonal) strategies for coping and adaptation. From Bowlby's perspective, the integrated functioning of these two levels is critical for optimal self-regulation.

This idea is consistent with extensive research on infants, children, and adults that demonstrates that, in order to understand the mechanisms through which social relationships shape emotional functioning across the lifespan, we must investigate biological, as well as psychological–behavioral, processes of emotion regulation (Repetti et al., 2002; Ryff et al., 2001; Taylor, Dickerson, & Klein, 2002). Such research has taken place across a range of different disciplines, employing divergent methods and aims, and yet the findings are remarkably consistent: Attachment-related processes—specifically, nurturance, caregiving, and support from emotionally primary relationships—fundamentally influence mental and physical functioning over the life course. When viewed collectively, we believe that this body of research indicates two independent (but interacting) pathways through which attachment influences physical health:

1. In infancy, early caregiving experiences establish enduring expectations and orientations regarding attachment figures and also "tune" the brain's sensitivity to stress, predisposing insecurely attached individuals to ineffective physiological and emotional regulation (i.e., ineffective mobilization and management of attentional and metabolic resources in response to environmental demands) and thus poorer long-term health.
2. From childhood to adulthood, attachment-related expectations and experiences shape individuals' cognitive, affective, and behavioral responses to environmental events and their willingness and ability to derive comfort and support from close social ties. As a result, insecurely attached individuals experience higher and more sustained levels of negative affect and lower levels of positive affect, which subsequently influence their long-term health through multiple biobehavioral pathways.

We posit that the joint functioning of these pathways explains the increasing—but as yet undertheorized—body of empirical findings linking attachment insecurity to health-related outcomes such as increased symptom reports and health complaints (reviewed in Feeney, 2000). Both of the aforementioned pathways posit that such links are mediated by emotion-related processes, and thus we begin by outlining the basis for this perspective.

EMOTIONS AS THE LINK BETWEEN ATTACHMENT AND HEALTH

As noted by Mikulincer and Florian (1998), although attachment theory has historically been viewed as a theory of interpersonal functioning, Bowlby (1973) placed considerable emphasis on the role of the attachment system in governing *overall* responses to danger and threat. This is reflected in the increasing attention paid by attachment researchers to the distress-alleviation and emotion-regulation functions of attachment (Feeney, 1995; Mikulincer & Florian, 1998; Mikulincer & Sheffi, 2000; Rholes, Simpson, & Orina, 1999). Specifically, regular contact with a supportive, secure attachment figure is theorized to help individuals sustain positive affect and attenuate negative affect on a day-to-day basis (reviewed in Diamond, 2001).

Individual differences in both infant (Ainsworth, Blehar, Waters, & Wall, 1978) and adult attachment style (Hazan & Shaver, 1987) have also been increasingly conceptualized as indexing different capacities and strategies for emotion regulation (reviewed in Mikulincer, Shaver, & Pereg, 2003). Briefly, infants who did not receive adequate "external" emotion regulation from their caregivers are thought to sustain developmental deficits in their "internal" self-regulatory capacities (see Glaser, 2000) and, consequently, to come to rely on secondary—and suboptimal—emotion-regulation strategies. Specifically, individuals with high attachment *anxiety* tend to maximize experiences of negative affect and to be hypervigilant to threat cues, whereas those with high attachment *avoidance* tend to minimize experiences of negative affect and to direct attention away from threat cues (Mikulincer et al., 2003). Both types of attachment insecurity are also thought to involve the inability and/or unwillingness to derive emotion-regulating benefits from contact with attachment figures (Feeney, 1999).

We address the specific consequences of these strategies in greater detail later. For now, we simply emphasize that adaptive emotional functioning lies at the heart of attachment theory's model of human health and development. Extensive research over the past 30 years has confirmed Bowlby's views in this regard. As researchers have increasingly investigated how and why social and environmental factors influence immediate and long-term health, they have collectively come to emphasize the beneficial effects of positive affectivity and the detrimental effects of negative affectivity for multiple physiological processes, particularly neuroendocrine, autonomic, and immune functioning. Because several detailed reviews of this literature are already available (Kiecolt Glaser et al., 2002; Repetti et al., 2002; Ryff & Singer, 2001; Taylor et al., 2002; Taylor, Repetti, & Seeman, 1997), we do not attempt to reiterate these findings. Rather, we highlight the specific role of attachment relationships and dynamics for health–emotion links.

Quite simply, not all emotional experiences are created equal. Multiple research reviews attest to the fact that the emotional context of one's most *intimate* and *important* relationships—parental ties in childhood and romantic ties in adulthood—has the greatest impact on both mental and physical well-being (Reis, 2001; Repetti et al., 2002; Ryff et al., 2001). This is not only because attachment relationships often precipitate some of our most intense positive and negative emotions, but also because the security we (ideally) derive from well-functioning attachments provides an organizing meta-emotional framework for the experience, interpretation, expression, and modulation of positive and negative emotions over the lifespan. Thus, although studies investigating interconnections among relationships, emotions, and health are not typically grounded in an attachment-theoretical framework, we believe that such a framework provides the most powerful and comprehensive unifying explanation for the overall pattern of "cradle-to-grave" associations among these domains.

Before we move on, it is important to note that most of the research we review focuses on negative rather than positive emotions, and particularly on psychological stress. This is not without cause, given that chronic experiences of stress, anxiety, and depression have particularly deleterious physical and mental health consequences (reviewed in Kiecolt Glaser et al., 2002; Repetti et al., 2002). However, research has increasingly focused on the important and independent effects of *positive* emotions on physical and mental functioning (Taylor et al., 2002). For example, positive emotions have been theorized to broaden individuals' thought–action repertoires and build their intrapsychic and interpersonal resources (Fredrickson, 2001), partly through facilitating creative and flexible cognition and adaptive problem solving (reviewed in Isen, 2003). Such conceptualizations have not yet been systematically integrated into attachment-theoretical perspectives on emotion regulation (with some exceptions, such as Mikulincer et al., 2003); clearly, this is a critical priority for future research.

PATHWAY 1: EARLY ATTACHMENT RELATIONSHIPS "TUNE" STRESS-REGULATORY SYSTEMS

Bowlby's lifelong inquiry into the nature of infant–caregiver bonds was prompted by his observation that orphans *deprived* of such bonds during their earliest years developed stark psychosocial deficits. Voluminous research on both animals and humans has since demonstrated that these deficits are linked to alterations in multiple neurobiological processes that appear to be "tuned" in the early years of life by normative maternal care (see Glaser, 2000; Repetti et al., 2002; Schore, 1996; Taylor et al., 2002). To briefly summarize, early infant–caregiver interactions provide for effective and reliable activation and deactivation of stress-regulatory systems in the orbitofrontal cortex that provide the foundation for effective emotion regulation. Understanding these early-developing stress-regulatory systems helps to clarify how and why *adults'* attachment experiences and histories shape their long-term health status. We focus here on those systems for which there is the greatest evidence regarding the impact of early attachment experiences.

Corticotropin-Releasing Factor

The synthesis and release of corticotropin-releasing factor (CRF) from the hypothalamus plays a critical role in mediating behavioral, emotional, autonomic, and endocrine responses to stress, and thus central CRF systems have been extensively investigated as sites for the development and expression of individual differences in stress reactivity (Francis, Caldji, Champagne, Plotsky, & Meaney, 1999; Meaney, 2001). To briefly summarize, environmental demands are processed in the central nervous system by neocortical and limbic centers, and in response the hypothalamus releases CRF and vasopressin into the anterior pituitary, stimulating synthesis and release of adrenocorticotropin (ACTH). This triggers the immediate release of catecholamines (epinephrine and norepinephrine) and subsequent release of adrenal glucocorticoids (most notably, cortisol). The catecholamines and glucocorticoids operate in concert to increase blood glucose levels and influence the specific type, magnitude, and duration of immunological response to environmental demands.

Importantly, increasing levels of glucocorticoids eventually feed back to inhibit CRF synthesis and release, helping to down-regulate (i.e., attenuate or shut down) stress-related hypothalamic–pituitary–adrenocortical (HPA) activation once an adequate neuroendocrine response has been mounted. Notably, however, animal research indicates that these feedback mechanisms—as well as initial CRF gene expression and release—are substantially shaped by early social experiences. Specifically, physical handling of rat pups (by humans) is associated with decreased stress-induced CRF activity and *increased* feedback sensitivity to glucocorticoids, which may account for handled rats' reduced HPA reactivity to stress, reduced behavioral reactivity, and reduced fearfulness (reviewed in Meaney, 2001). In contrast, rat pups that are repeatedly deprived of maternal contact show exactly the opposite effects, and these patterns persist into adulthood (Plotsky & Meaney, 1993).

Of course, both maternal deprivation and human handling are non-normative rearing conditions for rats; yet additional research has found that variations *within the normal range* of rodent caregiver behavior also influence CRF and HPA functioning. Specifically, pups raised by mothers who exhibited low frequencies of licking, grooming, and arched-back nursing developed heightened CRF, HPA, and behavioral activation in response to stress, whereas pups raised by mothers with high frequencies of licking, grooming, and nursing showed the opposite pattern (Francis et al., 1999). Interestingly, some of these effects might be mediated by opioid mechanisms. Animal research has found that endogenous opioid peptides are released in response to social—and especially physical—contact, whereas social isolation is associated with reduced brain opioid levels (reviewed in Nelson & Panksepp, 1998). Some research suggests that brain opioids may down-regulate CRF activity (McCubbin, 1993), with attendant down-regulation of HPA and sympathetic nervous system (SNS) activity, thereby suggesting another mechanism through which early infant–caregiver interactions shape the CRF system and its interrelated stress-regulatory processes.

The Hypothalamic–Pituitary–Adrenocortical Axis

Multiple studies of animals and humans have documented individual differences in HPA reactivity to stress (Kirschbaum et al., 1995; Nachmias, Gunnar, Mangelsdorf, Parritz, & Buss, 1996; Suomi, 1991), and these individual differences correspond to behavioral and self-report measures of emotion regulation. For example, individuals with exaggerated HPA reactivity (indexed by heightened and prolonged cortisol levels) show deficient coping strategies and exaggerated experiences of negative affect (reviewed in Scarpa & Raine, 1997; Stansbury & Gunnar, 1994), and those whose HPA reactivity fails to habituate to *repeated* stressor administration are characterized by low self-esteem, high introversion, high neuroticism, and multiple physical complaints (Kirschbaum et al., 1995).

Such individual differences have direct implications for physical and mental health over the lifespan. As reviewed by Sapolsky (1996), the excess cortisol secretion associated with exaggerated HPA reactivity is associated with neural degeneration in the hippocampus. Negative effects of HPA hyperreactivity on hippocampal function have been detected as early as 12 months of age in humans and have direct implications for memory, attention, and cognition (reviewed in Gunnar, 1998). HPA hyperreactivity is also associated with impaired immune functioning (Coe, Rosenberg, & Levine, 1988; Webster, Elenkov, & Chrousos, 1997), impaired memory and attentional process (Lupien et al., 1994), and increased risks for a variety of pathophysiological processes and outcomes, including cardiovascular disease, diabetes, hypertension, and cancer (Brindley & Rolland, 1989; Henry, 1983; Krantz & Manuck, 1984; McEwen & Stellar, 1993; Truhan & Ahmed, 1989).

Interindividual differences in HPA activity are partially heritable (Kirschbaum, Wust, Faig, & Hellhammer, 1992; Wuest, Federenko, Hellhammer, & Kirschbaum, 2000) but are also influenced by early experiences with stress and caregiving (see also the review in Gunnar & Donzella, 2002; Liu et al., 1997). For example, maternal separation in rhesus monkeys leads to HPA hyperreactivity, along with passive and withdrawn behavior (Suomi, 1991). HPA activity in human children and adolescents varies as a function of multiple family factors, but the most important of these appears to be the quality of maternal care (Flinn & England, 1995). Such effects are long lasting: Children who have lost one of their parents show exaggerated HPA stress reactivity as adults (Luecken, 1998).

Correspondingly, *high* levels of physical affection and infant–caregiver warmth during stressful periods is associated with normal HPA activation profiles (Chorpita & Barlow, 1998; Hertsgaard, Gunnar, Erickson, & Nachmias, 1995). Specifically, secure attachment—as measured by the Strange Situation—has been linked to attenuated HPA reactivity in response to environmental challenges (Gunnar, Brodersen, Krueger, & Rigatuso, 1996; Nachmias et al., 1996). Thus studies of the HPA axis provide some of the strongest evidence for the health implications of early infant–caregiver attachment.

Autonomic Nervous System Functioning

The cascade of neuroendocrine responses to stress, described previously, is also responsible for triggering activation of the sympathetic and parasympathetic branches of the autonomic nervous system, producing the increased heart rate, blood pressure, and sweat production that are the classic hallmarks of stress. Importantly, the parasympathetic nervous system (PNS) and the sympathetic nervous system (SNS) have antagonistic effects on autonomic functioning, and thus stress responses such as heart rate acceleration can be brought about by activation of the SNS, withdrawal of the PNS, or some combination of the two. The specific balance of SNS and PNS control over cardiovascular functioning varies from situation to situation (Berntson, Cacioppo, & Fieldstone, 1996), as well as from person to person (Cacioppo, Uchino, & Berntson, 1994).

These patterns have important health implications. Cardiovascular responses to stress that are more SNS driven than PNS driven are associated with exaggerated HPA stress reactivity (Cacioppo et al., 1995), hypertension (Grossman, Brinkman, & de Vries, 1992) and other long-term cardiovascular health risks (Kristal-Boneh, Raifel, Froom, & Rivak, 1998) and immune deficits (Irwin, Hauger, & Brown, 1992). PNS-driven stress responses appear to be more rapid, more flexible, and easier to disengage than SNS-driven responses (Saul, 1990), and thus robust PNS functioning, typically measured and described as "vagal tone," has been viewed as a key substrate for the development of effective emotion regulation (Porges et al., 1994).

This view is supported by research demonstrating that infants with greater vagal tone are better able to sustain attention to stimuli and to avoid distraction (Porges, 1992; Richards & Casey, 1992), whereas infants with low vagal tone show poor emotional control (Fox, 1989; Porges, 1991) and high behavioral inhibition (Snidman, 1989). Studies of older children have found that vagal tone at ages 4–5 predicts effective emotion regulation 3 years later (Gottman, Katz, & Hooven, 1996) and buffers 8- to 12-year-old children from the negative physical health effects associated with high exposure to marital conflict (El Sheikh, Harger, & Whitson, 2001). In adults, greater vagally mediated heart rate variability is associated with more effective emotional and behavioral responses to stress (Fabes & Eisenberg, 1997), whereas lower levels are associated with depression, anger, mental stress, generalized anxiety, and panic anxiety (reviewed in Brosschot & Thayer, 1998; Friedman & Thayer, 1998; Horsten et al., 1999).

Although the origin and lifetime stability of these interindividual differences have not been definitively established, some researchers have suggested that early distress-alleviating interactions between infants and their caregivers may shape autonomic functioning through their influence on the secretion of oxytocin, a neuropeptide hormone that is critically implicated in both attachment processes and the down-regulation of HPA and autonomic nervous system (ANS) stress reactivity (reviewed in Carter, 1998; Knox & Uvnas-Moberg, 1998; Taylor et al., 2002). One might therefore hypothesize that insecurely attached infants experience less oxytocin-mediated distress alleviation and subsequently develop less PNS-driven patterns of stress reactivity. There is mixed support for this possibility from research on infants and adults (reviewed in Diamond & Hicks, 2004; Fox & Card, 1999); clearly, this is an important area for future developmental research.

Summary and Caveats Regarding Pathway 1

The preceding review is certainly not comprehensive—early social experiences also have lasting influences on dopamine (Depue & Collins, 1999), oxytocin and vasopressin (Uvnäs-Moberg, 1998; Young, 2002), serotonin (reviewed in Glaser, 2000; Repetti et al., 2002), and catecholamines (reviewed in Taylor et al., 2002), which space constraints preclude us from covering in depth. Note, too, that not all "early rearing" effects are best conceptualized as "attachment" effects—rather, the degree to which such influences are *specifically* attributable to attachment-related dynamics (i.e., those revolving around emotional security) awaits further study.

Along the same lines, we do not mean to suggest that *all* insecurely attached infants and adults suffer from biologically based regulatory deficits. Rather, we expect that correspondences between attachment insecurity and biobehavioral dysregulation depend on the *degree* and *timing* of infant–caregiver relational deficits, in combination with the initial, genetically based psychobiological characteristics of the infant. Thus, for example, infants with a basic predisposition for HPA hyperreactivity who *also* experience inconsistent and unresponsive caregiving should be most likely to manifest both attachment insecurity and biobehavioral dysregulation.

Then, of course, there is the question of longitudinal continuity: Might certain childhood and adult experiences "repair" (or worsen) regulatory patterns? With regard to attachment style, the answer appears to be "yes." Longitudinal data demonstrate that life events can precipitate developmental discontinuities in attachment style from infancy to adolescence and adulthood (Lewis, Feiring, & Rosenthal, 2000; Weinfield, Sroufe, & Egeland, 2000), and thus researchers must take account of ongoing, evolving interactions between infant–caregiver "legacies" and later interpersonal experiences in order to appropriately model links between attachment style and health over the life course. With respect to biobehavioral regulatory patterns, there are mixed findings regarding the stability of individual differences in HPA (Lewis & Ramsay, 1995) and PNS functioning (Bornstein & Suess, 2000; Stifter & Jain, 1996) over the first 12–15 months of life, but we know little about longitudinal stability after that point. This is clearly a critical area for future research, particularly with regard to the possibility that positive and negative life experiences have concurrent, parallel influences on both biobehavioral stress-regulatory systems and attachment representations.

PATHWAY 2: ATTACHMENT AND THE PHYSIOLOGICAL EFFECTS OF CHRONIC EMOTIONAL EXPERIENCES

There has been extensive research on the affective, cognitive, and behavioral manifestations of attachment insecurity and their implications for social functioning and mental health (Cooper, Shaver, & Collins, 1998; Mickelson, Kessler, & Shaver, 1997). Yet over the lifespan these manifestations also impair physical health through their influence on many of the same physiological systems implicated in Pathway 1. Here we outline how this occurs by detailing (1) how attachment-related expectations and experiences shape cognitive processes in a manner that predisposes individuals to certain types of chronic emotional experiences and (2) how these emotional experiences influence multiple endocrinological, autonomic, and immunological processes that directly influence health.

First, however, the relative importance of attachment *histories* versus *current* experiences bears discussion. Interestingly, whereas adult attachment research has historically emphasized the former at the expense of the latter, research on social support and health has historically emphasized the latter at the expense of the former. Of course, the two constructs are fundamentally interrelated (Feeney & Noller, 1990), and researchers have therefore increasingly called for their simultaneous assessment (La Guardia, Ryan, Couchman, & Deci, 2000). Accordingly, one might best interpret the dimensions of "security" versus "insecurity" discussed here as *cumulative* constellations of individuals' specific attachment histories, generalized attachment-related expectations, and current experiences of need fulfillment.

Attachment, Appraisal, and Emotion

Attachment theory maintains that, through repeated, emotionally relevant interactions with their caregivers, individuals develop stable expectations about themselves and others that come to organize the encoding, storage, retrieval, and manipulation of affect-laden information, particularly information regarding interpersonal experiences (reviewed in Mikulincer et al., 2003). For example, adults with secure attachment styles (as assessed with self-report measures) make more positive and benign interpretations of others' facial expressions (Magai, Hunziker, Mesias, & Culver, 2000), endorse more positive and less negative interpretations of both hypothetical and actual relationship events (Collins, 1996; Mikulincer & Florian, 1998; Simpson, Ickes, & Grich, 1999), make less hostile attributions of others' motives (Mikulincer, 1998), and make more positive interpretations of others' supportive behavior (Lakey, McCabe, Fisicaro, & Drew, 1996). They also make more positive appraisals of their own coping resources (Berant, Mikulincer, & Florian, 2001).

These patterns of cognitive appraisal subsequently shape individuals' day-to-day patterns of emotional activity and reactivity. For example, securely attached individuals report more frequent and intense positive emotions and less frequent and intense negative emotions than insecurely attached individuals (Feeney, 1995, 1999; Simpson, 1990), both in response to everyday events (Pietromonaco & Feldman-Barrett, 1997; Tidwell, Reis, & Shaver, 1996) and to naturally occurring and laboratory-induced stressors (Magai & Cohen, 1998; Mikulincer, 1998; Rholes et al., 1999).

These patterns of emotional experience not only influence social competence, adjustment, and adult affective disorders (Cooper et al., 1998; Mickelson et al., 1997; Repetti et al., 2002) but also provide the gateway through which social and environmental experiences "get under our skin" (Seeman, 2001) to shape our physical functioning. As reviewed by Seeman (2001), both interpretations of environmental demands and one's resources (social and nonsocial) for meeting these demands are processed first by the neocortex and then fed to the amygdala and hippocampus, leading to systemwide neuroendocrine activation (LeDoux, 1995). Thus information-processing biases that consistently favor negative and threat-related interpretations of environmental events can consistently overstimulate physiological regulatory systems. Here we discuss several systems for which there is the greatest evidence for the deleterious effects of chronic negative emotionality.

Emotions and Hypothalamic–Pituitary–Adrenocortical Reactivity

As we have reviewed, individual differences exist in HPA reactivity that reflect both genetic and early environmental influences. Yet one's HPA response to a particular stressor is also influenced by a constellation of situational factors, particularly those revolving around experiences of negative affect and the extent to which the stressor is appraised as a threat rather than a challenge (reviewed in Blascovich & Tomaka, 1996). Thus attachment experiences and expectations can directly influence individuals' exposure to the cumulative deleterious physiological effects of sustained HPA hyperreactivity through their influence on such emotions and appraisals.

Evidence in support of this view comes from research demonstrating that adults' HPA activity is negatively associated with overall social support (Seeman et al., 1994; Turner Cobb, Sephton, Koopman, Blake Mortimer, & Spiegel, 2000) and positively associated with chronic experiences of negative affect (reviewed in Scarpa & Raine, 1997). Also, whereas most individuals' HPA reactivity demonstrates habituation on repeated administration of a stressor, individuals who perceive themselves to have inadequate coping resources (Kirschbaum & Hellhammer, 1994) or who continue to appraise a particular stressor as threatening (Stansbury & Gunnar, 1994) will fail to show this habituation response, hence heightening the cumulative toll taken on their stress-regulatory systems.

Correspondingly, studies in which individuals' social support perceptions and experiences were specifically manipulated have detected significant effects on HPA functioning. One study of HIV-positive and HIV-negative men found that plasma cortisol levels decreased significantly among those who participated in a structured social support intervention group compared with a control group of nonparticipants (Goodkin et al., 1998). Another study of HIV-positive men (Cruess, Antoni, Kumar, & Schneiderman, 2000) found that over a 10-week period, those who were randomly assigned to a stress management program showed reductions in both HPA activity and negative moods. On the basis of such findings, one might hypothesize that secure, supportive attachment relationships can attenuate chronic HPA reactivity—and its attendant health risks—through facilitating positive emotions and buffering against negative appraisals of major and minor stressors.

Emotions and Autonomic Nervous System Reactivity

Extensive research has also demonstrated consistent relations between positive and negative emotions and ANS reactivity. For example, studies comparing experimental inductions of positive and negative affect have found that negative affective states are associated with heightened cardiovascular reactivity (Gendolla & Kruesken, 2001), whereas positive affect is associated with enhanced cardiovascular recovery (Fredrickson, Mancuso, Branigan, & Tugade, 2000). Other studies have focused on the degree to which autonomic stress reactivity is sympathetically versus parasympathetically driven. Negative emotions such as anger, hostility, and anxiety are associated with greater sympathetic and less parasympathetic control over heart rate (Sloan et al., 1994), and individuals with SNS-driven patterns of reactivity describe themselves as being chronically nervous and emotionally reactive and as having difficulty dealing with their feelings. Notably, researchers have found that the negative long-term health implications associated with this constellation of emotional and autonomic functioning are moderated by the degree to which such individuals are also socially isolated (Orth-Gomer & Unden, 1990), suggesting the continuing importance of social "buffering" against stress reactivity throughout life. As a further example of this point, Horsten and colleagues (1999) found that among adult women, reduced parasympathetic control over heart rate was associated with being single, living alone, and having low social support.

Other evidence for links between ANS functioning and chronic emotional states comes from research documenting that structured interventions aimed at altering emotional states or reactivity have corresponding effects on autonomic functioning. Positive therapy outcomes for anxiety have been shown to be associated with corresponding increases in parasympathetic control (Friedman, Thayer, & Borkovec, 1993; Middleton & Ashby, 1995), and other studies have found similar effects as a result of structured relaxation tasks (Sakakibara, Takeuchi, & Hayano, 1994) and cognitive interventions aimed at shifting attention *away* from negative and *toward* positive feeling states (McCraty, Atkinson, Tiller, Rein, & Watkins, 1995). Such findings provide further evidence that attachment experiences can directly shape individuals' health trajectories by modulating their day-to-day experiences of negative and positive affect.

Emotions and Immune Functioning

Finally, there is substantial evidence for effects of chronic negative and positive emotions on immune functioning (reviewed in Cohen & Herbert, 1996; Kiecolt Glaser et al., 2002). Studies have assessed a diverse array of markers of immune function, including total numbers of immune lymphocytes, the ratio of different types of lymphocytes, secretion of proinflammatory cytokines and subsequent inflammatory response, cellular response to inoculations, likelihood and duration of illness in responses to infection exposure, and healing speed for minor, controlled wounds. Notably, effects on one parameter do not necessarily extend to others, and the duration and clinical relevance of immunological changes is often not clear.

Nonetheless, the findings consistently demonstrate that emotional states influence immunological functioning (reviewed in Cohen, Miller, & Rabin, 2001). For example, stress and anxiety have been found to be negatively related—and social support positively related—to medical students' immunological responses to hepatitis B inoculations (Glaser et al., 1992). Notably, certain individuals appear more prone to such immunological changes than others. Individuals with SNS-dominated patterns of stress reactivity (Uchino, 1995) or high basal levels of HPA activity (Petitto et al., 2000) are more likely to show stress-related declines in immune functioning. Chronic levels of and predispositions toward positive and negative affect are both related to antibody responses to immunizations (reviewed in Cohen et al., 2001), and research on clinical populations has found that the intensity of depressive affect appears linearly related to immunological effects (Herbert & Cohen, 1993). Correspondingly, studies involving *changes* in positive and negative affect have documented corresponding immunological changes. A 10-week bereavement support group for HIV-positive and HIV-negative men produced significant increases (assessed at a 6-month follow-up) in several different markers of immune functioning and decreases in numbers of physician visits, compared with control group members (Goodkin et al., 1998), and even laboratory-based inductions of negative and positive affect have been shown to influence immune function (Futterman, Kemeny, Shapiro, & Fahey, 1994).

The specific role of social relationships—and the unique provisions afforded by attachment relationships—holds particular promise for future study. Studies of primates have detected both transient and long-lasting changes in multiple parameters of immune function as a consequence of sustained maternal separation or other atypical rearing conditions in infancy (reviewed in Coe et al., 1988). Given the role of CRF in rearing effects on HPA functioning, it is notable that CRF secretion mediates some stress-induced declines in immune functioning, both through direct influences on proinflammatory immune cells and indirectly through its influences on HPA (Webster et al., 1997) and SNS activity (Friedman & Irwin, 1995). Finally, one intriguing study of HIV-positive teenagers found that those receiving massage therapy over a 12-week period showed increases in certain parameters of immune functioning, as well as reductions in anxiety and depression, compared with a control group that received muscle relaxation therapy (Diego et al., 2001). Given the aforementioned findings regarding the roles of early maternal contact on the development of infants' stress-regulatory systems, this suggests that the types of interactions and behaviors most commonly observed among individuals' most intimate and important relationships—such as regular and prolonged physical contact—might affect immune functioning not only through their emotion effects but perhaps also as a result of touch-induced secretion of neurochemicals such as endogenous opiods and oxytocin and their antistress effects (reviewed in Knox & Uvnas-Moberg, 1998; Taylor et al., 2000, 2002).

Summary and Caveats Regarding Pathway 2

Clearly, the types of day-to-day positive and negative emotional experiences that are shaped by attachment-related experiences and expectations influence not only our overall happiness and relationship quality but also multiple parameters of physiological functioning. This multiplicity of influences is important. Many researchers have argued that, in the modeling of links among stress, emotion, social relationships, and health over the life course, the chronic and combined activation of multiple stress-regulatory systems is more predictive of long-term health status than hyperactivation of any one system in isolation. The collective, cumulative impact of such repeated stress-related activation on the body has been referred to as "allostatic load" (McEwen & Stellar, 1993; Seeman, Singer, Rowe, Horwitz, & McEwen, 1997) and conceptualized as the accumulated wear and tear on multiple organ systems and tissues that results from the body's ongoing physiological adjustments to environmental demands. Over time, high allostatic load is thought to accelerate the aging process by dysregulating cardiovascular reactivity and recovery, blood pressure regulation, HPA axis functioning, parasympathetic nervous system activation, and serotonergic functioning (reviewed in Ryff et al., 2001).

One of the strengths of this conceptualization is its emphasis on *cumulative* risk factors, which necessitates a life-course approach to researching links between social relationships and health. This is certainly consistent with attachment theory's emphasis on lifetime trajectories of security and insecurity and is empirically supported by Ryff and colleagues' (2001) finding that long-term health status is best predicted by considering individuals' *overall* pathways of positive versus negative relationship experiences and the ways in which they build on—or compensate for—one another over time. Along these lines, one important direction for future research concerns the extent to which particular attachment relationships can single-handedly redirect either negative or positive emotion trajectories, thereby changing an individual's long-term health risks. In other words, just how detrimental is a consistently negative, unsupportive, conflictual marriage for an otherwise securely attached individual who generally adopts positive and instrumental appraisals of major and minor stressors? Conversely, how beneficial is a consistently positive and supportive marriage for an otherwise insecurely attached individual?

As noted earlier, longitudinal research that provides coordinated assessments of biobehavioral regulatory processes, relationship experiences, cognitive appraisal processes, day-to-day emotional experiences, and health status would produce invaluable information on the development and maintenance of interconnections among these domains at different stages of the life course and their long-term health implications. It will be particularly informative to try and pinpoint exactly where individuals' information processing biases come into play and the direct and immediate relevance of such biases for physiological processes. For example, one study found that rumination about an emotional task (but not, notably, about an unemotional task) resulted in heightened blood pressure reactivity, and this effect could be successfully extinguished by introducing manipulations that prevented participants from engaging in rumination (Carels, Blumenthal, & Sherwood, 2000). Of course, attachment phenomena are not the only potential influences on such cognitive–affective processes, and thus, in order to appropriately model the relevance of attachment-specific processes, future research must take a variety of individual-difference dimensions (for example, extraversion, hostility, anxiety) into account.

Finally, as discussed earlier, most research in this area has focused disproportionately on the detrimental impact of negative cognitions and emotional experiences, insufficiently theorizing and investigating the specific cognitive, emotional, behavioral, and physiological benefits associated with positive relational experiences and expectations. Thus attachment researchers should consider embarking on future investigations with an eye toward elucidating the role of emotional security in health maintenance and promotion rather than the role of insecurity in health risk and disease.

CONCLUSION

Reflecting on animal research that documents the coordinated coregulation of biological functions between infants and caregivers, Pipp and Harmon (1987) speculated, "it may be that throughout the lifespan we are biologically connected to those with whom we have close relationships. . . . [H]omeostatic regulation between members of a dyad is a stable aspect of all intimate relationships throughout the lifespan" (p. 651). This model of enduring psychobiological linkage between intimate social partners has yet to be systematically and specifically validated in humans, but it provides a compelling framework for conceptualizing the multiple associations between attachment phenomena and health-related biological processes outlined herein. Most notably, such a model highlights the fact that interpersonal effects on biological functioning may be for either good or ill—just as positive and supportive relationships may continuously optimize our emotional and biological functioning, so too may negative, hostile, and neglectful bonds have the opposite effect. A laudable goal for future research is to trace these biobehavioral processes over the lifespan across multiple functional domains, helping to map the psychobiological processes through which our most intimate and important affectional tics progressively shape our physical, as well as mental, health over the lifespan.

REFERENCES

Ainsworth, M. D. S., Blehar, M. C., Waters, E., & Wall, S. (1978). *Patterns of attachment: A psychological study of the Strange Situation.* Hillsdale, NJ: Erlbaum.

Berant, E., Mikulincer, M., & Florian, V. (2001). The association of mothers' attachment style and their psychological reactions to the diagnosis of infant's congenital heart disease. *Journal of Social and Clinical Psychology, 20,* 208–232.

Berntson, G. G., Cacioppo, J. T., & Fieldstone, A. (1996). Illusions, arithmetic, and the bidirectional modulation of vagal control of the heart. *Biological Psychology, 44,* 1–17.

Blascovich, J., & Tomaka, J. (1996). The biopsychosocial model of arousal regulation. In M. Zanna (Ed.), *Advances in experimental social psychology* (Vol. 28, pp. 1–51). New York: Academic Press.

Bornstein, M. H., & Suess, P. E. (2000). Child and mother cardiac vagal tone: Continuity, stability, and concordance across the first 5 years. *Developmental Psychology, 36,* 54–65.

Bowlby, J. (1973). *Attachment and loss: Vol. 2: Separation: Anxiety and anger.* New York: Basic Books.

Brindley, D. N., & Rolland, Y. (1989). Possible connections between stress, diabetes, obesity, hypertension and altered lipoprotein metabolism that may result in atherosclerosis. *Clinical Science, 77,* 453–461.

Brosschot, J. F., & Thayer, J. F. (1998). Anger inhibition, cardiovascular recovery, and vagal function: A model of the link between hostility and cardiovascular disease. *Annals of Behavioral Medicine, 20,* 326–332.

Cacioppo, J. T., Malarkey, W. B., Kiecolt Glaser, J. K., Uchino, B. N., Sgoutas-Emch, S. A., Sheridan, J. F., et al. (1995). Heterogeneity in neuroendocrine and immune responses to brief psychological stressors as a function of autonomic cardiac activation. *Psychosomatic Medicine, 57,* 154–164.

Cacioppo, J. T., Uchino, B. N., & Berntson, G. G. (1994). Individual differences in the autonomic origins of heart rate reactivity: The psychometrics of respiratory sinus arrhythmia and preejection period. *Psychophysiology, 31,* 412–419.

Carels, R. A., Blumenthal, J. A., & Sherwood, A. (2000). Emotional responsivity during daily life: Relationship to psychosocial functioning and ambulatory blood pressure. *International Journal of Psychophysiology, 36,* 25–33.

Carter, C. S. (1998). Neuroendocrine perspectives on social attachment and love. *Psychoneuroendocrinology, 23,* 779–818.

Chorpita, B. F., & Barlow, D. H. (1998). The development of anxiety: The role of control in the early environment. *Psychological Bulletin, 124,* 3–21.

Coe, C. L., Rosenberg, L. T., & Levine, S. (1988). Immunological consequences of psychological disturbance and maternal loss in infancy. *Advances in Infancy Research, 5,* 97–134.

Cohen, S., & Herbert, T. B. (1996). Health psychology: Psychological factors and physical disease from the perspective of human psychoneuroimmunology. *Annual Review of Psychology, 47,* 113–142.

Cohen, S., Miller, G. E., & Rabin, B. S. (2001). Psychological stress and antibody response to immunization: A critical review of the human literature. *Psychosomatic Medicine, 63,* 7–18.

Collins, N. L. (1996). Working models of attachment: Implications for explanation, emotion, and behavior. *Journal of Personality and Social Psychology, 71,* 810–832.

Cooper, M. L., Shaver, P. R., & Collins, N. L. (1998). Attachment styles, emotion regulation, and adjustment in adolescence. *Journal of Personality and Social Psychology, 74,* 1380–1397.

Cruess, D. G., Antoni, M. H., Kumar, M., & Schneiderman, N. (2000). Reductions in salivary cortisol are associated with mood improvement during relaxation training among HIV seropositive men. *Journal of Behavioral Medicine, 23,* 107–122.

Depue, R. A., & Collins, P. F. (1999). Neurobiology of the structure of personality: Dopamine, facilitation of incentive motivation, and extraversion. *Behavioral and Brain Sciences, 22,* 491–569.

Diamond, L. M. (2001). Contributions of psychophysiology to research on adult attachment: Review and recommendations. *Personality and Social Psychology Review, 5,* 276–295.

Diamond, L. M., & Hicks, A. M. (2004). *Attachment style, current relationship security, and negative emotions.* Manuscript submitted for publication.

Diego, M. A., Field, T., Hernandez Reif, M., Shaw, K., Friedman, L., & Ironson, G. (2001). HIV adolescents show improved immune function following massage therapy. *International Journal of Neuroscience, 106,* 35–45.

El Sheikh, M., Harger, J., & Whitson, S. M. (2001). Exposure to interparental conflict and children's adjustment and physical health: The moderating role of vagal tone. *Child Development, 72,* 1617–1636.

Fabes, R. A., & Eisenberg, N. (1997). Regulatory control in adults' stress-related responses to daily life events. *Journal of Personality and Social Psychology, 73,* 1107–1117.

Feeney, J. A. (1995). Adult attachment and emotional control. *Personal Relationships, 2,* 143–159.

Feeney, J. A. (1999). Adult romantic attachment and couple relationships. In J. Cassidy & P. R. Shaver (Eds.), *Handbook of attachment: Theory, research, and clinical applications* (pp. 355–377). New York: Guilford Press.

Feeney, J. A. (2000). Implications of attachment style for patterns of health and illness. *Child: Care, Health and Development, 26,* 277–288.

Feeney, J. A., & Noller, P. (1990). Attachment style as a predictor of adult romantic relationships. *Journal of Personality and Social Psychology, 58,* 281–291.

Flinn, M. V., & England, B. G. (1995). Childhood stress and family environment. *Current Anthropology, 36,* 854–866.

Fox, N. A. (1989). Psychophysiological correlates of emotional reactivity during the first year of life. *Developmental Psychology, 25,* 495–504.

Fox, N. A., & Card, J. A. (1999). Psychophysiological measures in the study of attachment. In J. Cassidy & P. R. Shaver (Eds.), *Handbook of attachment: Theory, research, and clinical applications* (pp. 226–245). New York: Guilford Press.

Francis, D. D., Caldji, C., Champagne, F., Plotsky, P. M., & Meaney, M. J. (1999). The role of corticotropin-releasing factor-norepinephrine systems in mediating the effects of early experience on the development of behavioral and endocrine responses to stress. *Biological Psychiatry, 46,* 1153–1166.

Fredrickson, B. L. (2001). The role of positive emotions in positive psychology: The broaden-and-build theory of positive emotions. *American Psychologist, 56,* 218–226.

Fredrickson, B. L., Mancuso, R. A., Branigan, C., & Tugade, M. M. (2000). The undoing effect of positive emotions. *Motivation and Emotion, 24,* 237–258.

Friedman, B. H., & Thayer, J. F. (1998). Autonomic balance revisited: Panic anxiety and heart rate variability. *Journal of Psychosomatic Research, 44,* 133–151.

Friedman, B. H., Thayer, J. F., & Borkovec, T. D. (1993). Heart rate variability in generalized anxiety disorder [Abstract]. *Psychophysiology, 30,* S28.

Friedman, E. M., & Irwin, M. R. (1995). A role for CRH and the sympathetic nervous system in stress-induced immunosuppression. *Annals of the New York Academy of Sciences, 771,* 396–418.

Futterman, A. D., Kemeny, M. E., Shapiro, D., & Fahey, J. L. (1994). Immunological and physiological changes associated with induced positive and negative mood. *Psychosomatic Medicine, 56,* 499–511.

Gendolla, G. H. E., & Kruesken, J. (2001). Mood state and cardiovascular response in active coping with an affect-regulative challenge. *International Journal of Psychophysiology, 41,* 169–180.

Glaser, D. (2000). Child abuse and neglect and the brain: A review. *Journal of Child Psychology and Psychiatry and Allied Disciplines, 41,* 97–116.

Glaser, R., Kiecolt-Glaser, J. K., Bonneau, R. H., Malarkey, W., Kennedy, S., & Hughes, J. (1992). Stress-induced modulation of the immune response to recombinant hepatitis B vaccine. *Psychosomatic Medicine, 54,* 22–29.

Goodkin, K., Feaster, D. J., Asthana, D., Blaney, N. T., Kumar, M., Baldewicz, T., et al. (1998). A bereavement support group intervention is longitudinally associated with salutary effects on the CD4 cell count and number of physician visits. *Clinical and Diagnostic Laboratory Immunology, 5,* 382–391.

Gottman, J. M., Katz, L. F., & Hooven, C. (1996). Parental meta-emotion philosophy and the emotional life of families: Theoretical models and preliminary data. *Journal of Family Psychology, 10,* 243–268.

Grossman, P., Brinkman, A., & de Vries, J. (1992). Cardiac autonomic mechanisms associated with borderline hypertension under varying behavioral demands: Evidence for attenuated parasympathetic tone but not for enhanced beta-adrenergic activity. *Psychophysiology, 29,* 698–711.

Gunnar, M. R. (1998). Quality of early care and buffering of neuroendocrine stress reactions: Potential effects on the developing human brain. *Preventive Medicine, 27,* 208–211.

Gunnar, M. R., Brodersen, L., Krueger, K., & Rigatuso, J. (1996). Dampening of adrenocortical responses during infancy: Normative changes and individual differences. *Child Development, 67,* 877–889.

Gunnar, M. R., & Donzella, B. (2002). Social regulation of cortisol levels in early human development. *Psychoneuroendocrinology, 27,* 199–220.

Hazan, C., & Shaver, P. R. (1987). Romantic love conceptualized as an attachment process. *Journal of Personality and Social Psychology, 52,* 511–524.

Henry, J. P. (1983). Coronary heart disease and arousal of the adrenal cortical axis. In T. M. Dembroski, T. H. Schmidt, & G. Blumchen (Eds.), *Biobehavioral bases of coronary heart disease* (pp. 365–381). Basel, Switzerland: Karger.

Herbert, T. B., & Cohen, S. (1993). Depression and immunity: A meta-analytic review. *Psychological Bulletin, 113,* 472–486.

Hertsgaard, L., Gunnar, M., Erickson, M. F., & Nachmias, M. (1995). Adrenocortical responses to the Strange Situation in infants with disorganized/disoriented attachment relationships. *Child Development, 66,* 1100–1106.

Horsten, M., Ericson, M., Perski, A., Wamala, S. P., Schenck-Gustafsson, K., & Orth-Gomér, K. (1999). Psychosocial factors and heart rate variability in healthy women. *Psychosomatic Medicine, 61,* 49–57.

Irwin, M., Hauger, R., & Brown, M. (1992). Central corticotropin-releasing hormone activates the sympathetic nervous system and reduces immune function: Increased responsivity of the aged rat. *Endocrinology, 131,* 1047–1053.

Isen, A. M. (2003). Positive affect as a source of human strength. In L. A. Aspinwall & U. M. Staudinger (Eds.), *A psychology of human strengths: Fundamental questions and future directions for a positive psychology* (pp. 179–195). Washington, DC: American Psychological Association.

Kiecolt Glaser, J. K., McGuire, L., Robles, T. F., & Glaser, R. (2002). Emotions, morbidity, and mortality: New perspectives from psychoneuroimmunology. *Annual Review of Psychology, 53,* 83–107.

Kirschbaum, C., & Hellhammer, D. H. (1994). Salivary cortisol in psychoneuroendocrine research: Recent developments and applications. *Psychoneuroendocrinology, 19,* 313–333.

Kirschbaum, C., Prussner, J. C., Stone, A. A., Federenko, I., Gaab, J., Lintz, D., et al. (1995). Persistent high cortisol responses to repeated psychological stress in a subpopulation of healthy men. *Psychosomatic Medicine, 57,* 468–474.

Kirschbaum, C., Wust, S., Faig, H. G., & Hellhammer, D. H. (1992). Heritability of cortisol responses to human corticotropin-releasing hormone, ergometry, and psychological stress in humans. *Journal of Clinical Endocrinology and Metabolism, 75,* 1526–1530.

Kitigawa, E. M., & Hauser, P. M. (1973). *Differential mortality in the United States: A study in socio-economic epidemiology.* Cambridge, MA: Harvard University Press.

Knox, S. S., & Uvnas-Moberg, K. (1998). Social isolation and cardiovascular disease: An atherosclerotic pathway? *Psychoneuroendocrinology, 23,* 877–890.

Krantz, D. S., & Manuck, S. B. (1984). Acute psychophysiologic reactivity and risk of cardiovascular disease: A review and methodologic critique. *Psychological Bulletin, 96,* 435–464.

Kristal-Boneh, E., Raifel, M., Froom, P., & Rivak, J. (1998). Heart rate variability in health and disease. *Scandinavian Journal of Work and Environmental Health, 21,* 85–95.

La Guardia, J. G., Ryan, R. M., Couchman, C. E., & Deci, E. L. (2000). Within-person variation in security of attachment: A self-determination theory perspective on attachment, need fulfillment, and well-being. *Journal of Personality and Social Psychology, 79,* 367–384.

Lakey, B., McCabe, K. M., Fisicaro, S. A., & Drew, J. B. (1996). Environmental and personal determinants of support perceptions: Three generalizability studies. *Journal of Personality and Social Psychology, 70,* 1270–1280.

LeDoux, J. E. (1995). In search of an emotional system in the brain: Leaping from fear to emotion and consciousness. In M. S. Gazzaniga (Ed.), *The cognitive neurosciences* (pp. 1049–1062). Cambridge, MA: MIT Press.

Lewis, M., Feiring, C., & Rosenthal, S. (2000). Attachment over time. *Child Development, 71,* 707–720.

Lewis, M., & Ramsay, D. S. (1995). Stability and change in cortisol and behavioral response to stress during the first 18 months of life. *Developmental Psychobiology, 28,* 419–428.

Liu, D., Diorio, J., Tannenbaum, B., Caldji, C., Francis, D., Freedman, A., et al. (1997). Maternal care, hippocampal glucocorticoid receptors, and hypothalamic–pituitary–adrenal responses to stress. *Science, 277,* 1659–1662.

Luecken, L. J. (1998). Childhood attachment and loss experiences affect adult cardiovascular and cortisol function. *Psychosomatic Medicine, 60,* 765–772.

Lupien, S., Lecours, A. R., Lussier, I., Schwartz, G., Nair, N. P., & Meaney, M. J. (1994). Basal cortisol levels and cognitive deficits in human aging. *Journal of Neuroscience, 14,* 2893–2903.

Magai, C., & Cohen, C. I. (1998). Attachment style and emotion regulation in dementia patients and their relation to caregiver burden. *Journals of Gerontology: Series B. Psychological Sciences and Social Sciences, 53,* P147–154.

Magai, C., Hunziker, J., Mesias, W., & Culver, L. C. (2000). Adult attachment styles and emotional biases. *International Journal of Behavioral Development, 24,* 301–309.

McCraty, R., Atkinson, M., Tiller, W. A., Rein, G., & Watkins, A. D. (1995). The effects of emotions on short-term power spectrum analysis of heart rate variability. *American Journal of Chronology, 76,* 1089–1093.

McCubbin, J. A. (1993). Stress and endogenous opioids: Behavioral and circulatory interactions. *Biological Psychology, 35,* 91–122.

McEwen, B. S., & Stellar, E. (1993). Stress and the individual: Mechanisms leading to disease. *Archives of Internal Medicine, 153,* 2093–2101.

Meaney, M. J. (2001). Maternal care, gene expression, and the transmission of individual differences in stress reactivity across generations. *Annual Review of Neuroscience, 24,* 1161–1192.

Mickelson, K. D., Kessler, R. C., & Shaver, P. R. (1997). Adult attachment in a nationally representative sample. *Journal of Personality and Social Psychology, 73,* 1092–1106.

Middleton, H. C., & Ashby, M. (1995). Clinical recovery from panic disorder is associated with evidence of changes in cardiovascular regulation. *Acta Psychiatrica Scandinavica, 91,* 108–113.

Mikulincer, M. (1998). Adult attachment style and individual differences in functional versus dysfunctional experiences of anger. *Journal of Personality and Social Psychology, 74,* 513–524.

Mikulincer, M., & Florian, V. (1998). The relationship between adult attachment styles and emotional and cognitive reactions to stressful events. In J. A. Simpson & W. S. Rholes (Eds.), *Attachment theory and close relationships* (pp. 143–165). New York: Guilford Press.

Mikulincer, M., Shaver, P. R., & Pereg, D. (2003). Attachment theory and affect regulation: The dynamics, development, and cognitive consequences of attachment-related strategies. *Motivation and Emotion, 27,* 77–102.

Mikulincer, M., & Sheffi, E. (2000). Adult attachment style and cognitive reactions to positive affect: A test of mental categorization and creative problem solving. *Motivation and Emotion, 24,* 149–174.

Nachmias, M., Gunnar, M., Mangelsdorf, S., Parritz, R. H., & Buss, K. (1996). Behavioral inhibition and stress reactivity: The moderating role of attachment security. *Child Development, 67,* 508–522.

Nelson, E. E., & Panksepp, J. (1998). Brain substrates of infant-mother attachment: Contributions of opioids, oxytocin, and norepinephrine. *Neuroscience and Biobehavioral Reviews, 22,* 437–452.

Orth-Gomer, K., & Unden, A. L. (1990). Type A behavior, social support, and coronary risk: Interaction and significance for mortality in cardiac patients. *Psychosomatic Medicine, 52,* 59–72.

Petitto, J. M., Leserman, J., Perkins, D. O., Stern, R. A., Silva, S. G., Gettes, D., et al. (2000). High versus low basal cortisol secretion in asymptomatic, medication free HIV infected men: Differential effects of severe life stress on parameters of immune status. *Behavioral Medicine, 25,* 143–151.

Pietromonaco, P. R., & Feldman Barrett, L. (1997). Working models of attachment and daily social interactions. *Journal of Personality and Social Psychology, 73,* 1409–1423.

Pipp, S., & Harmon, R. J. (1987). Attachment as regulation: A commentary. *Child Development, 58,* 648–652.

Plotsky, P. M., & Meaney, M. J. (1993). Early, postnatal experience alters hypothalamic corticotropin-releasing factor (CRF) mRNA, median eminence CRF content and stress-induced release in adult rats. *Molecular Brain Research, 18,* 195–200.

Porges, S. W. (1991). Vagal tone: An autonomic mediator of affect. In J. Garber & K. A. Dodge (Eds.), *The development of emotion regulation and dysregulation* (pp. 111–128). New York: Cambridge University Press.

Porges, S. W. (1992). Autonomic regulation and attention. In B. A. Campbell, H. Hayne, & R. Richardson (Eds.), *Attention and information processing in infants and adults* (pp. 201–223). Hillsdale, NJ: Erlbaum.

Porges, S. W., Doussard-Roosevelt, J. A., & Maiti, A. K. (1994). Vagal tone and the physiological regulation of emotion. In N. Fox (Ed.), The development of emotion regulation: Biological and behavioral considerations. *Monographs of the Society for Research in Child Development, 59*(2–3, Serial No. 240), 167–186.

Reis, H. T. (2001). Relationship experiences and emotional well-being. In C. D. Ryff & B. H. Singer (Eds.), *Emotion, social relationships, and health* (pp. 57–85). New York: Oxford University Press.

Repetti, R. L., Taylor, S. E., & Seeman, T. E. (2002). Risky families: Family social environments and the mental and physical health of offspring. *Psychological Bulletin, 128,* 330–366.

Rholes, W. S., Simpson, J. A., & Oriña, M. M. (1999). Attachment and anger in an anxiety-provoking situation. *Journal of Personality and Social Psychology, 76,* 940–957.

Richards, J. E., & Casey, B. J. (1992). Development of sustained visual attention in the human infant. In B. A. Campbell, H. Hayne, & R. Richardson (Eds.), *Attention and information processing in infants and adults* (pp. 30–60). Hillsdale, NJ: Erlbaum.

Ross, C. E. (1995). Reconceptualizing marital status as a continuum of social attachment. *Journal of Marriage and the Family, 57,* 129–140.

Ryff, C. D., & Singer, B. H. (Eds.). (2001). *Emotions, social relationships, and health.* New York: Oxford University Press.

Ryff, C. D., Singer, B. H., Wing, E., & Love, G. D. (2001). Elective affinities and uninvited agonies: Mapping emotion with significant others onto health. In C. D. Ryff & B. H. Singer (Eds.), *Relationship experiences and emotional well-being* (pp. 133–174). New York: Oxford University Press.

Sakakibara, M., Takeuchi, S., & Hayano, J. (1994). Effect of relaxation training on cardiac parasympathetic tone. *Psychophysiology, 31,* 223–228.

Sapolsky, R. (1996). Why stress is bad for your brain. *Science, 273,* 749–750.

Saul, J. P. (1990). Beat-to-beat variations of heart rate reflect modulation of cardiac autonomic outflow. *News in Psychological Science, 5,* 32–37.

Scarpa, A., & Raine, A. (1997). Psychophysiology of anger and violent behavior. *Psychiatric Clinics of North America, 20,* 375–394.

Schore, A. N. (1996). Effects of a secure attachment relationship on right brain development, affect regulation, and infant mental health. *Infant Mental Health Journal, 22,* 269–276.

Seeman, T. E. (2001). How do others get under our skin? Social relationships and health. In C. D. Ryff & B. H. Singer (Eds.), *Emotion, social relationships, and health* (pp. 189–209). New York: Oxford University Press.

Seeman, T. E., Charpentier, P. A., Berkman, L. F., Tinetti, M. E., Guralnik, J. M., Albert, M., et al. (1994). Predicting changes in physical performance in a high-functioning elderly cohort. MacArthur studies of successful aging. *Journal of Gerontology, 49,* M97–108.

Seeman, T. E., Singer, B. H., Rowe, J. W., Horwitz, R. I., & McEwen, B. S. (1997). Price of adaptation: Allostatic load and its health consequences. MacArthur studies of successful aging. *Archives of Internal Medicine, 157,* 2259–2268.

Simpson, J. A. (1990). Influence of attachment styles on romantic relationships. *Journal of Personality and Social Psychology, 59*(5), 971–980.

Simpson, J. A., Ickes, W., & Grich, J. (1999). When accuracy hurts: Reactions of anxious–ambivalent dating partners to a relationship-threatening situation. *Journal of Personality and Social Psychology, 76,* 754–769.

Sloan, R. P., Shapiro, P. A., Bagiella, E., Boni, S. M., Paik, M., Bigger, J. T. J., et al. (1994). Effect of mental stress throughout the day on cardiac autonomic control. *Biological Psychology, 37,* 89–99.

Snidman, N. (1989). Behavioral inhibition and sympathetic influence on the cardiovascular system. In J. S. Reznick (Ed.), *Perspectives on behavioral inhibition* (pp. 51–70). Chicago: University of Chicago Press.

Stack, S., & Eshleman, J. R. (1998). Marital status and happiness: A 17-nation study. *Journal of Marriage and the Family, 60,* 527–536.

Stansbury, K., & Gunnar, M. R. (1994). Adrenocortical activity and emotion regulation. In N. Fox (Ed.), The development of emotion regulation: Biological and behavioral considerations. *Monographs of the Society for Research in Child Development, 59*(2–3, Serial No. 240) 108–134.

Stifter, C. A., & Jain, A. (1996). Psychophysiological correlates of infant temperament: Stability of behavior and autonomic patterning from 5 to 18 months. *Developmental Psychobiology, 29,* 379–391.

Suomi, S. J. (1991). Up-tight and laid-back monkeys: Individual differences in response to social challenges. In S. Brauth, W. Hall, & R. Dooling (Eds.), *Plasticity of development* (pp. 27–56). Cambridge, MA: MIT Press.

Taylor, S. E., Dickerson, S. S., & Klein, L. C. (2002). Toward a biology of social support. In C. R. Snyder & S. J. Lopez (Eds.), *Handbook of positive psychology* (pp. 556–569). London: Oxford University Press.

Taylor, S. E., Klein, L. C., Lewis, B. P., Gruenewald, T. L., Gurung, R. A. R., & Updegraff, J. A. (2000). Biobehavioral responses to stress in females: Tend-and-befriend, not fight-or-flight. *Psychological Review, 107,* 411–429.

Taylor, S. E., Repetti, R. L., & Seeman, T. E. (1997). Health psychology: What is an unhealthy environment and how does it get under the skin? *Annual Review of Psychology, 48,* 411–447.

Tidwell, M. O., Reis, H. T., & Shaver, P. R. (1996). Attachment, attractiveness, and social interaction: A diary study. *Journal of Personality and Social Psychology, 71,* 729–745.

Truhan, A. P., & Ahmed, A. R. (1989). Corticosteroids: A review with emphasis on complications of prolonged systemic therapy. *Annals of Allergy, 62,* 375–391.

Turner Cobb, J. M., Sephton, S. E., Koopman, C., Blake Mortimer, J., & Spiegel, D. (2000). Social support and salivary cortisol in women with metastatic breast cancer. *Psychosomatic Medicine, 62,* 337–345.

Uchino, B. N. (1995). Individual differences in cardiac sympathetic control predict endocrine and immune responses to acute psychological stress. *Journal of Personality and Social Psychology, 69,* 736–743.

Uvnäs-Moberg, K. (1998). Oxytocin may mediate the benefits of positive social interaction and emotions. *Psychoneuroendocrinology, 23,* 819–835.

Webster, E. L., Elenkov, I. J., & Chrousos, G. P. (1997). The role of corticotropin-releasing hormone in neuroendocrine-immune interactions. *Molecular Psychiatry, 2,* 368–372.

Weinfield, N. S., Sroufe, L. A., & Egeland, B. (2000). Attachment from infancy to early adulthood in a high-risk sample: Continuity, discontinuity, and their correlates. *Child Development, 71,* 695–702.

Wuest, S., Federenko, I., Hellhammer, D. H., & Kirschbaum, C. (2000). Genetic factors, perceived chronic stress, and the free cortisol response to awakening. *Psychoneuroendocrinology, 25,* 707–720.

Young, L. J. (2002). The neurobiology of social recognition: Approach and avoidance. *Biological Psychiatry, 51,* 18–26.

PART IV

INTERPERSONAL ASPECTS OF ATTACHMENT

Intimacy, Conflict, Caregiving,
and Satisfaction

CHAPTER 9

Conflict in Adult Close Relationships
An Attachment Perspective

PAULA R. PIETROMONACO
DARA GREENWOOD
LISA FELDMAN BARRETT

Relationship researchers have focused on the frequency of conflict in couples' relationships and the manner in which couples engage in and try to resolve conflicts. Three generalizations arise from this work. First, conflict occurs regularly in most close relationships (Brehm, Miller, Perlman, & Campbell, 2002). Second, dealing with conflict, under some conditions, may facilitate the development and maintenance of intimacy and satisfaction in a relationship (Canary & Cupach, 1988; Fincham & Beach, 1999; Gottman, 1994; Holmes & Boon, 1990). Third, in unhappy marriages, conflict is associated with patterns of behavior (e.g., negative affect reciprocity, demand–withdraw) and thought that tend to escalate conflict and make it more difficult to negotiate a resolution (Bradbury & Fincham, 1990; Fincham & Beach, 1999). Whether conflict facilitates intimacy or exacerbates distress may depend on individual differences in the way in which people interpret and respond to conflict.

Attachment theory (e.g., Bowlby, 1973), as applied to adult relationships (Hazan & Shaver, 1987), provides a framework for understanding different responses to conflict. People are thought to differ in their working models of attachment, which include expectations, beliefs, and goals about the self in relation to others (Bartholomew & Horowitz, 1991; Collins & Read, 1994; Pietromonaco & Feldman Barrett, 2000). These working models are likely to shape people's thoughts, feelings, and behavior during conflict. For example, a person who expects close others to be generally responsive and available is likely to interpret and respond to conflict very differently from a person who expects close others to be rejecting and unavailable. Attachment theory may be able to inform the literature on conflict in close relationships by suggesting how individuals might differ in how they construe conflict.

267

At the same time, the study of relationship conflict provides a useful context for testing important aspects of attachment theory. Conflict may be particularly likely to reveal attachment processes because (1) it may act as a stressor on the relationship and thereby activate the attachment system (Simpson, Rholes, & Phillips, 1996); (2) it challenges partners' abilities to regulate their emotions and behavior (Kobak & Duemmler, 1994), which are thought to be connected to attachment processes; and (3) it may trigger behaviors (e.g., personal disclosures) that typically promote intimacy, thereby providing evidence relevant to different attachment goals, such as achieving intimacy or maintaining self-reliance (Pietromonaco & Feldman Barrett, 1997).

In this chapter, we first discuss how conflict can be conceptualized within an attachment framework. Specifically, we propose that conflict may pose a threat to the attachment bond, but that it also may provide an opportunity for perceiving or experiencing greater intimacy. Furthermore, the degree to which people perceive conflict as a threat, opportunity, or both will depend on the content (e.g., expectations, beliefs, goals) of their working models of attachment. Next, we identify a set of predictions that follow from this framework and evaluate the extent to which empirical findings support these predictions; in particular, we attempt to integrate divergent findings in the empirical literature. Finally, we outline several critical issues that will need to be addressed in future work.

THE SIGNIFICANCE OF CONFLICT FOR ADULT ATTACHMENT PROCESSES

Since the goal of attachment behaviour is to maintain an affective bond, any situation that seems to be endangering the bond elicits action designed to preserve it; and the greater the danger of loss appears to be the more intense and varied are the actions elicited to prevent it
—BOWLBY (1980, p. 42)

Once his attachment behaviour has become organised mainly on a goal-corrected basis, the relationship developing between a child and his mother becomes much more complex. Whilst true collaboration between the two then becomes possible, so also does intractable conflict.... Since each partner has his own personal set-goals to attain, collaboration between them is possible only so long as one is prepared, when necessary, to relinquish, or at least adjust, his own set-goals to suit the other's.
—BOWLBY (1969, pp. 354–355)

Although the original formulation of attachment theory (Bowlby, 1969, 1973, 1979, 1980) does not offer a detailed theoretical analysis of the link between conflict and attachment, these quotes suggest two important ways in which conflict might be tied to attachment processes.

First, if individuals perceive conflict as a potential threat to an attachment bond, then conflict should activate attachment behavior (e.g., protest, proximity seeking). Second, interactions involving conflict require relationship partners to attend to each other's goals and to adjust their behavior accordingly; this process offers an opportunity to enhance intimacy and communication because partners learn about each other's goals and feelings and because they may engage in collaborative strategies to try to resolve the conflict. Several researchers (Kobak & Duemmler, 1994; Pietromonaco & Feldman Barrett, 1997, 2000; Rholes, Simpson, & Stevens, 1998; Simpson, Rholes, & Phillips, 1996) have extended these two theoretical ideas.

Conflict as a Threat to the Attachment Bond

According to Bowlby (1980), any situation that threatens an attachment bond will activate attachment behaviors (e.g., clinging, crying) that are designed to reestablish and maintain the bond. Such situations can include a range of threats, such as fears about physical harm, illness, failures at work, loss of a loved one, and interactions involving conflict (Kobak & Duemmler, 1994; Simpson & Rholes, 1994; Simpson, Rholes, & Phillips, 1996). Individuals may experience interactions involving conflict as a threat to attachment security if such interactions raise questions about the partner's availability (e.g., evoke concerns about the partner leaving; Kobak & Duemmler, 1994; Simpson et al., 1996) or about the degree to which the partner is willing or able to listen, understand, and respond sensitively to their concerns. This point suggests that it is important to distinguish between conflicts about issues that are central to attachment (e.g., about the proximity and availability of the partner) and those that are less central to attachment (e.g., about finances). Conflicts that focus on attachment concerns are more likely to evoke threat, but if they can be resolved successfully, they also are likely to promote stronger attachment bonds. Determining whether a conflict evokes attachment concerns, however, may be a difficult task. Although some types of content (e.g., a conflict about finances) may be normatively less central to attachment concerns, some individuals (e.g., those with a preoccupied attachment style) may perceive such conflicts as a threat to the attachment bond. Thus even issues that are normatively less central to attachment may evoke attachment concerns for some individuals.

Attachment Style Differences

Although conflict may be somewhat aversive for everyone, the degree to which conflict evokes an attachment-relevant threat and the precise nature of the threat will vary depending on the content of working models of attachment. People who hold a secure attachment style, who expect their partners to be responsive and available and who therefore are not overly concerned with their partner's availability, may not perceive conflict as a threat to the relationship. As a consequence, securely attached individuals should be able to communicate openly during conflicts, and they should be able to apply a variety of strategies to negotiate with their partner (Kobak & Duemmler, 1994; Simpson et al., 1996).

In contrast, people with either a preoccupied (anxious–ambivalent) or a dismissing–avoidant attachment style are likely to experience conflict as a threat to the relationship, but for different reasons. For people with a preoccupied style, conflict may trigger concerns about being abandoned by the partner or about the partner's responsiveness to their needs, leading to hyperactivation of the attachment system (Kobak & Duemmler, 1994; Simpson et al., 1996). As a result, people with a preoccupied attachment style may respond to conflict by displaying intense emotions and excessively focusing on their own concerns, and they may have difficulty attending to the information conveyed by their partners. For people with a dismissing–avoidant style, conflict may pose a threat because it impinges on their preference for independence and self-reliance, a preference that may reflect a belief that others will be emotionally unavailable and unresponsive. During conflict, dismissing–avoidant individuals might be pressured to engage in behaviors that are connected to establishing emotional closeness, such as revealing personal thoughts and feelings, a process that may threaten their need to maintain their independence. Thus people with a dismissing–avoidant attachment style may respond to conflict by deactivating the attachment system, leading them to withdraw or downplay the significance of conflict (Kobak & Duemmler, 1994). Finally, people with a fearful–avoidant attachment style show aspects of both preoccupation with attachment and dismissing avoidance. Thus they may experience conflict as a threat for both of the reasons outlined.

This analysis points out that different attachment-related expectations and goals may determine perceptions of threat and that the behaviors following from such perceptions depend on the nature of the threat perceived (e.g., a threat that the partner will become unavailable or a threat to self-reliance through revealing one's inner thoughts and feelings).

Conflict as an Opportunity for Communication and Intimacy

Although conflict is likely to be associated with negative feelings and, under some circumstances, to be perceived as a potential threat, conflict also may provide an opportunity for enhancing intimacy and for improving communication. First, disagreements allow partners to express personal thoughts and feelings, which may lead to greater feelings of intimacy. Theorists (Reis & Patrick, 1996; Reis & Shaver, 1988) focusing on adult close relationships have suggested that interactions in which partners disclose their thoughts and feelings, listen and respond to each other, and feel accepted and understood promote relationship intimacy, and empirical evidence (Laurenceau, Feldman Barrett, & Pietromonaco, 1998; Laurenceau, Rivera, Schaffer, & Pietromonaco, 2004) supports this view. If interactions about a conflict include one or more of these components (e.g., disclosing feelings), then individuals might perceive the interaction as enhancing intimacy.

Second, disagreements may give partners a chance to learn and establish constructive strategies for adjusting to each other's needs and for resolving conflict. The literature on parent–child attachment relationships suggests that effective parents provide a model for constructive conflict resolution. As Bowlby (1979) points out, children can learn how to peacefully resolve conflicts if their parents behave in a gentle, nonpunitive fashion when handling disputes with the child. Kobak and Duemmler (1994) have elaborated this idea by proposing that, as children develop more complex language skills, conversations provide a context in which children learn to understand differences between their own perspectives and those of their partners (e.g., their parents). If parents respond in ways that promote harmonious interactions, these conversations may help children to learn constructive strategies (e.g., compromising, creating a mutually acceptable plan) for handling areas of disagreement (Kobak & Duemmler, 1994).

Processes similar to those observed between parents and children are thought to occur in adult romantic relationships (Kobak & Duemmler, 1994; Rholes et al., 1998; Simpson et al., 1996). In adult relationships, conversations about a conflict may promote security when (1) partners are able to maintain open communication despite differences, (2) partners learn new information about each other, and (3) partners are able to articulate their goals and feelings and, as a result, to consider revising them (see Kobak & Duemmler, 1994).

Attachment Style Differences

The ideas presented here suggest that attachment style differences might occur in perceptions of intimacy, as well as in actual intimacy-promoting behaviors. We first discuss differences in perceptions of intimacy and then turn to differences in behavior.

Just as perceptions of threat should vary as a function of individuals' attachment styles, perceptions of the intimacy-promoting aspects of conflict also should depend on individuals' underlying working models of attachment and their associated attachment goals. In particular, chronic goals to achieve intimacy and to maintain independence and self-reliance are likely to guide perceptions of interactions involving conflict, and the degree to which people hold each of these goals should differ as a function of attachment style (Pietromonaco & Feldman Barrett, 1997, 2000). People with a secure attachment style desire both intimacy and independence, but they are able to balance these two goals and to show flexibility in applying them. Thus their perceptions of conflict may be determined more by the nature of the interaction than by prior goals.

In contrast, people with a preoccupied attachment style appear to have an overriding goal to achieve intimacy that directs their perceptions and leads them to be sensitive to cues (e.g., personal disclosures) that are about their partner's responsiveness. During conflict, adults with a preoccupied style initially may interpret disclosures of thoughts and feelings by the partner as evidence of intimacy, because the partner is responding to them rather than avoiding or ignoring them. Thus, although people with a preoccupied style may perceive conflict as threatening, they also may see it as an opportunity for becoming closer to their partner. In considering this hypothesis, two issues need to be addressed. First, this idea may appear to be inconsistent with some findings (e.g., Collins, 1996) that indicate that preoccupied individuals view their partners as less responsive to their needs. However, preoccupied individuals are characterized by ambivalence in their views of others; although their global expectations about others tend to be negative (e.g., Collins & Read, 1990; Hazan & Shaver, 1987), they also tend to idealize their partners and relationships (Feeney & Noller, 1991). This tendency to idealize their partner and to hope that he or she will be responsive may lead them to interpret a disclosure as responsiveness. We propose that this kind of interpretation occurs close in time to the event and therefore would be more likely to appear in their immediate, online responses; over time, however, these initially hopeful perceptions may become more negative (e.g., if no real change actually occurs in the relationship) and thus would be reflected in their retrospective, global responses. Second, although we propose that both secure and preoccupied individuals have a goal to obtain intimacy, the two groups are likely to differ in how they attempt to achieve this goal (Pietromonaco & Feldman Barrett, 2000). Secure individuals may attempt to achieve intimacy through mutual sharing and open communication. In contrast, preoccupied individuals may attempt to achieve intimacy by obtaining self-regulatory assistance from their partners (Pietromonaco & Feldman Barrett, 2003), a process that may not lead to true intimacy in the relationship.

In contrast to preoccupied individuals, people with a dismissing–avoidant attachment style appear to hold an overriding goal to maintain independence, thereby protecting themselves from partners who are unresponsive and rejecting. Conflict generally will be aversive for those with a dismissing–avoidant attachment style, and they will attempt to withdraw from the situation. People with a fearful–avoidant style may hold goals to achieve intimacy and to maintain independence, and if both goals are activated at the same time, they may be caught in an approach–avoidance conflict, leading them to display patterns characteristic of both preoccupied and dismissing–avoidant individuals.

It is important to note that perceptions of conflict may or may not reflect the reality of the situation. That is, a woman might feel closer to her partner after the two have talked about their differences; if the partner actually feels closer to her as well, the woman's feelings are an accurate reflection of reality. However, it also is possible that she will interpret an interaction in which she and her partner disclosed as evidence of closeness, whereas her partner resents being pressured to reveal his inner feelings and actually feels more distant, a dynamic that may serve to increase, rather than decrease, the impact of conflict within the relationship. The extent to which such perceptions map onto reality is apt to depend on the quality of the behaviors enacted during conflict.

Attachment style also should be associated with behavioral differences in responses to conflict. We would expect behaviors that promote security (e.g., those involving open communication and negotiation) to be most common in interactions involving at least one secure partner. Repeated interactions in which partners listen and respond to each other's needs and concerns should form the basis for the development and maintenance of intimacy in the relationship (e.g., Reis & Shaver, 1988). Thus, in the long term, the relationships of secure individuals should be characterized by greater intimacy and satisfaction than those of insecure individuals. Indeed, this pattern has been repeatedly found in empirical work (for a review, see Mikulincer, Florian, Cowan, & Cowan, 2002).

THEORETICAL PREDICTIONS AND EMPIRICAL EVIDENCE

A number of theoretical predictions follow from the preceding analysis, but only some have received empirical attention. Indeed, two key theoretical assumptions have not yet been tested, but they form the basis for other predictions that have been tested. The first assumption is that people with an insecure attachment style (i.e., anxious–ambivalent or avoidant) are more likely to perceive conflict as a threat than those with a secure style. The second assumption is that people with different attachment styles are guided by different goals (e.g., goals for achieving intimacy or maintaining self-reliance) during conflict. The predictions that have been addressed in the empirical literature seem to follow from these assumptions. In the next sections, we review and evaluate the findings relevant to these predictions. Table 9.1 summarizes the methods and main findings of the studies considered here.

TABLE 9.1. Studies of Attachment Style and Conflict

Study	Participants	Attachment measure	Task	Conflict measure	Main findings
				Retrospective self-report studies of conflict strategies	
Levy & Davis (1988)	n = 234 (Study 2)	H & S (continuous ratings for each prototype)	Questionnaire	Conflict/ambivalence; ROCI	Ax & Av associated with > conflict. Ax & Av associated with < compromising & < integrating. Ax associated with > dominating. S associated with > compromising & > integrating.
Pistole (1989)	Students M & F (n = 137)	H & S (categorical)	Questionnaire	ROCI Assessed own use of conflict styles (e.g., compromising, obliging, integrating).	S > Ax & Av on integrating. S > Ax on compromising. Ax > Av on obliging.
Senchak & Leonard (1992)	Newlywed couples (n = 322 pairs)	H & S (categorical)	Questionnaire	MCI Assessed frequency of partner's problem solving, withdrawal, verbal aggression during conflict.	Couple effects: S–S < I–I & S(husband)–I(wife) on withdrawal & verbal aggression. S(wife)–I(husband) did not differ from other groups.
Carnelley et al. (1994) Study 1	College F in dating relationships (n = 163)	Multi-item: Anxiety & Avoidance (continuous)	Questionnaire	CSQ Assessed own degree of compromising, collaborating, accommodating, avoiding, demanding.	Av associated with < constructive conflict style. Ax n.s.
Study 2	Married F (recovering from	Same as above	Same as above	Same as above	Same as above

Study	Sample	Attachment measure	Method	Conflict measure	Findings
	clinical depression & nondepressed) (n = 48)				
Feeney (1994)	Married couples (n = 361 pairs)	H & S Revised to statements; 2 factors = Comfort with Closeness & Anxiety Over Relationships (continuous)	Questionnaire	CPQ Assessed own & partner's strategies of mutuality, coercion, destructive process, postconflict distress.	Comfort associated with > mutuality & < coercion, < destructiveness, & < distress. Ax associated with < mutuality & > coercion, > destructiveness, & > distress.
Creasey, Kershaw, & Boston (1999)	College women (n = 140)	RSQ (continuous)	Questionnaire	MADS Assessed positive (e.g., affection, validation) & negative (e.g., escalation, withdrawal) communication strategies.	Ax & Av associated with poorer conflict management skills, > negative escalation, & > withdrawal in romantic relationship.
O'Connell Corcoran & Mallinckrodt (2000)	Parents (n = 124) (94 F)	ASQ (continuous)	Questionnaire	ROCI-II Assessed own style (i.e., compromising, integrating, obliging, dominating, avoiding) in an important love relationship.	More confidence in attachments associated with > integration, > compromising, & < avoiding. More discomfort with closeness associated with > avoiding, < integration, & < compromising.
Creasey & Hesson-McInnis (2001)	Students in romantic dating relationship (n = 357) (273 F)	RSQ (continuous)	Questionnaire	MADS	More Ax with > negative emotions, > difficulty coping with negative emotions. More Ax or more Av with > difficulty inhibiting behavior, < positive tactics, > escalation, > withdrawal.

(continued)

TABLE 9.1. (continued)

Study	Participants	Attachment measure	Task	Conflict measure	Main findings
			Behavioral interaction studies		
Kobak & Hazan (1991)	Married couples (n = 40 pairs)	Marital Q sort (continuous)	Discussed & tried to resolve major disagreement.	Coded behavior for rejection and support/validation.	Wives who were more able to rely on their partners and/or who viewed partners as more available showed < rejection. Husbands who viewed partners as more available showed < rejection and > support/validation. Partner effects for husband only: The more he saw wife as available, the less she showed rejection and the more she showed support/validation.
Kobak et al. (1993), Study 2	Teens & their mothers (n = 48 pairs)	Q-sort: secure–anxious; hyperactivation–deactivation (continuous)	Discussed & tried to resolve major disagreement.	Coded behavior for support/validation, dysfunctional anger, assertiveness, avoidance of problem solving.	More secure male teens showed < avoidant problem solving. Males with a deactivating strategy (i.e., > dismissing) showed > dysfunctional anger. More secure females showed < dysfunctional anger. Mothers of female teens with a deactivating strategy (i.e., > dismissing) showed > dominance in the interaction.
Cohn et al. (1992)	Married couples with a preschool child (n = 27 pairs)	AAI (categorical)	Couple with child interaction in lab & natural interactions at home.	Interviewer ratings of observed conflict, positive interaction, marital functioning.	Couple effects: S–S > I–I positive interactions. SS < I–I in conflict. S(husband)–I(wife) < I–I in conflict. SS = S(husband)–I(wife) in conflict.
Simpson et al. (1996)	Dating couples (n = 123 pairs)	AAQ (continuous)	Discussed & tried to resolve major or minor problem.	Self-reported distress & perceptions of change in the partner/relationship from before to after conflict;	Men & women who were more Ax reported more distress in both conditions. Men & women for major problem only: More Ax reported less positive

Study	Sample	Attachment measure	Task	Behavioral measure	Findings
				coded behavior (e.g., stress, warmth, support, synchrony).	perception of change. More Av men showed less warmth & support, especially in major problem condition. More Ax women showed more stress/anxiety, especially in major problem condition.
Paley, Cox, Burchinal, & Payne (1999)	Married couples prior to birth of 1st child (n = 138 pairs)	AAI (categorical)	Discussed & tried to resolve major conflict.	Coded behavior (positive & negative affect; withdrawal).	Wives: P < S (continuous or earned) positive affect. D > S (continuous or earned) withdrawal. Husbands: n.s. Partner effects: Wives with D husbands less positive affect, more negative affect than those with cont. S husbands. Wives of earned S husbands less positive affect than wives of cont. S husbands.
Bouthillier, Julien, Dube, Belanger, & Hamelin (2002)	Cohabiting French Canadian couples (78%) married (n = 40 pairs)	AAQ (translated continuous) & AAI (categorical)	Discussed and tried to resolve most salient marital problem.	Coded behavior (IDCS) (e.g., conflict, withdrawal, support/validation, synchrony, escalation).	Men: S > P & D support, self-disclosure. Women: S > P & D support. Couple effect: S > I synchrony. S < I dominance.
Creasey (2002)	Student couples (n = 145 pairs)	AAI (categorical)	Discussed top 2 problems & tried to resolve; also, waiting-room conversation.	Coded behavior (SPAFF)—negative emotional expression (e.g., contempt, belligerence) & positive emotional expression (e.g., validation, affection).	Men, conflict condition: S < P & D for negative behavior. P = D for negative behavior. Women: S > P & D positive behavior, both conditions. S < P & D negative behavior, conflict condition. P = D. Partner effects: Couple with S woman > couple with I woman, positive behavior, both conditions. Couple with I man > couple with S man, negative behavior, conflict condition.

(continued)

TABLE 9.1. *(continued)*

Study	Participants	Attachment measure	Task	Conflict measure	Main findings
		Daily diary studies and cognitive study			
Tidwell et al. (1996)	Students M & F (*n* = 125)	H & S (categorical)	RIR	Perceived conflict in daily social interactions.	n.s.
Pietromonaco & Feldman Barrett (1997)	Students M & F (*n* = 70)	B & H (categorical)	RIR	Number & intensity of conflict interactions. Perceptions of partner & quality of interaction	n.s. For high-conflict interactions, P < S & D in negative perceptions of partner & interaction & own emotions. (This pattern was not found for lower conflict interactions.)
Fishtein et al. (1999)	Students involved in a dating relationship (*n* = 145) (72 M)	B & H (categorical)	Relationship Complexity Task	DAS conflict items	At higher levels of relationship conflict, Ps showed > positive complexity than S, D, or F. Individuals from all groups showed > negative complexity at higher levels of conflict.

Retrospective self-report studies of conflict frequency or intensity

Collins & Read (1990), Study 3	Dating couples	Multi-item: Close, Anxiety, Depend (continuous)	Questionnaire	Frequency, severity of conflict	Women: Comfort with closeness associated with < conflict. Men: n.s. Partner effect: Women with partner who is comfortable with closeness report < conflict. Men with more Ax partner report > conflict.
Kirkpatrick & Davis (1994)	Dating couples (n = 354 pairs)	H & S (categorical)	Questionnaire	Conflict/ambivalence	Women: Ax & Av > S. Men: n.s. Partner effect: W & M with Ax partners > W & M with S or Av partners.

Note. M, male; F, female; Ax, anxious–ambivalent or anxious ambivalence; Av, avoidant or avoidance; I, insecure; S, secure; P, preoccupied; F, fearful–avoidant; D, dis-missing–avoidant.

Attachment measures: AAI, Adult Attachment Interview (George, Kaplan, & Main, 1996), three categories (secure, preoccupied, and avoidant) and an additional desig-nation of unresolved/disorganized; ASQ, Attachment Style Questionnaire (Feeney, Noller, & Hanrahan, 1994), five subscales (Confidence in Attachment; Discomfort with Closeness; Relationships as Secondary to Achievement; Need for Approval; Preoccupation with Relationships); AAQ, Adult Attachment Questionnaire (Simpson, Rholes, & Nelligan, 1992), two dimensions (anxiety and avoidance); B & H, Bartholomew and Horowitz (1991), four categories (secure, preoccupied, fearful–avoidant, dismissing–avoidant); H & S, Hazan and Shaver (1987), three categories (secure, anxious–ambivalent, avoidant); RSQ, Relationship Scales Questionnaire (Griffin & Bartholomew, 1994), two dimensions (avoidance, anxious–ambivalent).

Conflict Measures: CSQ, Conflict Style Questionnaire (Levinger & Pietromonaco, 1989); CPQ, Communication Patterns Questionnaire (Christensen & Sullaway, 1984); DAS, Dyadic Adjustment Scale (Spanier, 1976); IDCS, Interactional Dimensions Coding System (Julien et al., 1989); MADS, Managing Affect and Differences Scale (Arellano & Markman, 1995); MCI, Margolin Conflict Inventory (Margolin, 1980); RIR, Rochester Interaction Record (Reis & Wheeler, 1991); ROCI, Rahim Or-ganizational Conflict Inventory (Rahim, 1983); ROCI-II, Rahim Organizational Conflict Inventory II (Rahim, 1990); SPAFF, Specific Affect Coding System (Gottman, 1996).

279

Prediction 1: People with insecure attachment styles will show less constructive behavior during conflict than those with a secure style. In particular, people high in anxious–ambivalence will use maladaptive approach tactics (e.g., coercion), whereas those high in avoidance will use withdrawal tactics.

Although difficulty handling conflict might follow from perceiving conflict as a threat, these studies do not provide direct evidence for this proposition. The first sections of Table 9.1 present studies that are relevant to this prediction—studies that use participants' retrospective self-reports of their typical behavioral strategies during conflict and studies that directly assess behavior during conflict.

Self-Reported Conflict Strategies

Consistent with Prediction 1, people who evidence greater attachment security on either categorical or multi-item self-report measures report using more constructive strategies, whereas those who evidence attachment insecurity (i.e., either higher anxious–ambivalence, avoidance, or both) report using less constructive strategies (Carnelley, Pietromonaco, & Jaffe, 1994; Creasey & Hesson-McInnis, 2001; Creasey, Kershaw, & Boston, 1999; Feeney, 1994; Levy & Davis, 1988; O'Connell Corcoran & Mallinckrodt, 2000; Pistole, 1989). People high in either form of insecure attachment report poorer conflict management skills, including greater difficulty understanding their partner's perspective, behaving in ways that escalate the conflict (e.g., attacking the partner, using coercion), withdrawing, and using fewer positive tactics such as validation or maintaining a focus on the topic (Creasey & Hesson-McInnis, 2001; Creasey et al., 1999; Feeney, 1994). These patterns of self-reported conflict tactics appear to generalize across samples of students (e.g., Creasey et al., 1999; Pistole, 1989), married women (Carnelley et al., 1994, Study 2), married couples (Feeney, 1994), and individual parents (O'Connell Corcoran & Mallinckrodt, 2000).

Many of the findings (Creasey et al., 1999; Creasey & Hesson-McInnis, 2001; O'Connell Corcoran & Mallinckrodt, 2000) show similarities in the self-reported conflict tactics of those high in anxious–ambivalence or avoidance; for example, people high in either anxious–ambivalence or avoidance report strategies related to conflict escalation and conflict avoidance or withdrawal. The exception is that anxious–ambivalence is associated with being more willing to oblige the partner (O'Connell Corcoran & Mallinckrodt, 2000; Pistole, 1989), whereas avoidance is not. Thus self-report studies consistently support the idea that insecure attachment is associated with poorer conflict resolution skills but that, in general, the strategies associated with anxious–ambivalence are similar to those for avoidance.

Self-reports of conflict strategies, like self-reports in general, are limited because people must calculate in some way how they typically behave during conflict. People may not always be aware of their behavioral patterns, and their reports may not accurately reflect what they actually do. For example, self-reports may be biased by how participants feel at the moment, by their most salient recent experience, or by a desire to appear socially competent (see Ross, 1989; Schacter, 1996).

Observations of Behavior during Interactions: Effects of Own Attachment Style

Studies in which partners' behaviors are observed and coded address this limitation of self-report studies and thereby better test whether behavior during conflict varies as a function of attachment style. The first study (Kobak & Hazan, 1991) to demonstrate a link between romantic attachment (assessed using a marital Q-sort) and conflict found that wives who were more secure (i.e., who were able to rely on their partner and/or who viewed their partner as psychologically available) were less likely to show rejection when discussing a disagreement in their relationship. Furthermore, husbands who were more secure (i.e., who viewed their partners as psychologically available) were less likely to show rejection and more likely to provide support and validation during the discussion. Similarly, in a study (Kobak et al., 1993) of mother–teen dyads, teens who were more secure displayed more constructive strategies (e.g., expressed less dysfunctional anger) when discussing a conflict with their mother, and teens who relied on an avoidance strategy (i.e., who were characterized as "deactivating the attachment system") engaged in less constructive behaviors, although the nature of the behaviors differed for males and females. Thus these studies suggest that security is associated with more constructive behaviors during conflict in both romantic relationships and parent–child relationships.

Studies (Bouthillier, Julien, Dube, Belanger, & Hamelin, 2002; Simpson et al., 1996) using self-reported adult attachment styles have examined whether anxious–ambivalence and avoidance predict unique sets of behaviors during conflict. One study (Simpson et al., 1996) examined the link between attachment scores on the Adult Attachment Questionnaire (AAQ; Simpson, Rholes, & Nelligan, 1992) and dating couple members' behavior during a discussion in which they tried to resolve either a major or minor problem in their relationship. Observer ratings of behavior in the interaction indicated that more anxious–ambivalent women who discussed a major problem evidenced greater stress and anxiety and poorer quality (e.g., showed less synchrony and less ease with the interaction) discussions. Men who showed greater attachment avoidance who discussed a major problem displayed less warmth and support, especially when discussing a major problem. In addition, across both major and minor problems, observers rated the discussions of men who showed greater avoidance as lower in quality. (Anxious–ambivalent men showed patterns similar to those of avoidant men, but the findings did not reach conventional levels of significance.)

Another study (Bouthillier et al., 2002) used the same self-report measure (AAQ) as did Simpson and colleagues (1996) but did not replicate the pattern of results. As in the Simpson and colleagues study, couples engaged in an interaction in which they tried to resolve a major problem in their relationship, and observers coded a variety of communication behaviors (e.g., assertiveness, support–validation, withdrawal, conflict, problem solving, negative escalation, synchrony). In contrast to Simpson and colleagues' findings, the self-report measure of attachment was not associated with any of the communication behaviors. The difference in findings between the two studies could be accounted for by multiple differences between the samples. The samples in the Bouthillier and colleagues (2002) study versus the Simpson and colleagues study, respectively, differed in relationship status (married/cohabiting vs. dating), age ($M = 44$ vs. $M = 19$), size (40 couples vs. 123 couples), and culture (French Canadian vs. American).

However, Bouthillier and colleagues (2002) did find that attachment style based on childhood relationships with parents, assessed using the Adult Attachment Interview (AAI; e.g., Main, Kaplan, & Cassidy, 1985; for a full description, see Hesse, 1999), predicted some differences in behavior. Husbands who received an AAI classification of preoccupied or dismissing evidenced less supportive behaviors and less self-disclosure and more withdrawal than those classified as secure. Wives classified as dismissing or preoccupied showed fewer supportive behaviors than those classified as secure. (AAI classifications were not associated with scores on the self-report measure of romantic attachment.)

Three additional studies (Cohn, Silver, Cowan, Cowan, & Pearson, 1992; Creasey, 2002; Paley, Cox, Burchinal, & Payne, 1999) have demonstrated that attachment assessed via the AAI predicts behavior during conflict. Similar to the Bouthillier and colleagues (2002) study, an investigation (Creasey, 2002) of dating couples showed that preoccupied and dismissing men and women displayed more negative behavior when discussing a conflict than did those who were secure. In addition, preoccupied and dismissing women showed less positive behavior than did secure women across both waiting-room and conflict interactions, but men's positive behavior did not differ by attachment style.

Similarly, a study (Paley et al., 1999) of married men and women found that wives classified as preoccupied showed less positive affect than those classified as either continuous secure (individuals who provide coherent reports of mainly positive childhood experiences) or earned secure (individuals who experienced adversity in childhood but who provide coherent and thoughtful reports of their experiences). Furthermore, wives classified as dismissing showed withdrawal more often than wives classified as either form of secure. Husbands' attachment styles, however, were not significantly associated with their own behavior.

In other work (Cohn et al., 1992), however, it was husbands classified as insecure, in comparison with those classified as secure, who showed more conflict and fewer positive exchanges when interacting with their wife and child on a challenging task and who evidenced poorer functioning (e.g., clearer communication, more respect, less blaming and hostility) in interactions at home. Wives' AAI scores, however, were not associated with their own behavior.

Overall, behavioral observation studies have found that securely attached individuals display more constructive behavior during conflict than do insecurely attached individuals. These studies have relied primarily on the AAI to assess attachment, and only two studies (Bouthillier et al., 2002; Simpson et al., 1996) have examined behavior using self-report measures of romantic attachment. We might expect assessments of attachment based specifically on romantic relationships to be a more precise predictor of behavior during conflict with a romantic partner than assessments based on the caregiver–child relationship. The single study that included both measures found effects for the AAI but not for the self-report measure of romantic attachment (Bouthillier et al., 2002). Unfortunately, the two measures differ not only in focus (i.e., caregiver–child relationship vs. romantic relationship) but also in method (i.e., interview vs. self-report). In general, the interview and self-report measures of attachment are not highly correlated, especially when they focus on different domains (e.g., a parent–child relationship vs. a romantic relationship), and findings from studies using the interview method do not necessarily match those of studies using a self-report method (e.g., Bartholomew & Shaver, 1998; Crowell, Fraley, & Shaver, 1999).

Summary

Both self-report and behavioral observation studies generally support the prediction that securely attached individuals behave more constructively during conflict than do insecurely attached individuals, and these more constructive interactions may facilitate the development of intimacy. The idea that people with a preoccupied attachment style will show different behavior patterns from those with a dismissing attachment style received little support. Although a few findings (e.g., Paley et al., 1999; Simpson et al., 1996) suggest that anxious–ambivalence and avoidance may trigger somewhat different patterns of behavior, these patterns were not consistent across studies. In addition, men and women do not always show similar or equally strong patterns, suggesting that gender may moderate the way in which attachment behavior is manifested during conflict. One possibility is that behaviors that are more closely linked to gender-role stereotypes are most likely to show differences during conflict. For example, one study (Simpson et al., 1996) found that men who were more avoidant showed less warmth and support when discussing a major problem, and these behaviors are more consistent with stereotypically masculine behavior. In contrast, women who were more anxious showed greater stress and anxiety, which is more consistent with stereotypically feminine behavior. Similarly, other work (Creasey, 2002; Paley et al., 1999) suggests that secure women show differences that are consistent with the stereotype that women must appear agreeable or pleasant, even during conflict; in both of these studies, secure women (but not secure men) expressed more positive affect or positive behavior during conflict than did insecure women. Although gender differences appear in only a subset of studies, it seems reasonable to assume that the precise behaviors that vary as a function of attachment during conflict may depend, in part, on the fit between the behavior and gender-role expectations.

Prediction 2: People high in anxious ambivalence will show more negative emotion during conflict than those who are high in either avoidance or security.

This prediction follows from the assumption that people with an anxious–ambivalent attachment style perceive conflict as a threat, leading to hyperactivation of the attachment system; as a result, they will be more likely to show emotional distress (Kobak et al., 1993; see also Mikulincer & Shaver, in press).

Several studies (Creasey & Hesson-McInnis, 2001; Feeney, 1994; Simpson et al., 1996) have found that people higher in anxious ambivalence report experiencing more negative emotion during conflict. One study (Simpson et al., 1996) found that men and women higher in anxious ambivalence reported more distress after discussing either a minor or major relationship conflict. Other work has indicated that people higher in anxious ambivalence report that they generally experience more postconflict distress (Feeney, 1994) or more negative emotions and difficulty coping with negative emotions during arguments (Creasey & Hesson-McInnis, 2001).

These findings are open to several interpretations. People high in anxious ambivalence may show more negative emotion during conflict because (1) they wish to convey their distress to their partner, (2) they actually feel more distress, or (3) they are simply more willing to report negative feelings in general. People higher in anxious ambivalence generally appear more willing to report distress, particularly when they provide global, memory-based reports of their experiences (e.g., Collins & Read, 1990; Pietromonaco & Carnelley, 1994; Pietromonaco & Feldman Barrett, 1997). It is interesting that, in the one study (Pietromonaco & Feldman Barrett, 1997) in which anxious ambivalence was not associated with reports of greater negative emotion, participants provided reports of their emotions immediately following social interactions, thereby reducing the likelihood that memory played a role in their responses; instead, the immediate reports of dismissing–avoidant individuals evidenced more negative emotion following high-conflict interactions than did those of secure individuals.

It may be that people high in avoidance will show sensitivity to threat on measures that require less conscious, reflective processing. People high in avoidance are thought to deal with the threat posed by conflict by shutting down the attachment system. Because this process is likely to occur below conscious awareness, their efforts to regulate emotions may not be evident in their self-reports, but they may be revealed by more covert measures (e.g., behavioral or physiological measures). The scant evidence from behavioral measures of emotional expression during conflict is mixed. For example, some work (Simpson et al., 1996) has found that people high in anxious ambivalence display more anger and hostility during conflict, and other work (Kobak et al., 1993) indicates that individuals with more avoidant strategies evidence more dysfunctional anger during conflict. Still other work (Creasey, 2002) found that both preoccupied and dismissing–avoidant individuals expressed more negative emotion than secure individuals. No studies have examined the link between physiological reactivity and attachment during conflict, but some work (Dozier & Kobak, 1992; Feeney & Kirkpatrick, 1996; Mikulincer, 1998) suggests that avoidance may be associated with greater physiological reactivity under some circumstances (for an exception, see Fraley & Shaver, 1997).

Summary

Self-report evidence is consistent with the prediction: People characterized by an anxious–ambivalent attachment style report more negative emotion during conflict than those characterized by a secure or dismissing–avoidant style. It is not clear, however, whether this evidence reflects a greater willingness on the part of anxious–ambivalent individuals to report distress or whether they actually experience greater distress. The few studies using measures other than retrospective self-reports do not reveal a consistent pattern; findings variously indicate that anxious ambivalence, avoidance, or both are associated with greater negative emotion. Overall, this hypothesis needs to be examined more fully in studies using both self-report and more covert measures of emotion. Research has yet to adequately answer the key theoretical question underlying this prediction: Is attachment associated with differences in the need to regulate emotion in the face of conflict and in the strategies (e.g., deactivation or hyperactivation) people use?

Prediction 3: People high in anxious ambivalence will hold less negative (or even more positive) perceptions about their partner and relationship following conflict than those high in either avoidance or security.

This prediction follows from the idea that, for people high in anxious ambivalence, conflict activates their goal to achieve intimacy, and therefore they will focus on cues that suggest that they have obtained intimacy and responsiveness from a partner. Three studies (Fishtein, Pietromonaco, & Feldman Barrett, 1999; Pietromonaco & Feldman Barrett, 1997; Simpson et al., 1996) provide evidence relevant to this prediction about perceptions of conflict. One study (Pietromonaco & Feldman Barrett, 1997) relied on an event-contingent daily diary method (Reis & Wheeler, 1991) to examine perceptions and feelings following everyday interactions. The advantage of this method is that participants report on their thoughts and feelings immediately after an interaction occurs, making their self-reports less subject to the usual memory biases associated with global retrospective self-reports. Participants, who had been preselected on the basis of the attachment prototype choices (i.e., secure, preoccupied, fearful–avoidant, dismissing–avoidant; Bartholomew & Horowitz, 1991), recorded their responses to the majority of their social interactions for 1 week. We found that people with a preoccupied attachment style held more positive (or less negative) perceptions of high-conflict interactions (i.e., those rated as 4 or 5 on a 5-point scale). When rating their high-conflict interactions, preoccupied individuals reported feeling greater intimacy and satisfaction than did either secure or dismissing–avoidant individuals and reported greater self-disclosure than did those in any of the other attachment groups. Furthermore, preoccupied individuals also evidenced more positive perceptions of their partners following high-conflict interactions; they reported higher esteem for their partners than did secure or fearful–avoidant individuals; and they perceived their partners as disclosing more and as experiencing more positive emotion than did either secure or dismissing–avoidant individuals. Further analyses examining the associations between the full range of conflict ratings (i.e., from low to high) and perceptions of the quality of the interaction and of the partner indicated that preoccupied individuals generally reported more positive or less negative perceptions of the interaction and/or partner as conflict increased and did so to a greater extent than individuals in other attachment groups.

Overall, this study suggests that—despite their difficulties with managing conflict and negative emotions—under some conditions preoccupied individuals may view conflict as an opportunity to reveal themselves, to learn about their partners, and ultimately to achieve greater intimacy. It is important to note, however, that this study examined perceptions of interactions across a range of interaction partners (e.g., romantic partners, friends, strangers) and that, unlike much of the other research, it did not focus exclusively on romantic relationships.

Another study (Fishtein et al., 1999) provides further evidence that, for preoccupied individuals, conflict in romantic relationships might be connected to both positive and negative feelings. Although this study did not examine responses to a specific conflict, it did investigate how people involved in high- versus low-conflict romantic relationships think about and organize information about their relationship. In this study, college men and women were preselected on the basis of their attachment prototype choices (Bartholomew & Horowitz, 1991), and all were involved in a stable romantic relationship. Participants completed a relationship complexity task, a modified version of Linville's (1985) self-complexity task, in which they selected positive (e.g., "accepting," "close," "mature") and negative (e.g., "controlling," "uncomfortable," "dull") descriptors from a deck of 100 cards and organized them into as many or as few groups needed to describe their romantic relationship. Relationship complexity is defined as the degree to which people describe a relationship using many distinct, nonoverlapping attributes. We were particularly interested in the degree to which people showed complexity in describing the positive attributes and the negative attributes of their relationship, and therefore we examined both positive and negative complexity. Participants also completed the Dyadic Adjustment Scale (DAS; Spanier, 1976), which provided information about the degree of conflict in their relationship.

We predicted that preoccupied individuals, who desire a high degree of intimacy and responsiveness, would hold more complex knowledge about the positive aspects of their relationship, when the relationship was high in conflict. We also anticipated that preoccupied individuals, as well as individuals with other attachment styles, would hold more complex knowledge about the negative aspects of their relationship when they were high in conflict. The results indicated that, as relationship conflict increased, people with a preoccupied attachment style showed greater positive relationship complexity, whereas people with other attachment styles showed less positive relationship complexity. Furthermore, greater conflict was associated with greater negative relationship complexity, and this was true for people of all attachment styles. These findings suggest that people with a preoccupied attachment style may not only attend to the negative aspects of conflict but also may see the more positive, potentially intimacy-promoting aspects of conflict.

Although the findings of these two studies are consistent with Prediction 3, it is noteworthy that another study (Simpson et al., 1996) in which couples discussed and tried to resolve either a minor or a major relationship conflict yielded findings in the direction opposite to the prediction. Men and women who were higher in anxious ambivalence reported (1) more distress when discussing either a minor or a major problem and (2) less positive perceptions of their partner or relationship when they explicitly compared their feelings after the discussion with their feelings before the discussion (e.g., reported on the degree to which they perceived change in the amount of love or commitment felt toward the partner or relationship), but only in the major-problem condition.

The methods and measures used in the three studies described in this section varied considerably. For example, the task used in the Simpson and colleagues (1996) study may have been particularly threatening for people high in anxious ambivalence because they were (1) asked to try to resolve a conflict and (2) asked to "tell the other what it is about his or her attitudes, habits, or behaviors that bothers you," increasing the likelihood that anxious–ambivalent individuals received feedback that threatened their fragile self-views. In contrast, the event-contingent diary study (Pietromonaco & Feldman Barrett, 1997) examined interactions that participants designated as high in conflict (4–5 on a 5-point scale), did not specify a particular structure for the conflict, and examined interactions across a range of partners (e.g., romantic and nonromantic). The other study (Fishtein et al., 1999) focused on the general level of conflict in the romantic relationship rather than conflict in a particular interaction. In addition, the dependent measures differed greatly across the three studies.

It will be important for future work to examine this question using methods and measures that are more comparable across studies. The current findings suggest that, under some conditions, people who are anxious–ambivalent may view conflict both as a threat and as an opportunity for intimacy, but attention to the intimacy-promoting aspects may be limited by the magnitude of the threat and the degree to which it evokes negative feelings about oneself. Future investigations that manipulate the magnitude and focus of the threat will help to address this issue.

Summary

This prediction has not received much empirical attention, and the evidence is mixed. Furthermore, the three studies that provide relevant evidence differ greatly in their methods, making it difficult to compare the findings. Nevertheless, these studies raise the possibility that people with an anxious–ambivalent attachment style may perceive both positive and negative sides of conflict.

MODERATING EFFECT OF THE RELATIONAL CONTEXT

Partner and Couple Effects

Although the predictions following from attachment theory focus on the link between a person's attachment style and his or her own perceptions and behavior, attachment behavior occurs in the context of a relationship to which two partners each bring their own attachment histories. Attachment relationships have been conceptualized as goal-corrected partnerships in which partners attend to and adjust to the goals and needs of the other (Bowlby, 1969), but few theoretical statements specify how one partner's attachment style might contribute to the other partner's behavior (i.e., partner effects) or how the match between two partners' attachment styles might shape behavior during conflict (i.e., couple effects).

Although attachment theorists have not developed clear predictions about the influence of one partner's attachment style on the other partner's perceptions or behavior or about the joint effects of couple members' attachment styles, two expectations seem reasonable. First, when both partners are secure, they should be better able to handle conflict than when one or both partners have an insecure style. Second, individuals in relationships in which at least one partner is secure will be better able to handle conflict than those in which both partners are insecure.

In line with the first expectation, couples including two secure partners evidence the most constructive conflict styles. In a self-report questionnaire study (Senchak & Leonard, 1992), newly married couples in which both partners were secure reported less withdrawal and verbal aggression during conflict than couples made up of two insecure partners or an insecure wife with a secure husband; couples with a secure wife and an insecure husband did not differ from any of the other couple types. In addition, behavioral observation studies (Bouthillier et al., 2002; Cohn et al., 1992) have shown that couples made up of two secure partners (assessed using the AAI) generally communicate better during conflict than couples with two insecure partners.

In line with the second expectation, couples in which only one partner is secure appear to resolve conflict better than those in which both partners are insecure. Four studies (Cohn et al., 1992; Creasey, 2002; Kobak & Hazan, 1991; Paley et al., 1999) have demonstrated that couples that include one secure partner, especially when the secure partner was the husband, show more constructive behavior during conflict than those that include two insecure partners. One study (Cohn et al., 1992) found that couples made up of a secure husband and an insecure wife evidenced less conflict and better functioning than those made up of two insecure partners, but this study did not include a comparison group with a secure wife and insecure husband.

Two additional studies (Kobak & Hazan, 1991; Paley et al., 1999), however, suggest that husband's attachment security contributes to wives' behavior during conflict, whereas wives' attachment security does not show a similar effect on husbands' behavior. For example, wives of continuously secure husbands evidenced more positive and less negative affect than those with dismissing husbands, and they showed more positive affect than wives of earned secure husbands; wives' attachment, however, did not predict husbands' behavior (Paley et al., 1999). Similarly, other work (Kobak & Hazan, 1991) has found that the more the husband viewed his wife as psychologically available (i.e., the more the husband showed secure attachment), the less his wife displayed rejection and the more she provided support and validation during a problem-solving task. As in the Paley and colleagues (1999) study, wives' attachment scores (on reliance and on seeing the partner as psychologically available) were not associated with husbands' behaviors. One additional study (Creasey, 2002) also found that couples in which the man was secure displayed less negative behavior when discussing a conflict than those in which the man was insecure; however, couples in which the woman was secure also showed more positive behavior in both a waiting room (warm-up) interaction and when discussing a conflict. In addition, the two studies (Creasey, 2002; Paley et al., 1999) that tested for interactions between partners' attachment styles did not find any significant joint effects.

Overall, studies examining partner and couple effects suggest three patterns. First, couples that include two secure partners show the most constructive conflict resolution styles. Second, couples that include one secure partner are generally more adept at dealing with conflict than those with two insecure partners. Third, the way in which couples handle conflict may depend more on the husband's attachment security than on the wife's attachment security. This pattern parallels many studies (see Maushart, 2002) that suggest that husbands' perceptions are better predictors of marital satisfaction than wives' perceptions, and it further highlights the importance of taking into account gender (or gender roles) when evaluating attachment patterns. It is important to note that some studies (Kobak & Hazan, 1991; Rholes, Simpson, Campbell, & Grich, 2001) have found that wives' attachment better predicted behavior in interactions involving support giving and receiving. These findings suggest that the context of the interaction may influence the degree to which the attachment style of the husband or wife contributes to the quality of the interaction.

Level of Conflict in the Relationship

Theoretical perspectives on attachment and conflict do not necessarily predict differences in the amount or intensity of conflict, but this question is important because any differences in perceptions, emotions, and behavior might follow from differences in the frequency or intensity of conflict. Although people with a secure attachment style generally are more satisfied in their relationships than those with an insecure attachment style (e.g., Carnelley et al., 1994; Cohn et al., 1992; Collins & Read, 1990; Kirkpatrick & Davis, 1994), they do not necessarily experience less conflict in their relationships than those with an insecure attachment style. In retrospective self-report studies, women who were less comfortable with closeness (Collins & Read, 1990, Study 3) or who endorsed either an anxious–ambivalent or an avoidant style (Kirkpatrick & Davis, 1994) reported more conflict in their relationships, but men did not show significant associations between their own style and reported conflict in either study. In both studies, however, men's reports of conflict were associated with their partner's attachment style; specifically, men paired with an anxious–ambivalent partner reported more conflict.

In contrast to retrospective self-report studies, event-contingent diary studies in which participants report on conflict on an interaction-by-interaction basis have not found attachment differences in perceived degree of conflict (Pietromonaco & Feldman Barrett, 1997; Tidwell, Reis, & Shaver, 1996) or in the number of interactions rated as high in conflict (Pietromonaco & Feldman Barrett, 1997).

In addition, two studies (Collins & Read, 1990; Kirkpatrick & Davis, 1994) found that men's reports of conflict were associated with their partner's attachment style; men reported more conflict when they were paired with a woman who evidenced anxious ambivalence. One of these studies (Kirkpatrick & Davis, 1994) also found a similar partner effect for women; that is, women paired with an anxious–ambivalent man also reported more conflict than those paired with either an avoidant or secure man.

Overall, these studies suggest that the association between attachment style and amount of conflict is not straightforward. Men and women do not show the same patterns in retrospective self-report studies, and immediate perceptions of conflict intensity appear to be unrelated to attachment style. Furthermore, one partner's attachment style contributes to the other person's perceptions of conflict, suggesting that it will be important for future work to examine the relationship context (i.e., the partner's characteristics, interactions between both partners' characteristics) in which perceptions of conflict arise.

CONSIDERATIONS FOR FUTURE RESEARCH AND CONCLUSIONS

Several basic assumptions about the link between attachment and conflict have yet to be directly tested. The first untested assumption is that attachment style predicts whether conflict is perceived as a threat. Many studies have shown that people who evidence insecure attachment are more likely to have difficulty handling conflict, but these problems may arise because conflict represents a threat or for other, equally plausible reasons. For example, people who are insecurely attached may show less constructive behavior during conflict because they have poorer social skills than those who are securely attached, rather than because they perceive conflict as a threat. In addition, in examining the assumption that conflict evokes a threat for some people, it will be useful to move beyond defining conflict in broad terms (i.e., as an area of major disagreement) and to take into account the focus of the disagreement. Some people may perceive a threat when the conflict focuses on intimacy and partner availability, but they may not do so when the conflict focuses on another issue (e.g., how to spend money). Distinguishing among different areas of conflict may reveal the conditions under which people high in anxious ambivalence versus those high in avoidance perceive conflict as a threat.

Furthermore, although threat is likely to be important in activating the attachment system (e.g., Bowlby, 1980; Simpson & Rholes, 1994), it is not clear whether a threat that originates within an attachment relationship (e.g., from conflict) differs from threats that originate outside of the relationship (e.g., threat from a physical, nonhuman source). For threats arising outside of the relationship, an attachment figure may serve as a safe haven who is not associated with the cause of the distress. For threats arising within the relationship (e.g., a conflict with a romantic partner), the attachment figure may be perceived both as the source of the threat and as a potential safe haven, presenting an approach–avoidance dilemma. To our knowledge, no studies have compared responses to these two classes of threat, but we would expect attachment style differences to be more pronounced when threat arises from within the relationship. A related issue is whether threat arising from conflict between relationship partners activates not only the attachment system but also the caregiving system; partners must deal with their own fears by using the other as a secure base, but at the same time, they also need to be able to serve as a secure base for their partner. Research on attachment differences in support seeking and caregiving (e.g., Carnelley, Pietromonaco, & Jaffe, 1996; Collins & Feeney, 2000; Feeney & Collins, 2001; Kobak & Hazan, 1991;

Simpson et al., 1992) can inform further work on attachment and conflict because good conflict resolution skills may require the ability to balance between using a partner as a secure base (i.e., seeking support) and serving as a secure base (i.e., giving support) for the partner.

The second untested assumption is that people with different attachment styles are guided by different goals during conflict; specifically, people high in anxious ambivalence seek to achieve intimacy during conflict interactions, whereas those high in avoidance seek to remain self-reliant. Our own work suggests that anxious ambivalence (preoccupation) is associated with perceiving not only the negative side of conflict but also its potential to promote intimacy, but whether this pattern results from differences in interpersonal goals during conflict remains to be determined.

In addition to testing these basic assumptions, several other issues need to be addressed. First, it will be important to assess whether perceptions during conflict accurately reflect the reality of the situation; for example, if a person with a preoccupied attachment style experiences greater intimacy after conflict, does that person's partner also report greater intimacy, or does the partner feel less intimacy? Studies examining both partners' perceptions after conflict will help to address this issue. Second, the long-term effects of conflict on perceptions of intimacy and communication need to be explored. It may be that preoccupied individuals show less negative perceptions in the short run, but, over time, it may be secure individuals who show less negative perceptions. Furthermore, research along these lines might help to resolve the puzzling findings of some longitudinal studies (see Fincham & Beach, 1999) that have shown that negative conflict behavior predicts enhanced marital satisfaction over time. Perhaps couples with two (or at least one) secure partner accrue benefits over time from conflict, whereas other couples do not.

Third, an attachment perspective on conflict should integrate ideas about partner and couple effects. The few studies that examine both partners' attachment security suggest that behavior during conflict is improved by the presence of at least one secure partner, and this is especially true when the secure partner is the husband. These findings highlight the importance of examining attachment within the context of the partnership, in addition to considering it as an individual difference variable (see Pietromonaco & Feldman Barrett, 2000).

Fourth, attachment effects associated with conflict need to be considered within the context of gender. Husbands' attachment security appears to dictate the quality of interactions during conflict, a pattern that is consistent with other work showing that men's outcomes better predict the status of the marriage (see Maushart, 2002). The process underlying these patterns remains to be determined, but it is possible either that men are more likely to dominate the interactions and thereby set the tone or that women, who tend to hold more relational, interdependent self-views (e.g.,

Cross & Madson, 1997), are more likely to attend to the partner's behavioral cues and to modulate their own behavior accordingly. Thus a theoretical framework for understanding the connection between attachment and conflict will need to specify when gender-related differences might occur.

Fifth, future investigations may benefit from examining each partner's perceptions and behavior over the time frame of the conflict. Behaviors that occur at the beginning of the conflict may not be the same as those toward the end. For example, people with a preoccupied attachment style might begin with constructive tactics, but if their needs are not met, they might engage in coercion or attack as the conflict progresses.

Overall, attachment theory provides a framework for understanding how people will think, feel, and behave during conflict. In particular, it suggests that people's working models will shape their perceptions of threat and their goals during conflict, resulting in distinct response profiles. The empirical work so far supports the idea that attachment security (or insecurity) contributes to how people respond to conflict in a general way, but as our review has pointed out, several key assumptions of an attachment perspective on conflict remain to be tested, and the role of contextual variables (e.g., the relationship as a whole; gender roles) needs to be integrated into the theoretical account. It is clear that conflict situations provide a unique context in which to test critical predictions following from attachment theory. A closer examination of these predictions offers the potential to enrich knowledge about attachment processes in general in close relationships and to organize diverse findings about relationship conflict within an overarching theoretical framework.

REFERENCES

Arellano, C., & Markman, H. (1995). The Managing Affect and Differences Scale (MADS): A self-report measure assessing conflict management in couples. *Journal of Family Psychology, 9,* 319–334.

Bartholomew, K., & Horowitz, L. M. (1991). Attachment styles among young adults: A test of a four-category model. *Journal of Personality and Social Psychology, 61,* 226–244.

Bartholomew, K., & Shaver, P. R. (1998). Methods of assessing adult attachment: Do they converge? In J. A. Simpson & W. S. Rholes (Eds.), *Attachment theory and close relationships* (pp. 25–45). New York: Guilford Press.

Bouthillier, D., Julien, D., Dube, M., Belanger, I., & Hamelin, M. (2002). Predictive validity of adult attachment measures in relation to emotion regulation behaviors in marital interactions. *Journal of Adult Development, 9,* 291–305.

Bowlby, J. (1969). *Attachment and loss: Vol. 1. Attachment.* New York: Basic Books.

Bowlby, J. (1973). *Attachment and loss: Vol. 2. Separation: Anxiety and anger.* New York: Basic Books.

Bowlby, J. (1979). *The making and breaking of affectional bonds.* London: Tavistock.

Bowlby, J. (1980). *Attachment and loss: Vol. 3. Loss: Sadness and depression.* New York: Basic Books.

Brehm, S. S., Miller, R. S., Perlman, D., & Campbell, S. M. (2002). *Intimate relationships.* Boston: McGraw-Hill.

Bradbury, T. N., & Fincham, F. D. (1990). Attributions in marriage: Review and critique. *Psychological Bulletin, 3,* 3–33.

Canary, D. J., & Cupach, W. R. (1988). Relational and episodic characteristics associated with conflict tactics. *Journal of Social and Personal Relationships, 5,* 305–325.

Carnelley, K. B., Pietromonaco, P. R., & Jaffe, K. (1994). Depression, working models of others, and relationship functioning. *Journal of Personality and Social Psychology, 66,* 127–140.

Carnelley, K. B., Pietromonaco, P. R., & Jaffe, K. (1996). Attachment, caregiving, and relationship functioning in couples: Effects of self and partner. *Personal Relationships, 3,* 257–277.

Christensen, A., & Sullaway, M. (1984). *Communication Patterns Questionnaire.* Unpublished manuscript, University of California, Los Angeles.

Cohn, D. A., Silver, D. H., Cowan, C. P., Cowan, P. A., & Pearson, J. (1992). Working models of childhood attachment and couple relationships. *Journal of Family Issues, 13,* 432–449.

Collins, N., & Read, S. J. (1990). Adult attachment, working models, and relationship quality in dating couples. *Journal of Personality and Social Psychology, 58,* 644–663.

Collins, N. L. (1996). Working models of attachment: Implications for explanation, emotion, and behavior. *Journal of Personality and Social Psychology, 17,* 810–832.

Collins, N. L., & Feeney, B. C. (2000). A safe haven: An attachment theory perspective on support seeking and caregiving in intimate relationships. *Journal of Personality and Social Psychology, 78,* 1053–1073.

Collins, N. L., & Read, S. J. (1994). Cognitive representations of attachment: The structure and function of working models. In K. Bartholomew & D. Perlman (Eds.), *Advances in personal relationships: Vol. 5. Attachment processes in adulthood* (pp. 53–90). London: Kingsley.

Creasey, G. (2002). Associations between working models of attachment and conflict management behavior in romantic couples. *Journal of Counseling Psychology, 49,* 365–375.

Creasey, G., & Hesson-McInnis, M. (2001). Affective responses, cognitive appraisals, and conflict tactics in late adolescent romantic relationships: Associations with attachment orientations. *Journal of Counseling Psychology, 48,* 85–96.

Creasey, G., Kershaw, K., & Boston, A. (1999). Conflict management with friends and romantic partners: The role of attachment and negative mood regulation expectancies. *Journal of Youth and Adolescence, 28,* 523–543.

Cross, S. E., & Madson, L. (1997). Models of the self: Self-construals and gender. *Psychological Bulletin, 122,* 5–37.

Crowell, J. A., Fraley, R. C., & Shaver, P. R. (1999). Measurement of individual differences in adolescent and adult attachment. In J. Cassidy & P. R. Shaver

(Eds.), *Handbook of attachment: Theory, research, and clinical applications* (pp. 434–465). New York: Guilford Press.

Dozier, M., & Kobak, R. R. (1992). Psychophysiology in attachment interviews: Converging evidence for deactivating strategies. *Child Development, 63,* 1473–1480.

Feeney, B. C., & Collins, N. L. (2001). Predictors of caregiving in adult intimate relationships: An attachment theoretical perspective. *Journal of Personality and Social Psychology, 80,* 972–994.

Feeney, B. C., & Kirkpatrick, L. A. (1996). Effects of adult attachment and presence of romantic partners on physiological responses to stress. *Journal of Personality and Social Psychology, 70,* 255–270.

Feeney, J. A. (1994). Attachment style, communication patterns, and satisfaction across the life cycle of marriage. *Personal Relationships, 1,* 333–348.

Feeney, J. A., & Noller, P. (1991). Attachment style and verbal descriptions of romantic partners. *Journal of Social and Personal Relationships, 8,* 187–215.

Feeney, J. A., Noller, P., & Hanrahan, M. (1994). Assessing adult attachment. In M. B. Sperling & W. H. Berman (Eds.), *Attachment in adults: Clinical and developmental perspectives* (pp. 128–152). New York: Guilford Press.

Fincham, F. D., & Beach, S. R. (1999). Marital conflict: Implications for working with couples. *Annual Review of Psychology, 50,* 47–77.

Fishtein, J., Pietromonaco, P. R., & Feldman Barrett, L. (1999). The contribution of attachment style and relationship conflict to the complexity of relationship knowledge. *Social Cognition, 17,* 228–244.

Fraley, R. C., & Shaver, P. R. (1997). Adult attachment and the suppression of unwanted thoughts. *Journal of Personality and Social Psychology, 73,* 1080–1091.

George, C., Kaplan, N., & Main, M. (1996). *Adult Attachment Interview protocol* (3rd ed.). Unpublished manuscript. University of California at Berkeley.

Gottman, J. M. (1994). *Why marriages succeed or fail.* New York: Simon & Schuster.

Gottman, J. M. (1996). *What predicts divorce: The measures* [Unpublished coding manuals]. Mahwah, NJ: Erlbaum.

Griffin, D. W., & Bartholomew, K. (1994). The metaphysics of measurement: The case of adult attachment. In K. Barthlomew & D. Perlman (Eds.), *Advances in personal relationships: Vol. 5. Attachment processes in adulthood* (pp. 17–52). London: Kingsley.

Hazan, C., & Shaver, P. R. (1987). Romantic love conceptualized as an attachment process. *Journal of Personality and Social Psychology, 52,* 511–524.

Hesse, E. (1999). The Adult Attachment Interview: Historical and current perspectives. In J. Cassidy & P. R. Shaver (Eds.), *Handbook of attachment: Theory, research, and clinical applications* (pp. 395–433). New York: Guilford Press.

Holmes, J. G., & Boon, S. D. (1990). Developments in the field of close relationships: Creating foundations for intervention strategies. *Personality and Social Psychology Bulletin, 16,* 23–41.

Julien, D., Markman, H. J., & Lindhal, K. M. (1989). A comparison of a global and a microanalytic coding system: Implications for future trends in studying interactions. *Behavioral Assessment, 11,* 81–100.

Kirkpatrick, L. A., & Davis, K. E. (1994). Attachment style, gender, and relationship stability: A longitudinal analysis. *Journal of Personality and Social Psychology, 66,* 502–512.

Kobak, R. R., Cole, H. E., Ferenz-Gillies, R., Fleming, W. S., & Gamble, W. (1993). Attachment and emotion regulation during mother–teen problem solving: A control theory analysis. *Child Development, 64,* 231–245.

Kobak, R. R., & Duemmler, S. (1994). Attachment and conversation: Toward a discourse analysis of adolescent and adult security. In K. Bartholomew & D. Perlman (Eds.), *Advances in personal relationships: Vol. 5. Attachment processes in adulthood* (pp. 121–149). London: Kingsley.

Kobak, R. R., & Hazan, C. (1991). Attachment in marriage: Effects of security and accuracy of working models. *Journal of Personality and Social Psychology, 60,* 861–869.

Laurenceau, J. P., Feldman Barrett, L., & Pietromonaco, P. R. (1998). Intimacy as an interpersonal process: The importance of self-disclosure, partner disclosure, and perceived partner responsiveness in interpersonal exchanges. *Journal of Personality and Social Psychology, 74,* 1238–1251.

Laurenceau, J. P., Rivera, L. M., Schaffer, A. R., & Pietromonaco, P. R. (2004). Intimacy as an interpersonal process: Current status and future directions. In D. Mashek & A. Aron (Eds.), *Handbook of closeness and intimacy* (pp. 61–78). Mahwah, NJ: Erlbaum.

Levinger, G., & Pietromonaco, P. (1989). *Conflict Style Inventory.* Unpublished scale, University of Massachusetts, Amherst.

Levy, M. B., & Davis, K. (1988). Lovestyles and attachment styles compared; Their relations to each other and to various relationship characteristics. *Journal of Social and Personal Relationships, 5,* 439–471.

Linville, P. W. (1985). Self-complexity and affective extremity: Don't put all your eggs in one cognitive basket. *Social Cognition, 3,* 94–120.

Main, M., Kaplan, N., & Cassidy, J. (1985). Security in infancy, childhood, and adulthood: A move to the level of representation. *Monographs of the Society for Research in Child Development, 50* (1–2, Serial No. 209), 66–104.

Margolin, G. (1980). *The Conflict Inventory.* Unpublished manuscript.

Maushart, S. (2002). *Wifework: What marriage really means for women.* New York: Bloomsbury.

Mikulincer, M. (1998). Adult attachment style and individual differences in functional versus dysfunctional experiences of anger. *Journal of Personality and Social Psychology, 74,* 513–524.

Mikulincer, M., Florian, V., Cowan, P. A., & Cowan, C. P. (2002). Attachment security in couple relationships: A systematic model and its implications for family dynamics. *Family Process, 41,* 405–434.

Mikulincer, M., & Shaver, P. R. (in press). The attachment behavioral system in adulthood: Activation, psychodynamics, and interpersonal processes. In M. Zanna (Ed.), *Advances in experimental social psychology.* New York: Academic Press.

O'Connell Corcoran, K., & Mallinckrodt, B. (2000). Adult attachment, self-efficacy, perspective taking, and conflict resolution. *Journal of Counseling and Development, 78,* 473–483.

Paley, B., Cox, M. J., Burchinal, M. R., & Payne, C. C. (1999). Attachment and marital functioning: Comparison of spouses with continuous–secure, earned–secure, dismissing, and preoccupied attachment stances. *Journal of Family Psychology, 13,* 580–597.

Pietromonaco, P. R., & Carnelley, K. B. (1994). Gender and working models of attachment: Consequences for perceptions of self and romantic relationships. *Personal Relationships, 1,* 63–82.

Pietromonaco, P. R., & Feldman Barrett, L. (1997). Working models of attachment and daily social interactions. *Journal of Personality and Social Psychology, 73,* 1409–1423.

Pietromonaco, P. R., & Feldman Barrett, L. (2000). The internal working models concept: What do we really know about the self in relation to others? *Review of General Psychology, 4,* 155–175.

Pietromonaco, P. R., & Feldman Barrett, L. (2003). *What can you do for me?: Attachment style and motives underlying esteem for partners.* Manuscript submitted for publication.

Pistole, M. C. (1989). Attachment in adult romantic relationships: Style of conflict resolution and relationship satisfaction. *Journal of Social and Personal Relationships, 6,* 505–510.

Rahim, M. A. (1983). A measure of styles of handling interpersonal conflict. *Academy of Management Journal, 26,* 368–376.

Rahim, M. A. (1990). *The Rahim Organizational Conflict Inventory–II.* Palo Alto, CA: Consulting Psychologists Press.

Reis, H. T., & Patrick, B. C. (1996). Attachment and intimacy: Component processes. In E. T. Higgins & A. W. Kruglanski (Eds.), *Social psychology: Handbook of basic principles* (pp. 523–563). New York: Guilford Press.

Reis, H. T., & Shaver, P. (1988). Intimacy as an interpersonal process. In S. W. Duck & D. F. Hay (Eds.), *Handbook of personal relationships* (pp. 367–389). Chichester, UK: Wiley.

Reis, H. T., & Wheeler, L. (1991). Studying social interaction with the Rochester Interaction Record. In M. P. Zanna (Ed.), *Advances in experimental social psychology* (Vol. 24, pp. 269–318). San Diego, CA: Academic Press.

Rholes, W. S., Simpson, J. A., Campbell, L., & Grich, J. (2001). Adult attachment and the transition to parenthood. *Journal of Personality and Social Psychology, 81,* 421–435.

Rholes, W. S., Simpson, J. A., & Stevens, J. G. (1998). Attachment orientations, social support, and conflict resolution in close relationships. In J. A. Simpson & W. S. Rholes (Eds.), *Attachment theory and close relationships* (pp. 166–188). New York: Guilford Press.

Ross, M. (1989). Relation of implicit theories to the construction of personal histories. *Psychological Review, 96,* 341–357.

Schacter, D. L. (1996). *Searching for memory: The brain, the mind, and the past.* New York: Basic Books.

Senchak, M., & Leonard, K. E. (1992). Attachment styles and marital adjustment among newlywed couples. *Journal of Social and Personal Relationships, 9,* 51–64.

Simpson, J. A., & Rholes, W. S. (1994). Stress and secure base relationships in adulthood. In K. Bartholomew & D. Perlman (Eds.), *Advances in personal relationships: Vol. 5. Attachment processes in adulthood* (pp. 181–204). London: Kingsley.

Simpson, J. A., Rholes, W. S., & Nelligan, J. S. (1992). Support seeking and support giving within couples in an anxiety-provoking situation: The role of attachment styles. *Journal of Personality and Social Psychology, 62,* 434–446.

Simpson, J. A., Rholes, W. S., & Phillips, D. (1996). Conflict in close relationships: An attachment perspective. *Journal of Personality and Social Psychology, 71,* 899–914.

Spanier, G. B. (1976). Measuring dyadic adjustment: New scales for assessing the quality of marriage and similar dyads. *Journal of Marriage and the Family, 38,* 15–28.

Tidwell, M. O., Reis, H. T., & Shaver, P. R. (1996). Attachment, attractiveness, and social interaction: A diary study. *Journal of Personality and Social Psychology, 71,* 729–745.

CHAPTER 10

Interpersonal Safe Haven and Secure Base Caregiving Processes in Adulthood

BROOKE C. FEENEY
NANCY L. COLLINS

Attachment theory describes caregiving as a basic component of human nature and essential for personal and relationship well-being (Bowlby, 1969/1982, 1973, 1988). Caregiving plays a central role in the nature and function of attachment relationships, and, according to the theory, it interacts in important ways with two other basic components of human nature—attachment and exploration. However, the caregiving aspects of adult attachment relationships have been understudied relative to the attachment aspects. Also, since Bowlby's theoretical contribution, very little empirical work or theoretical elaboration has been advanced regarding the interworkings of the attachment, exploration, and caregiving systems in adulthood. Thus our goal in this chapter is to elaborate on attachment theory's notions of how these three behavioral systems are likely to interact in adulthood, to highlight aspects of our program of research in this area, to integrate this work with the contributions of other researchers in this area, and to point to directions for future research.

INTERWORKINGS OF ATTACHMENT, EXPLORATION, AND CAREGIVING

We view attachment theory as providing an ideal framework for studying social support and caregiving processes in adulthood because it stipulates that the need for security is one of the most fundamental of all basic needs across the lifespan and because it provides a basis for understanding the complex interpersonal dynamics involved in three important and interrelated components of human nature: attachment (care seeking), caregiving, and exploration. All three systems are presumed to have survival value; thus the urges to engage in each form of behavior are likely to be preprogrammed to some degree. Bowlby (1988) argues that "to leave their development solely to the caprices of individual learning would be the height of biological folly" (p. 5). Because attachment theory considers the interworkings of these three systems, it points to interesting and important avenues for research on social support and caregiving processes that have previously gone unexplored in the social-support and relationship literatures. The three systems are briefly described as a backdrop for our in-depth discussion of caregiving processes, theory, and research.

Attachment

First, attachment theory regards the propensity to form strong emotional bonds with particular individuals as an innate human characteristic, present in all individuals from the cradle to the grave. The attachment system presumably functions to maintain an individual's safety and security through contact with nurturing caregivers. The attachment system becomes activated most strongly in adversity so that, when frightened, distressed, tired, or ill, the individual will feel an urge to seek protection, comfort, and support from a primary caregiver (Bowlby, 1973, 1969/ 1982; Bretherton, 1987).

Although attachment theory was originally developed to explain the nature of the relationship that develops between a parent and child, Bowlby has consistently emphasized that attachment behavior is in no way limited to children. Although it is likely to be less readily activated in adults than in children, attachment behavior can be seen in adults whenever they are feeling distressed. One of the most public and intense examples of attachment behavior in adults could be seen around the time of the terrorist attacks of September 11, 2001, during which time many individuals reported a strong desire to be in close proximity to their loved ones. However, attachment behavior in adults can be witnessed, perhaps with less intensity, in many other types of distressing situations—for example, adults often seek proximity to the significant people in their lives (often spouses) in response to stress resulting from physical pain, fatigue, fear of new situations, feelings of rejection by others, work problems, threat of loss, and so forth. Attachment behavior, and an associated increase in desire for care, is considered to be the norm in these situations (Bowlby, 1988).

An important postulate of attachment theory is that both adults and children tend to maintain relations to the significant people in their lives (attachment figures) within certain limits of distance or accessibility. Attachment behaviors can be regarded as a set of behavior patterns that have the effect of keeping the individual in close proximity to a nurturing caregiver, and the conditions that terminate activation of the attachment system depend on the intensity of its arousal. At low intensity, it may simply be the sight or sound of the caregiver; at higher intensity, clinging, prolonged embraces, and/or active problem solving may be necessary. Attachment theory emphasizes that adults' desire for comfort and support in adversity should not be regarded as childish or immature dependence; instead, it should be respected as being an intrinsic part of human nature that contributes to personal health and well-being. Moreover, research in both the child and adult attachment literatures supports the postulate that the particular way in which attachment behavior comes to be organized within an individual (e.g., how it is manifested by a particular individual) depends to a large extent on the individual's history of experiences with attachment figures or caregivers in distressing situations and on the general knowledge the individual possesses regarding the self and attachment figures—for example, their capabilities and likely responses as environmental conditions change.

Exploration

The urge to explore the environment—to work, play, discover, create, and take part in activities with peers—is regarded as another basic component of human nature (Bowlby, 1988). According to attachment theory, true exploration is likely to occur only when attachment needs have been satisfied (when the attachment system is deactivated). In this sense, exploration can be inconsistent with attachment behavior (Bowlby, 1988). That is, when an individual of any age is feeling safe and secure, he or she is likely to explore away from the attachment figure (or caregiver); however, when distressed in any way, he or she is likely to feel an urge toward proximity. According to the theory, when individuals are confident that an attachment figure (in adulthood often a romantic partner) will be available and responsive when needed and called upon, they should feel secure enough to explore the environment, take on challenges, and make discoveries. For adults, these exploratory activities may take many forms and may last for varying lengths of times. Examples of exploratory activities for adults include traveling, developing hobbies, visiting new places, working toward important personal goals, developing new friendships, working (Hazan & Shaver, 1990), engaging in leisure activities (Carnelley & Ruscher, 2000), and so forth. However, focused and productive exploratory activity is presumed to occur only when the individual (1) does not question the security and availability of his or her home base and (2) is not experiencing fear, distress, or any condition that would lead him or her to feel an urge to move toward his or her home base.

Caregiving

Caregiving is regarded by attachment theory as a major component of human nature, and it is the focus of this chapter. From an attachment theory perspective, caregiving includes a broad array of behaviors that complement a relationship partner's attachment behavior and exploration behavior. Thus it is viewed as serving two major functions: (1) providing a *safe haven* for the attached person by meeting his or her needs for security (e.g., by soothing and problem solving in stressful situations) and (2) providing a *secure base* for the attached person by supporting his or her autonomy and exploration in the environment. Although the concept of a secure base can be viewed more broadly as an attachment relationship that incorporates both safe haven and secure base dynamics (e.g., see Crowell et al., 2002; Waters & Cummings, 2000), we view the provision of a safe haven and a secure base as serving two different caregiving functions (on which we elaborate later).

In our work on caregiving processes in adult close relationships, we have been viewing caregiving, consistent with attachment theory, as part of an *interpersonal process*. Although both the attachment literature and social-support literature have become quite massive in the past couple of decades, there has been very little empirical work examining the caregiving processes that occur within adult close relationships, particularly as they unfold within the context of specific support and caregiving interactions. Bowlby (1969/1982) emphasized the need for additional research on caregiving processes and stated that caregiving should be studied systematically within a conceptual framework similar to that adopted for attachment behavior. However, theory regarding the development and functioning of the caregiving system was never developed in his writings in the same way that he detailed theory and evidence regarding the attachment system. George and Solomon (1989, 1999a, 1999b) have noted this as well and have launched a program of research in an effort to provide theoretical and empirical elaboration of maternal–infant caregiving dynamics (see also George & Solomon, 1996; Solomon & George, 1996). These researchers have presented a framework for conceptualizing and studying maternal caregiving in which parents are viewed as developing adults who possess an organized caregiving system that is linked developmentally and behaviorally to attachment yet remains distinct from it. A similar theoretical elaboration and intensive program of research regarding caregiving in adult relationships is needed.

Partly in response to this need, we began a program of research and conducted some in-depth investigations of caregiving processes in adulthood by considering important research questions such as the following:

1. What does it mean to be a good caregiver in adult relationships?
2. How are care seeking and caregiving behaviors coordinated in the context of specific support interactions?
3. Can we identify individuals who are effective and ineffective caregivers?
4. What types of skills, resources, and motivations are needed to be a good caregiver?
5. What are the personal and interpersonal mechanisms that might lead people to be responsive or unresponsive caregivers?
6. Do specific caregiving behaviors predict important outcomes, such as the quality and persistence of relationships over time?

Most of our work to date has centered on understanding the dynamics involved in responding to a relationship partner's expressions of distress. However, an element that, surprisingly, has been missing from research on support and caregiving in adult relationships is a comprehensive view of caregiving that considers not only the way that relationship partners provide each other with comfort, reassurance, and support in times of stress but also the ways in which relationship partners support each other's personal growth, autonomous exploration, and acceptance of intrinsically rewarding challenges. In accordance with attachment theory, our work in this area takes into account (1) the interpersonal nature of caregiving dynamics, (2) normative processes as well as individual differences in caregiving dynamics, and (3) the importance of considering subjective perceptions of behaviors, in addition to observing actual caregiving behaviors. In the following we describe the two major functions of caregiving in more depth, provide an integrating framework for examining the interpersonal processes involved in both caregiving functions, and describe some exciting research that has been and is currently being conducted in each caregiving domain. Finally, we point to some important directions for future work in this area.

SAFE HAVEN CAREGIVING PROCESSES

> To remain within easy access of a familiar individual known to be ready
> and willing to come to our aid in an emergency is clearly a good
> insurance policy—whatever our age.
> —BOWLBY (1988, p. 27)

Caregivers provide a safe haven for their relationship partners when they respond sensitively and appropriately to their partners' distress and resulting need for comfort, reassurance, and/or assistance. According to attachment theory, good caregivers are those who respond to attachment behavior by restoring "felt security"; that is, by facilitating problem resolution and alleviating distress. Attachment theory emphasizes the importance of responding flexibly, sensitively, and in a timely fashion to an attached person's needs as they arise.

The type and amount of support that is needed in any given situation is determined primarily by the care receiver (i.e., the degree to which he or she is distressed); however, various external contingencies (e.g., the dangers of a particular situation) are likely to be contributing factors. Bowlby (1969/1982, 1988) suggests that the particular type of attachment behavior emitted (e.g., crying, following, seeking), as well as the particular circumstances in which these behaviors are emitted (e.g., emergency vs. nonemergency situations), are important in determining the effects that each has on caregiving behavior. For example, pain cries and hunger cries of infants have been found to affect their caregiver's behavior very differently: Pain cries tend to elicit much faster and more alarmed caregiving behaviors, whereas hunger cries tend to elicit more relaxed responses from caregivers. The attachment behaviors of adults should similarly influence the caregiving behaviors of their partners. That is, when the attachment system has been activated with high intensity (as a result of experiencing very high levels of distress) and attachment behaviors are relatively intense (e.g., intense seeking, clinging), similarly intense caregiving behaviors, such as physical closeness, are necessary to restore feelings of security. However, attachment behaviors that have been activated with low intensity (e.g., expressed concern about an upcoming performance evaluation) are sufficiently appeased by more relaxed caregiving behaviors, such as verbal reassurance. Thus, in order for a caregiver to provide an adequate safe haven, he or she must sensitively and flexibly respond to attachment needs; be aware of the other's point of view, feelings, and intentions; encourage expression of feelings; and adjust his or her own behavior in response to the contingencies of the situation.

Although caregiving can take many positive or negative forms, Bowlby (1988) describes a sensitive caregiver as one who regulates his or her behavior so that it meshes with that of the person who is being cared for. A sensitive caregiver takes his or her cues from and allows his or her interventions to be paced by the care receiver, is attuned to the recipient's signals, attends to the details of the recipient's behavior, interprets the signals and behaviors correctly, discovers what response is most appropriate for the individual recipient, responds promptly and appropriately, and monitors the effects of his or her behavior on the recipient and modifies it accordingly. In response, the care receiver behaves in ways that take account of the caregiver's interventions. Thus, in a well-functioning partnership, each partner is adapting to the other. An insensitive caregiver, on the other hand, may not notice the care receiver's signals or may misinterpret or ignore them when they are noticed, interfere with activities in an arbitrary way, behave in a rejecting manner, and/or respond tardily, inappropriately, or not at all to a need for support.

Bowlby (1988) cautions, however, that adequate time and a relaxed atmosphere are necessary conditions in order for caregivers to behave in a sensitive manner. He also cautions that we have a strong tendency to treat others the same way that we ourselves have been treated. Although he postulates that caregiving behavior is, like attachment behavior, to some degree preprogrammed (meaning that it is ready to develop along certain lines when certain conditions elicit it), all the detail is learned. For example, research evidence indicates that abused individuals tend to be unsympathetic to the distress of others (Bowlby, 1988). Thus individuals are likely to learn either healthy or unhealthy caregiving patterns from the significant people who have previously been responsible for their care.

Bowlby (1988) further notes that good caregivers must have a genuine understanding and respect for the need for affection, intimacy, and support that is ingrained in all individuals. Although it requires some effort to provide an effective safe haven for a relationship partner, Bowlby notes that the rewards of such care are great: Individuals who are cared for in a sensitive, loving way are likely to be happy and trusting, develop confidence that others will be helpful when needed, become self-reliant and bold in their explorations of the world, be cooperative with others, and be sympathetic and helpful to others in distress. A particularly interesting aspect of this theory is that the sensitive acceptance of dependence when needed is likely to produce *less* neediness or dependence in the long run. This phenomenon has been observed in mother–infant dyads; for example, mothers who are sensitive and responsive to their baby's signals have babies who cry less than the babies of mothers who are less sensitive (Bowlby, 1988). According to attachment theory, a similar phenomenon may be characteristic of adult relationships.

SECURE BASE CAREGIVING PROCESSES

All of us, from the cradle to the grave, are happiest when life is organized as a series of excursions, long or short, from the secure base provided by our attachment figure(s).
                                                                     —BOWLBY (1988, p. 62)

Caregivers provide a secure base for their relationship partners when they respond sensitively and appropriately to their partners' exploratory behavior and to their need for encouragement in their exploratory activity. According to attachment theory, good caregivers are not only those who know how to intervene actively and respond appropriately to signals of distress, but they arc also those who know when to be encouraging, available, and noninterfering in support of their partner's personal growth and exploration (Bowlby, 1988). An important aspect of caregiving involves providing a secure base from which an attached person can make excursions into the outside world (by playing, working, learning, discovering, creating, making new friends), knowing that he or she can return for comfort, reassurance, and/or assistance should he or she encounter difficulties along the way. Bowlby (1988) describes the concept of a secure base as one in which caregivers create the conditions that enable the relationship partner to explore the world in a confident way:

> In essence this role is one of being available, ready to respond when called upon to encourage and perhaps assist, but to intervene actively only when clearly necessary. In these respects it is a role similar to that of the officer commanding a military base from which an expeditionary force sets out and to which it can retreat, should it meet with a setback. Much of the time the role of the base is a waiting one but it is none the less vital for that. For it is only when the officer commanding the expeditionary force is confident his base is secure that he dare press forward and take risks. (p. 11)

Bowlby (1988) suggested that individuals who are confident that their base is secure and ready to respond if called upon are likely to take it for granted. Yet, should the base suddenly become unavailable or inaccessible, the importance of the base to the "emotional equilibrium" of the individual is immediately apparent. In fact, it is a major postulate of attachment theory that individuals who thrive emotionally and socially and who make the most of their opportunities are those who have attachment figures, be they a parent in childhood or a spouse in adulthood, who, while always encouraging the individual's autonomy, are also available and responsive when called upon. As described previously with regard to safe haven caregiving, Bowlby emphasizes that no caregiver will be able to effectively provide a secure base for another person unless he or she understands and respects that attachment behavior is a part of human nature (even in adulthood) and is not a negative sign of dependency that should be outgrown.

Sensitive caregivers may function as a secure base for their relationship partners by facilitating exploration, responding to exploratory successes and difficulties in a way that is helpful and encouraging, promoting open communication regarding personal goals and desires, and variously fostering autonomy and providing assistance, depending on the partner's state of mind. In addition, sensitive caregivers promote the other's welfare by facilitating personal growth, encouraging the partner to take initiative, and recognizing the times when they should wait and not interfere versus step in and provide guidance. Encouraging behavior may involve drawing a partner's attention to an exploratory opportunity (whereas parents may draw their child's attention to a toy, a spouse may draw his or her partner's attention to a career opportunity) or giving tips on how to engage in an exploration activity that the partner may have difficulty initiating on his or her own. In contrast, insensitive caregivers who do not provide an adequate secure base for their relationship partners are likely to take little notice of the partner's goals and goal-related feelings, to intrude when a partner is trying to solve a problem on his or her own, to fail to respect the partner's desire for autonomy by discouraging or impeding exploration, to discourage bids for support and encouragement, or to respond in an ill-timed and unhelpful manner.

Whereas children use their parents as a secure base for exploration by keeping note of the parents' whereabouts, exchanging glances, and from time to time returning to the parents to share in enjoyable mutual contact, adults are likely to engage in similar yet more adult forms of these behaviors. For example, an adult is likely to keep track of a spouse's whereabouts, to maintain phone contact when exploring away from the spouse for an extended period of time, to share details of his or her explorations with the spouse, and so on. Adults who are less certain of their spouses' whereabouts—or of their availability and responsiveness when needed—are less likely to engage in exploratory activity. Although exploratory excursions in adulthood are longer than they are in childhood, attachment theory emphasizes that "throughout adult life the availability of a responsive attachment figure remains the source of a person's feeling secure" (Bowlby, 1988, p. 62). Thus the ability to confidently explore the environment stems from having a caregiver who both encourages and supports such exploration and who has proven to be readily available and responsive when comfort, assistance, and/or protection has been sought.

Because in well-functioning adult relationships, partners provide one another with a secure base from which they can explore and a safe haven to which they can retreat when distressed, caregiving appears to be an ongoing process that does not end when a partner's security is not being immediately threatened. From this perspective, taking care of a partner involves not only responding to expressions of distress and assisting in problem resolution but also in helping the partner to grow as an individual by encouraging autonomous exploration and the pursuit of personally rewarding challenges. Thus, if good caregivers are doing their job, they are "on duty" on a continual basis. This view of caregiving is somewhat different from the way social support and caregiving have been conceptualized in the relationship and social support literatures, and it has been an overlooked topic of research investigation.

INTEGRATIVE MODEL

Figure 10.1 depicts a theory-based model that is guiding some of our work in this area (originally proposed in Feeney, 2003). The general concept of this integrative model—which depicts the interpersonal processes involved in attachment, caregiving, and exploration, as well as the ways in which these three behavioral systems are likely to influence the functioning of one another—was inspired by a *Circle of Security* intervention,

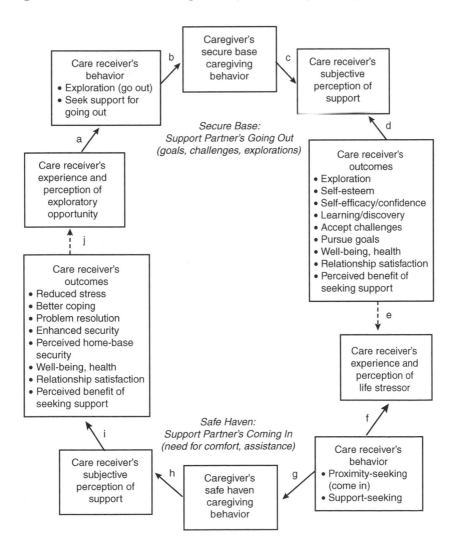

FIGURE 10.1. Circle of security in adulthood. Interpersonal model of support-seeking, caregiving, and exploration.

which was based on attachment theory and devised by Marvin, Cooper, Hoffman, and Powell (2002) in order to teach parenting skills. The specific details of the model presented here for adult relationships was inspired by attachment theory, as well as by previous empirical work examining caregiving processes in adult relationships (Collins & Feeney, 2000; Feeney & Collins, 2001; Hazan & Shaver, 1990) and by other relevant theories in the relationship and social-support literatures (e.g., Barbee, 1990; Cutrona, 1996; Reis & Shaver, 1988). We refer to the adult version of this model as the "Circle of Security in Adulthood."

For simplicity, the model refers to the member of the dyad who could potentially provide care in a given situation as the "caregiver" and to the person who could potentially benefit from support as the "care receiver." However, it is important to keep in mind that in adult relationships, the caregiving and care receiving roles are not exclusively assigned to particular couple members. Depending on the situation, adult partners are sometimes in the care giving role and sometimes in the care receiving role.

The bottom portion of the figure (beginning with the care receiver's experience and perception of a life stressor) depicts the *safe haven* function of caregiving, which is set into motion when an individual's *attachment* system is activated in response to a life stressor. As depicted in the model, the experience of a stressful event should lead an individual to desire proximity, support, and reassurance from an attachment figure (path *f*); this support-seeking behavior should motivate the caregiver to provide support (path *g*); the provision of support should lead the individual to feel supported (path *h*); and perceptions of being supported should contribute to the individual's overall sense of security and well-being (path *i*). Thus the safe haven aspect of care seeking and caregiving occurs when a caregiver supports his or her partner's attachment behavior or behavior that involves "coming in" toward the partner and the relationship. Some of these interpersonal processes involving safe haven caregiving have been established in previous empirical work with samples of dating couples (e.g., Collins & Feeney, 2000; Feeney & Collins, 2001; Simpson, Rholes, & Nelligan, 1992).

The top portion of the figure depicts the *secure base* function of caregiving, which is set into motion when an individual's *exploratory* system is activated in response to a potential exploratory opportunity. The secure base aspect of care seeking and caregiving occurs when a caregiver supports his or her partner's exploratory behavior or behavior that involves "going out" from the partner or the relationship. Because virtually no empirical work has been done on the secure base function of caregiving in adulthood, this is an important focus of current work (see Feeney, 2003).

According to attachment theory, an individual's overall perception that his or her home base is secure (based on many interactions involving the provision of safe haven caregiving) should lead him or her to (1) have a greater desire for exploration than would otherwise be the case and (2) perceive that exploratory opportunities (goals, challenges) are important, attainable, and worth the effort and risk (path *j*). In the next stage in the model, greater desires for exploration and greater perceptions that the pursuit of goals, explorations, discoveries, and challenges are worthwhile should predict (1) more exploratory behavior (efforts to identify and achieve personal goals, a desire to take on challenges, efforts to learn new skills, develop new competencies, and make new discoveries) and (2) a greater willingness to seek goal-relevant support (path *a*). It is important to note that not every personal goal or challenge will require support or assistance from others. Thus it is expected that challenges and goals that are perceived to be more daunting and difficult to obtain will increase one's desire for support from a significant other and lead one to solicit more active forms of secure base caregiving (e.g., assistance, encouragement; path *a*). In other cases, simply the perception that one's home base is secure and available *if needed* should suffice. Because the urge for exploration is such a basic component of human nature, seeking or desiring support from relationship partners for exploration (e.g., encouragement in the pursuit of goals) is expected to be a common occurrence.

In the next stage of the model, the behaviors of the caregiver and care receiver are expected to mesh in complementary ways. Adult caregivers function as a secure base for their romantic partners by (1) conveying a sense of confidence in their partners' abilities to handle challenging situations, (2) encouraging the partners to accept challenges and try new things, (3) showing interest in the partners' personal goals, plans, and desires for the future, (4) not interfering or intruding in the partners' explorations, and (5) balancing an acceptance of the partners' need for self-growth with the conveyance of a continued availability if needed. Thus clear and direct expressions of a need for support should be associated with more active secure base caregiving behavior (e.g., encouragement, assistance in removing obstacles), whereas exploratory behavior on the part of the care receiver should be associated with less active, non-interfering, nonintrusive secure base caregiving behavior (path *b*).

Next, the care receiver's subjective perception of the caregiver's behavior should depend on the degree to which the caregiver functions as a secure base. Caregiving behaviors that sensitively encourage the care receiver in his or her exploratory behavior, in the attainment of goals, and in the pursuit of personally rewarding challenges, as well as behaviors that convey availability if needed and that are appropriately contingent on the needs of the recipient, should be perceived by the care receiver as supportive. In contrast, intrusive, interfering, or discouraging behaviors should be viewed as unsupportive (path *c*).

Finally, to the extent that the care receiver perceives the caregiver to have effectively provided a secure base for exploration, he or she should experience both short-term and long-term benefits. Because each type of caregiving serves a different function, it is expected that secure base caregiving (the support of a partner's "going out" for exploration) will have important immediate and long-term consequences that are distinct from those that are likely to be afforded by safe haven caregiving (the support of a partner's "coming in" in times of stress). According to attachment theory, a secure base gives individuals the confidence and courage to explore the environment, accept challenges, and take risks (Bowlby, 1969/ 1982, 1988). Thus the unique consequences of receiving secure base caregiving (both immediately and over time) are expected to be higher levels of self-esteem, perceived competency, self-confidence, and self-efficacy and greater willingness and efforts to engage in exploratory activities involving the pursuit of goals, the acceptance of challenges, and attempts to learn new things and make new discoveries. Therefore, long-term improvements in the self (personal growth) are likely to be important consequences of secure base caregiving (path *d*). Self-esteem is especially likely to be improved or eroded over time as a function of the presence or absence of secure base caregiving in one's most significant relationship. For example, intrusive (overinvolved) caregiving, which discourages the recipient's exploratory behavior, is likely to result in less exploratory behavior, thus inhibiting the recipient's development of new competencies and eroding his or her self-esteem and perceptions of self-efficacy over time (path *d*).

Unique consequences of safe haven caregiving (both immediately and over time) are likely to be reduced stress and anxiety, improved coping capacity (greater perceived ability to cope), feelings of safety and security, and problem resolution (path *i*). Another important consequence of safe haven caregiving should be a general perception that one's home base is secure (path *i*). Because a secure base encourages autonomy and exploration *while being available to provide a safe haven if needed* (in the event that things go wrong), general perceptions of the security of one's home base should depend on one's experiences with the caregiver in times of stress.

Outcomes that are likely to result from both types of caregiving include (1) relationship stability (couples remaining together over time) and healthy relationship functioning (e.g., high levels of relationship satisfaction and trust, low levels of conflict, perceptions that the self is valued by the partner); (2) psychological well-being (e.g., life satisfaction, absence of depression); (3) physical well-being; and (4) general views that it is worthwhile to seek support from others. However, it is likely that secure base and safe haven caregiving influence physical and psychological well-being via different pathways. For example, secure base caregiving that results in personal growth and the development of new competencies should lead to increased self-esteem, happiness, and psychological well-being, which, in turn, may have implications for physical health. This speculation is consistent with evidence indicating that personal goal strivings are associated with both physical and emotional well-being (e.g., Emmons & King, 1988). However, safe haven caregiving (which involves the provision of comfort and support in times of stress) should result in stress reduction, better coping capacity, and greater feelings of security, which should, in turn, influence both physical and psychological well-being. It is also expected that individuals who reap the benefits of secure base caregiving (e.g., high self-esteem, perceptions of self-efficacy, increased sense of well-being) will be less likely than individuals who do not to perceive potentially stressful life events as threatening and beyond their ability to cope (path *e*)—a perception that should also contribute to psychological and physical well-being.

Individual Differences

Figure 10.1 depicts what are believed to be normative caregiving processes if all goes well. However, although they are not illustrated, individual-difference factors may influence any of the variables or moderate any of the paths in the model. For example, not all individuals are equally willing to engage in exploratory behavior, express distress, and seek support when needed, and not all caregivers are equally skilled and motivated to provide a secure base or a safe haven for their relationship partners. Moreover, preexisting beliefs and expectations that partners bring into their interactions may act as interpretative filters and shape the way they perceive one another's behavior. Thus a number of individual-difference factors may facilitate or interfere with each step in the model. One obvious individual-difference factor is the role of attachment style (which reflects general beliefs about oneself and others in attachment-relevant situations) in shaping the caregiving processes described herein.

Current research evidence for both normative caregiving processes and individual differences in these processes is described in the following sections. The review of research evidence is organized based on the research methodology used for addressing the specific caregiving process(es) depicted in Figure 10.1.

EMPIRICAL EVIDENCE FOR SAFE HAVEN PROCESSES

Observational Studies

Normative Processes

We began our research on safe haven caregiving processes by conducting an observational study with a sample of dating couples in order to examine some of the normative processes outlined in the bottom portion of

Figure 10.1 (Collins & Feeney, 2000). A laboratory paradigm was used in which couples were videotaped as one member of the couple (the "care receiver") disclosed a stressful problem (a recent personal concern or worry) to his or her partner. Prior to the discussion, couple members completed preliminary measures of personal and relationship characteristics. After the discussion, participants completed questionnaires that assessed their current (postinteraction) mood and their perceptions of the discussion. The videotaped interactions were coded for support-seeking and safe haven caregiving behaviors.

Results of this investigation supported attachment theory's proposition that individuals who experience distress (attachment-system activation) feel an urge toward proximity to a primary caregiver or attachment figure (path f in Figure 10.1). Specifically, care receivers who evaluated their problems as more distressing exhibited more support-seeking behavior during the discussion. Results also indicated that specific support-seeking behaviors were associated with specific caregiving behaviors (path g). For example, clear and direct expressions of need (emotional and instrumental disclosure) were strongly associated with the receipt of helpful forms of support (more responsiveness, more emotional and instrumental support), whereas indirect expressions of need were associated with unhelpful forms of support (less responsiveness and more negative support). Care-seeking and caregiving behaviors were also coordinated, such that the type of help offered was matched to the type of help sought. That is, when care receivers sought more emotional support, their partners provided both more emotional and instrumental support. However, when care receivers sought more instrumental support, their partners responded with more instrumental, but not more emotional, support. Thus the evidence suggests that safe haven caregiving and care-seeking behaviors are coordinated in complementary ways.

Results of this investigation also indicated that care receivers' perceptions of support are associated with their partners' observed caregiving behaviors (path h). Specifically, care receivers rated their interactions as more supportive when their partners provided more emotional and instrumental support and when their partners behaved in ways that were more responsive (e.g., by listening and communicating understanding). In contrast, care receivers whose partners engaged in negative support behaviors (e.g., dismissing the importance of the problem or blaming the care receiver) evaluated their interactions as much less supportive. These results provided some initial evidence that care receivers' subjective sense of being cared for is rooted in specific caregiving acts performed by the partner.

An important immediate outcome that was examined in this investigation (path i) was changes in the care receivers' mood from before to after the discussion. Presumably, the provision of a safe haven will lead to reduced distress (deactivation of the attachment system), and one useful index of this stress reduction is improvements in mood from before to after the discussion. Results of this investigation provided some evidence for the perceived support → reduced stress link (path *i*). Specifically, care receivers felt better after their interactions when their partners provided more responsive support (see Collins & Feeney, 2000, for additional details). These normative safe haven processes were also established in a replication study in which a stressor was introduced in the laboratory and the couples' spontaneous interactions were unobtrusively videotaped.

Further evidence for normative safe haven processes was also obtained in a daily diary study of romantic couples (Collins & Feeney, 2003). In this study, we asked couple members to complete a nightly diary for 3 weeks in which they recorded stressful life events, support-seeking and caregiving behaviors, mood and personal well-being, and thoughts and feelings about their relationship each day. Results indicated that individuals sought more support from their partner on days when they experienced more stressful life events (path *f*), and received more support on days when they expressed greater need (path *g*); these patterns were corroborated by their partners' reports. Moreover, on days when individuals perceived that their partners had been more supportive and responsive to their needs, they felt more loved and valued by their partners and more satisfied with their relationships (path *i*).

Individual Differences

Observational studies have also examined individual differences in some of the safe haven caregiving processes depicted in Figure 10.1. One of the most notable investigations in this regard is that of Simpson and colleagues (1992). These researchers introduced a stressor to the female members of romantic couples by telling them that they would be participating in a "set of experimental procedures that arouse considerable anxiety and distress in most people," then pretending to take their pulses and showing them a room that looked like an isolation chamber and that contained psychophysiological equipment. The procedure was designed to directly evoke distress and anxiety, thereby activating the attachment system. The couple members were unobtrusively videotaped as they interacted during a waiting period, and the couples' support-seeking and caregiving behaviors were later coded. Results of this investigation indicated that among more secure men, higher levels of partner distress were associated with greater support. In contrast, among more avoidant men, higher levels of partner distress were associated with lower levels of support. However, it is interesting and important to note that, when their female partners displayed lower levels of distress, more avoidant men provided *more* support than did more secure men. However, as their partners' levels of anxiety increased, more securely attached men offered greater reassurance and emotional support, and they made more supportive comments. These findings are consistent with the developmental literature indicating that avoidant mothers withdraw from interaction when their babies are distressed but engage in interaction when their babies are content (e.g., Escher-Graub & Grossman, 1983, as cited in Cassidy, 2001) and with a recent experimental study (described later) indicating that avoidant adults appear to provide less support when their partners need it most. Thus distress (attachment-system activation) appears to impede the provision of support and establishment of proximity in interactions involving avoidant individuals.

Simpson and colleagues (1992) also provided the first empirical demonstration of the effects of attachment styles on directly observable care-seeking behaviors in response to adult attachment-system activation. This is a theoretically important topic to investigate with regard to adult attachment–caregiving processes because the attachment system (and resulting attachment behavior) is postulated to become organized in different ways for different people, depending on their history of experiences with caregivers. For example, individuals who historically have not found support to be forthcoming when needed are likely to seek proximity and support in more subtle and indirect ways than those who have experienced a history of responsive caregiving.

The results of this investigation indicated that more secure women sought more support (emotional and physical comfort) from their partners as their levels of distress increased, whereas more avoidant women sought less support as they became more distressed. It appears that more securely attached women used their partners as sources of comfort and reassurance as their anxiety levels increased, whereas more avoidant women withdrew from their partners both emotionally and physically. It is interesting to note, however, that at lower levels of anxiety, more avoidant women sought *more* support from their partners than did secure women. Simpson and colleagues (1992) explained this finding in terms of the conflict model of avoidance (Ainsworth, Blehar, Waters, & Wall, 1978), which holds that the behavior of avoidant individuals is a product of conflicting motives—a desire for, yet a simultaneous fear of, proximity. These researchers speculate that the desire for proximity in adults is aroused more strongly than fear of proximity when environmental conditions are only moderately threatening and emotional distress is at lower levels. However, increases in perceived threat or distress sharply accelerate the onset of fear of proximity, resulting in decreased support seeking. Because the proximity needs of avoidant individuals have been frustrated in distressing situations, these individuals may overcompensate by seeking proximity under less threatening conditions.

It is also interesting to note that 16 of the 83 women in this study did not even mention the anxiety-provoking situation to their partners, and exploratory analyses revealed that these were the more avoidant women. Contrary to expectations, no significant effects emerged for individuals with a more anxious attachment style. Simpson and colleagues (1992) suggested that because anxiously attached adults strongly desire close, supportive relationships but typically are not involved in them, they may exhibit behavioral ambivalence in which tendencies to both approach and withdraw from the partner effectively counterbalance one another.

Another impressive study documenting the individual differences in caregiving processes depicted in Figure 10.1 was conducted by Westmaas and Silver (2001). In this investigation, participants interacted with a confederate who allegedly had cancer and whose attachment orientation had been manipulated prior to the interaction. Consistent with the results of Simpson and colleagues (1992), this study indicated that avoidant attachment predicted less supportive responses to the confederate, as assessed by observers' ratings and as reported by the participants themselves. Anxious attachment predicted greater participant-reported anxiety and self-criticism about the interaction with the confederate. Interestingly, this study demonstrated that the attachment characteristics of the interaction partner matter as well. That is, participants were more rejecting of an interaction partner who was perceived to be avoidant (fearful or dismissing) than of one who was perceived to be nonavoidant (secure or preoccupied). However, the degree of participants' rejection was partially determined by the participants' own attachment characteristics. It was the least avoidant participants who tended to feel more rejecting of an interaction partner who was perceived to be avoidant. The most avoidant participants were more rejecting of a nonavoidant (secure or preoccupied) partner and less rejecting of a similarly avoidant (fearful or dismissing) partner.

Collins and Feeney (2000) also examined attachment style differences in the safe haven caregiving processes depicted in Figure 10.1. Consistent with theory and prior research, we found that individuals who were higher in avoidance tended to use indirect support-seeking strategies and that individuals who were higher in attachment-related anxiety provided less instrumental support, were less responsive, and exhibited more negative caregiving behavior. Contrary to expectations, anxious attachment was not related to support-seeking behavior, and avoidant attachment was not significantly related to caregiving behavior in this investigation. However, attachment style did moderate some links in the model (paths f and g). Consistent with expectations, care receivers who were high in avoidance tended to seek relatively low levels of support regardless of how stressful they perceived their problems to be; however, those who were low in avoidance tended to seek more support the more stress they perceived. Another interactive effect revealed that caregivers who were high in attachment-related anxiety tended to provide relatively high levels of support when their partner's needs were clear and direct, but much lower levels when their partner's needs were less clear. In contrast, caregivers who were low in attachment-related anxiety (more secure) tended to provide relatively high levels of support regardless of whether their partners' support-seeking efforts were clear and direct. Taken together, these findings are consistent with the view that attachment insecurity limits one's ability to seek support effectively and to be a good caregiver.

Self-Report Studies

A number of self-report studies have been conducted examining various aspects of the safe haven caregiving process—in our labs and by other researchers in the field. This has been a useful method for investigating individual differences in care-seeking and caregiving behaviors, important predictors of effective or ineffective caregiving, and important mechanisms that underlie individual differences in caregiving behaviors.

Individual Differences in Caregiving

First, based on an extensive review of the literature describing caregiving behaviors associated with infant attachment styles, Kunce and Shaver (1994) developed an adult Caregiving Questionnaire that assesses four *relationship-specific* caregiving dimensions. These caregiving dimensions include (1) *proximity versus distance* (e.g., "When my partner seems to want or need a hug, I'm glad to provide it"); (2) *sensitivity versus insensitivity* (e.g., "I'm very good at recognizing my partner's needs and feelings, even when they're different from my own"); (3) *cooperation versus control* (e.g., "I tend to be too domineering when trying to help my partner"); and (4) *compulsive caregiving* (e.g., "I tend to get overinvolved in my partner's problems and difficulties").

   In a series of studies, these researchers found that each attachment style is associated with a unique pattern of caregiving. Specifically, individuals with a secure attachment style report relatively low levels of compulsive (overinvolved) and controlling caregiving, and they report relatively high levels of proximity (physical forms of comfort) and sensitivity. In contrast, preoccupied (anxious) individuals report relatively high levels of proximity and compulsive caregiving but relatively low levels of sensitivity and cooperation—suggesting that although they are capable of providing affectionate caregiving, their caregiving may be somewhat intrusive and out of sync with their partner's needs. Dismissing–avoidant individuals report the lowest levels of compulsive caregiving and provision of proximity, and they also report relatively low levels of sensitivity.

Finally, fearful–avoidant individuals report relatively low levels of provision of proximity and sensitivity while simultaneously reporting relatively high levels of compulsive caregiving.

In both dating and married couples, Carnelley, Pietromonaco, and Jaffe (1996) also examined the link between an individual's attachment characteristics and his or her self-reported caregiving activity within the relationship. They created a composite measure of caregiving activity on which higher scores reflected greater reciprocity (i.e., both partners give and receive about the same amount of care), greater engagement (i.e., partner is actively involved in providing care), and less neglect (i.e., partner does not ignore the other's needs). Their analyses focused on two composite attachment scales assessing fearful avoidance and preoccupation. Consistent with the results of Kunce and Shaver (1994), both married and dating individuals characterized by a fearful–avoidant attachment style reported less caregiving activity in their relationships. Among married couples, preoccupied respondents also reported less caregiving activity; however, in the dating sample, these individuals did not show more or less overall caregiving activity.

In a different sample of married couples, Feeney (1996) also examined the association between an individual's attachment characteristics and his or her caregiving style. Consistent with the findings described previously, secure individuals reported the most favorable style of caregiving, marked by high responsiveness (sensitivity, proximity, and cooperation) and a lack of compulsive caregiving. In contrast, fearful–avoidant individuals reported relatively low responsiveness and a more compulsive caregiving style, whereas dismissing–avoidant individuals reported intermediate levels of responsiveness and a lack of compulsive caregiving. Preoccupied (anxious) individuals generally fell in between secure and fearful individuals in their caregiving characteristics; however, preoccupied and secure wives reported similar levels of responsiveness. Feeney also observed a link between secure attachment and favorable caregiving using the two major dimensions underlying attachment styles—comfort with closeness and anxiety over relationships. Specifically, for both husbands and wives, responsive caregiving was associated with feeling more comfort with closeness and less anxiety over relationships. In contrast, compulsive caregiving was associated with feeling less comfort with closeness and more anxiety over relationships.

We also recently investigated the unique patterns of caregiving that are associated with each attachment style (Feeney & Collins, 2001). Our results indicated, consistent with prior research, that individuals who are high in attachment-related avoidance are less responsive and more controlling caregivers and that individuals who are high in attachment-related anxiety are more compulsive and controlling caregivers. Taken together, these studies reveal that insecure attachment is associated with less effective caregiving patterns, but the particular type of ineffective caregiving depends on the particular type of insecurity. Avoidant individuals appear to lack sensitivity, physical comfort, and nurturance, and when they do engage in any form of caregiving activity, it tends to be controlling. Anxious individuals, on the other hand, are not unresponsive, but they tend to be overinvolved caregivers in that they care for their partners in a way that is intrusive and controlling.

Individual Differences in Seeking Care

A number of self-report studies have examined individual differences in care seeking in stressful situations (e.g., Florian, Mikulincer, & Bucholtz, 1995; Mikulincer & Florian, 1995; Mikulincer, Florian, & Weller, 1993; Ognibene & Collins, 1998). As a whole, these studies reveal that attachment security is associated with a greater willingness to seek social support in response to stress. Specifically, adults with secure attachment characteristics report that they seek support from others as a primary method of coping with distress, whereas avoidant individuals report using more distancing strategies in order to cope with stress. However, the care-seeking behaviors exhibited by anxious or preoccupied individuals are less consistent. In some studies, these individuals report the use of care seeking as a coping strategy (Mikulincer & Florian, 1995; Ognibene & Collins, 1998); however, in other studies, they do not report seeking support from others as a way of coping with stress (Florian et al., 1995; Mikulincer et al., 1993).

Mechanisms Explaining Individual Differences in Caregiving

After helping to establish the caregiving patterns characteristic of each attachment style, we next attempted to explain why individuals with different attachment styles tend to be good or bad caregivers (Feeney & Collins, 2001). In other words, we wanted to identify the mediating mechanisms that underlie attachment-style differences in caregiving. Based on an extensive review of the helping and close relationships literatures, we reasoned that two broad categories of factors might mediate the link between attachment style and caregiving quality. First, certain chronic characteristics of the individual should mediate this link. For example, caregivers should differ with regard to the particular skills and abilities they bring with them into a relationship and with regard to their general orientation toward themselves and others. Therefore, we hypothesized that a caregiver's empathic abilities, general knowledge about how to support other people, chronic levels of self-focus, and communal and exchange orientation toward others would be important mediators. Next, certain characteristics of the particular relationship should be important mediating mechanisms. For example, caregivers should differ in the extent to which they feel committed to their relationships, in the extent to which they feel close to their partners, and in the degree to which they trust their partners. Caregivers should also differ in their specific motivations for taking care of their partners.

The results of this investigation suggest that avoidant adults' tendency to be unresponsive caregivers appears to be partially mediated by their lack of knowledge about how to support others, their lack of a prosocial orientation toward others, and their lack of relationship interdependence. In addition, avoidant adults' tendency to be controlling caregivers appears to be mediated by their lack of prosocial orientation toward others and their lack of relationship trust. Anxious adults' tendency to be compulsive caregivers appears to be partially mediated by their sense of relationship interdependence, their lack of relationship trust, and their relatively selfish motives for caring for their partners. And finally, the tendency of anxious adults to be controlling caregivers appears to be mediated by their lack of relationship trust and by their relatively selfish motives for caring for their partners. Taken together, current research is showing not only that there is more than one type of poor caregiving but also that unique patterns of motives, skills, and resources can help us understand why people with different attachment styles care for their partners in the particular ways that they do.

Motivations for Caregiving

Another question that we have been addressing in our research involves the degree to which specific motivations for providing support to one's partner influences caregiving behavior. Because the caregiving role often involves a good deal of responsibility, as well as substantial cognitive, emotional, and sometimes tangible resources, caregivers must be motivated to accept that responsibility and to expend the time and effort required to provide effective support. If caregivers are not sufficiently motivated, then it is likely that they will provide either low levels of support or ineffective forms of support that are out of sync with the partner's needs. Therefore, we conducted a study that focused explicitly on caregiving motivations as important mechanisms that might underlie the provision of responsive or unresponsive support.

As a first attempt at identifying the specific motivations that people have for providing or for not providing support to their close relationship partners, we developed a 40-item Motivations for Caregiving Questionnaire (see Feeney & Collins, 2003). We included items that reflect specific types of selfish or egoistic motives—such as helping a partner in order to avoid negative consequences—and we included items that reflect more altruistic motives—such as helping out of concern for one's partner. We also included items based on hypotheses about the types of motives that we thought would be characteristic of different types of people (e.g., people with different attachment styles or relationship characteristics). We factor analyzed the items on the motivations scale and found that they formed seven distinct dimensions. Thus we were able to identify seven specific motivations for the caregiving that occurs in adult romantic relationships. One factor involved motives reflecting feelings of love, concern, and responsibility for one's partner. Other motivations involved helping because the caregiver feels obligated to help, helping in order to get something in return (for some self-benefit), and helping for relationship reasons—for example, so that the partner will stay in the relationship or to make the relationship more equitable. Three other types of motivations that emerged from the factor analysis involved helping because the caregiver enjoys helping, helping because the caregiver feels capable of helping, and helping because the caregiver feels that his or her partner is incapable of handling problems on his or her own.

After identifying these specific motivations for caregiving in close relationships, we next addressed the question, From where do these motives come? Results revealed theoretically consistent links between the motive variables and a variety of personal and relationship characteristics. For example, avoidant caregivers (who are uncomfortable with intimacy) report that they help their partners for egoistic or selfish reasons: They report that when they help their partners, it is because they feel obligated to help or because they expect to get something in return. They are less likely to report helping because they feel love, concern, and responsibility for their partners or because they enjoy it. Anxious caregivers, on the other hand, report helping for both egoistic and altruistic reasons—because they enjoy it and feel love and concern for the partner and also because they feel obligated and hope to get something in return. It is interesting to note that these individuals, who are generally very concerned about other people's love and acceptance of them, also report helping their partners for relationship reasons—for example, to keep the partner in the relationship. Also noteworthy is the finding that people who report having had a supportive caregiving history with their parents when they were growing up are less likely to report that they help their partners for selfish reasons.

With regard to links between relationship characteristics and motives, results revealed that caregivers who are in satisfying relationships report helping their partners because they feel love and concern for them and because they enjoy helping. In contrast, caregivers who are in more conflictual relationships report helping their partners for selfish reasons—for relationship purposes, because they feel obligated, because they hope to get something in return, and because they perceive the partner to be needy and incapable of handling problems on his or her own. Thus it appears that both personality and relationship characteristics play a role in the development of different motivations that people have for providing care to their partners.

Next, we examined whether the specific motivations for caregiving are associated with three different types of caregiving behavior—responsive, compulsive (overinvolved), and controlling caregiving. Again, the reason we think it is important to study caregiving motivations is that they should influence the quality of care that is provided within a relationship. Consistent with expectations, responsive caregivers are those who report helping their partners because they feel love and concern for them, because they are good at helping, and because they enjoy helping. In contrast, the less responsive and more overinvolved and controlling caregivers are those who report helping because they feel obligated, because they want to get something in return, or because their partner is perceived to be needy and incapable. Interestingly, caregivers who report relationship motives for helping their partner also tend to be the more overinvolved caregivers. Taken together, these results provide support for the hypothesis that the underlying motivations that people have for providing care to their partners play an important role in determining the quality of care that is provided.

Experimental Studies

Another important goal of our work is to isolate and examine various components of the interpersonal caregiving process. Experimental studies are crucial for examining the microdynamics of this interpersonal process and for exploring causal relationships among variables. We began by conducting experimental studies that examine individual differences in safe haven caregiving behavior after manipulating the distress level of the care receiver (i.e., manipulating need for support; Collins, Ford, Guichard, & Feeney, 2003; Feeney & Collins, 2001), individual differences in perceptions of manipulated caregiving behavior (Collins & Feeney, in press), and individual differences in physiological responses to stressors (Carpenter & Kirkpatrick, 1996; Feeney & Kirkpatrick, 1996).

Predicting Caregiving

One recent study was conducted in order to examine individual differences in responsiveness to need (Feeney & Collins, 2001). From an attachment-theoretical perspective, good caregivers are able to effectively restore their partners' felt security *when it is needed* by alleviating distress and aiding in problem resolution. Thus caregiving behavior should be appropriately contingent on the partner's need. To examine individual differences in responsiveness to need, we created high and low need for support conditions by leading one member of the couple (the caregiver) to believe that his or her partner (the care receiver) was either extremely nervous about performing an upcoming speech task (high need condition) or not very nervous at all about the upcoming task (low need condition). The caregiver was then given an opportunity to write a note to his or her partner, which provided a behavioral measure of support and caregiving.

Overall, results revealed that caregiver notes were rated as being more supportive (by both independent observers and the recipients) when the caregivers believed that their partners were more distressed. With regard to individual differences, results revealed that avoidant caregivers (those who are uncomfortable with closeness and interdependence) tended to provide low levels of emotional support in both high and low need conditions and to provide less instrumental support in the low need condition than in the high need condition. Thus avoidant caregivers not only showed no evidence of responding to their partners' needs for support but also showed a tendency to provide less support in the condition in which their partners needed it the most. In contrast, individuals who are low in avoidance (those who are comfortable with closeness and interdependence) provided more instrumental support and were perceived by their partners as being more supportive in the high need condition than in the low need condition—providing evidence that these caregivers were responding to their partners' needs for support. In contrast to avoidant caregivers, anxious caregivers showed some evidence of responsiveness, although they were not always in sync with their partners' needs; they provided more instrumental support to their partners in the high need condition than in the low need condition, but they provided the same level of emotional support regardless of their partners' level of need. As a whole, this pattern of results reveals that there are indeed some theoretically consistent individual differences in the degree to which people respond to partners' expressions of distress (see Feeney & Collins, 2001, for additional details).

A second study using a similar methodology provides further evidence that anxious caregivers tend to be out of sync with their partners' needs (Collins et al., 2003). In this study, caregivers who were high in anxiety failed to increase their support in response to their partners' needs, and showed high levels of empathy, cognitive rumination, and partner focus regardless of their partners' level of distress, indicating a clear lack of sensitivity to their partners' emotional cues. They also made more negative dispositional inferences about their partners (e.g., perceiving their partners as emotionally weak) in the high need condition than in the low need condition. In contrast, caregivers who were low in anxiety were highly responsive to their partners' needs; when they believed that their partners were extremely distressed, they provided more support, experienced more empathy, were more cognitively focused on their partners, and made fewer negative dispositional inferences about their partners.

Taken together, our laboratory findings provide converging evidence that attachment-related avoidance and anxiety interfere with one's ability to be truly responsive to the needs of others. Avoidance is associated with a pattern of caregiving that is unresponsive and neglectful, whereas anxiety is associated with a pattern of caregiving that is not neglectful but that lacks sensitivity to the partners' expressed needs.

Predicting Perceptions of Caregiving

We also conducted an experimental study to examine individual (attachment style) differences in the link between the caregiver's provision of support and the care receiver's perception of the caregiver's behavior (path h; Collins & Feeney, in press, Study 1). Participants in this investigation were dating couples who were assigned to caregiver and care-receiver roles before arriving for the study. After completing background questionnaires, a stressor was introduced by telling one member of the couple (the "care receiver") that he or she would be giving a videotaped speech that would be rated by a group of his or her peers. After the stress induction, the couple's spontaneous interaction was unobtrusively videotaped, and the degree to which the caregiver provided support during this interaction was later coded by independent observers. The care receiver was then escorted to a quiet room to complete the speech activity, and support manipulations were delivered both before and after he or she gave the speech. Half of the care receivers received two highly supportive notes from their partners, and the other half received two ambiguous and relatively unsupportive notes. After receiving each note, the care receiver reported his or her perceptions of it. Finally, after completing the speech activity, the care receiver reported his or her perceptions of the caregiver's behavior during the interaction that had been videotaped.

First, we examined whether secure and insecure care receivers differed in their perceptions of the pre- and postspeech notes. Results indicated that secure and insecure recipients did, in fact, differ in their subjective appraisals of the same objective support experience. Although they did not differ in their appraisals when their partners were "objectively" supportive, they did differ in their appraisals when their partners were "objectively" less supportive. Overall, secure individuals made more benign appraisals of the low-support notes, even after controlling for relationship satisfaction, whereas insecure individuals tended to view these notes as less supportive and more upsetting, and they inferred more negative intent.

Next, we examined whether receiving a supportive or unsupportive note would influence care receivers' subjective perceptions of an interaction that took place *before* the notes were even sent. That is, we wanted to know if secure and insecure people would remember their earlier interaction as being more supportive or more unsupportive than it really was after having received two supportive or unsupportive notes. Results indicated that secure individuals' perceptions of their earlier interaction were unrelated to whether they received supportive or unsupportive notes, and this is how it should be: People's perceptions of their earlier interaction should be completely independent of the notes they received because the interaction happened *before* the experimental manipulation took place. However, a very different pattern emerged for the insecure people. When insecure people received two unsupportive notes from their partners, they rated their prior interaction as much less supportive.

This, of course, suggests that insecure people were remembering or perhaps reconstruing their earlier interaction as being more negative than it really was. Because people were randomly assigned to an experimental condition, there should be no relationship between the notes they received and the quality of their interactions. Because we had videotaped and coded the interactions, we were able to examine whether the interactions of insecure individuals who had received negative notes were really more unsupportive, and, as expected, the interactions of insecure people who received negative notes were *not* less supportive than the interactions of insecure people who received positive notes. Therefore, there does appear to be a negativity bias for insecure people who received negative notes from their partners; they appear to have remembered their earlier interaction as being unsupportive when it really had not been (see Collins & Feeney, in press, for additional details).

We found further evidence for biased perceptions of support in a conceptual replication (Collins & Feeney, in press, Study 2) in which we used a similar paradigm but allowed partners to write genuine notes (which were then rated by independent observers). Consistent with our experimental study, insecure support recipients tended to view their partners' notes as less supportive overall, but this effect only occurred when the notes were judged (by independent raters) to be somewhat less supportive. Taken together, these two studies suggest that insecure individuals will be predisposed to perceive their partners' support behavior as less supportive, but primarily when the support effort is more ambiguous and therefore more open to subjective construal.

Predicting Physiological Responses to Stressors

In another study, we experimentally manipulated the presence versus absence of a romantic partner during a stressful activity and found physiological evidence that insecure individuals react with more emotional distress than secure individuals to the same potentially stressful event (Feeney & Kirkpatrick, 1996). Specifically, female participants performed a standard psychological stress task both in the presence and in the absence of their male romantic partners. Results revealed that both avoidant and anxious women, relative to their more secure counterparts, displayed heightened physiological arousal (as indexed by measures of heart rate and blood pressure) when separated from their romantic partners just as they were about to face the stressful laboratory situation; however, their physiological reactivity did not differ from that of more secure women when they were not immediately separated from their romantic partners in the same situation. Anxious and avoidant women who were separated from their partners in the beginning of the study not only showed elevated physiological arousal during that part of the experiment, but they also continued to display heightened physiological arousal during the second half of the experiment—even after their partners had returned to the laboratory. In contrast, individuals whose partners were present during the first phase of the experiment did not evince elevated physiological arousal during that phase of the study, nor during the second part of the experiment, when their romantic partners left the room.

Carpenter and Kirkpatrick (1996) conducted a follow-up investigation that did not manipulate separation from a partner but instead manipulated whether or not a partner accompanied the participant to the study at all. Results revealed that for avoidant and anxious participants, physiological reactivity (heart rate, systolic blood pressure, and an aggregate arousal index) in response to the stressor was *greater* when the partner was present during the activity than when the partner was never present at all. However, partner proximity had no discernible effect on secure participants' psychophysiological responses to stress. It appears that, although insecure individuals find separation during a stressful event to be distressing, they also find a partner's presence during a stressful event to be more distressing than if the partner had not escorted the individual to the study and had no knowledge of the stressful event at all. Perhaps the psychological availability of the attachment figure (or caregiver) transcends physical separation in secure adult relationships. Taken together, these results are consistent with those of self-report studies indicating that insecure individuals appraise stressors as more threatening than secure individuals (Mikulincer & Florian, 1995; Ognibene & Collins, 1998).

Summary of Evidence for Safe Haven Processes

The results of the studies described here provide impressive evidence, using a variety of research methodologies and samples, for the normative safe haven processes depicted in paths *f* through *i* in Figure 10.1 and for individual-difference factors and mechanisms that are likely to influence these processes (e.g., attachment style, underlying motivations, relationship quality). As discussed in greater detail later, additional research is needed to continue to isolate and examine in greater depth each of the specific components of this process—particularly the long-term outcomes of receiving or not receiving safe haven caregiving from one's most significant relationship in adulthood.

EMPIRICAL EVIDENCE FOR SECURE BASE PROCESSES

Empirical investigations of secure base caregiving processes have been virtually ignored in the adult attachment literature. Surprisingly, investigations of similar processes have also been neglected in the broader social support and relationship literatures. This seems particularly surprising given that individuals routinely assign credit for their accomplishments and successes to the support of the significant people in their lives—people who have encouraged them to grow as individuals and strive to reach their full potential.

A few studies have examined links between adult attachment and exploratory behavior but have not examined or focused on related caregiving processes. Hazan and Shaver (1990) were the first to explore the interrelations between attachment and exploration in adulthood. They examined, in a large newspaper study, individual (attachment style) differences in feelings and approaches toward work—a major form of exploration in adulthood. Their results indicated that secure individuals approach their work with confidence, enjoy working, and are not burdened by fears of failure. Although they value work, they do not allow it to interfere with their relationships and do not use it as a means for meeting attachment needs or for avoiding social interaction. Anxious individuals, on the other hand, report that relationship concerns interfere with work performance; they fear poor performance evaluations; and they report a tendency to slack off after praise, suggesting that their primary work motivation is to gain the approval of others. In contrast, avoidant individuals report using work as a means of avoiding social interaction, and they report being less satisfied with their jobs than secure individuals. Comparable results were obtained in an investigation examining the links between attachment and one's approach to and engagement in leisure activities—another adult manifestation of exploratory behavior (Carnelley & Ruscher, 2000). Relatedly, a recent study examining exploration in adolescence revealed that secure adolescents are more likely than insecure adolescents to explore their emotional and cognitive independence in conversations with maternal attachment figures, most likely because their mothers support this exploration by validating the adolescents' viewpoints and remaining available and engaged in the interaction (Allen et al., 2003).

Taken together, these studies reveal important individual differences in exploratory behavior—individual differences that are consistent with attachment theory's predictions and with exploratory behaviors observed in the infant attachment literature. However, there have been no empirical investigations of secure base caregiving processes in adulthood—processes that support or hinder a relationship partner's exploration and that may help to explain some of these individual differences in exploratory behavior. One of our labs is currently focusing a great deal of research attention on this area.

A first in-depth investigation of normative secure base caregiving processes was conducted with a sample of couples who were in committed romantic relationships; they were married, engaged, or dating seriously. This investigation included both an observational and an experimental session, and the purpose was to provide a first examination of the basic interpersonal processes depicted the top portion of Figure 10.1. Detailed results of this investigation are reported in Feeney (2003).

Observational Session

First, secure base caregiving processes were examined in the context of discussions that couple members had about one member's personal goals and exploratory opportunities. Before arriving for the study, one member of the couple was randomly assigned to the role of a "care receiver," the person whose personal goals would be discussed, and the other member was assigned to the role of a "caregiver," the person who could potentially provide a secure base for his or her partner. The goal discussions were videotaped, and caregiver and care receiver behaviors were coded by independent observers. After the discussion, couple members completed postdiscussion questionnaires assessing their perceptions of the interaction, their mood and state self-esteem, and the care receiver's perceived likelihood of achieving his or her goals.

The first research question addressed was whether the care receivers' home-base security (operationally defined as the degree to which the caregiver is generally sensitive and responsive to signals of distress) is associated with the care receivers' perceptions of exploratory opportunities (path j). Results revealed that the more secure the recipients' home base (that is, the more sensitive caregivers are to their partners in times of distress), the more achievable the care receivers perceive their goals to be before the discussion, the more self-efficacy they report with regard to accomplishing goals, and the more willing they are to try new things and accept challenges. Thus the degree to which a caregiver provides an adequate safe haven for his or her partner plays some role in shaping the partner's perceptions of life opportunities that involve exploration away from the caregiver.

Next, this investigation provided evidence that care receivers' perceptions of exploratory opportunities are associated with the degree to which they engage in confident exploration of their goals and the degree to which they seek goal-relevant support during the discussion with their partners (path *a*). Specifically, the more achievable the care receivers perceived their goals to be before the discussion, and the more willing they were to try new things and accept challenges, the more they engaged in confident exploration of their goals during the discussion. Moreover, care receivers who are generally willing to accept challenges and try new things engaged in more support seeking during the discussion, whereas those who perceived their specific goals to be more achievable before their discussion exhibited less support seeking. Thus care receivers' perceptions of exploratory opportunities appear to influence, at least to some degree, the way they approach their goals and discuss them with their partners.

When the specific ways in which caregiver and care-receiver behaviors influence one another during secure base caregiving interactions (path *b*) were examined, results indicated that (as with safe haven caregiving dynamics) caregiver and recipient behaviors do appear to be meshed in complementary ways. For example, caregivers who were coded by observers as being supportive of and comfortable with their partners' goals had partners who discussed their goals openly, who confidently explored various avenues for achieving their goals, and who were receptive to support attempts. In contrast, caregivers who were coded by observers as avoiding discussion of the goals had partners who did not discuss their goals openly, who did not confidently explore avenues for achieving their goals, who were not receptive to support attempts (when they occurred), and who avoided discussion of the goals themselves. Interestingly, caregivers who were coded by observers as being intrusive and controlling during the discussion had partners who tended to modify their goals during the course of the discussion.

The next stage in the model (path *c*) indicates that caregiving behaviors exhibited during the discussion should predict the recipients' perceptions of having been supported. Consistent with this expectation, results revealed that caregivers who were observed as being encouraging and supportive of their partners' goals and comfortable with their partners' goals and autonomy were seen by their partners as being supportive, encouraging, and sensitive during the discussion. However, caregivers who were unsupportive of, discouraging of, and uncomfortable with their partners' goals were viewed by their partners as being insensitive, self-focused, and disappointing during the discussion.

Finally, this investigation permitted the examination of some immediate outcomes of secure base caregiving for the recipient. Interestingly, when recipients felt that their goals were supported by their partners during the discussion, they experienced increases in self-esteem and positive mood after the discussion (controlling for global self-esteem and mood before the discussion), and they rated their likelihood of achieving their goals to be greater after the discussion than they rated them to be before the discussion. Thus this initial investigation revealed that the support of a partner's goal strivings and explorations have some important implications for his or her happiness and self-esteem and for his or her perceptions of the likelihood of achieving specific goals, at least in the short term (Feeney, 2003).

Experimental Session

A second phase of the investigation was conducted in order to experimentally examine some immediate consequences of secure base caregiving behavior (and lack thereof) for recipients (paths c and d). As one member of the couple (the care receiver) worked on a computer puzzle game, secure base caregiving behavior was manipulated through the use of an instant messaging system. Before arriving for the study, care receivers were randomly assigned to one of four experimental conditions: (1) *intrusive/ controlling condition,* in which the care receiver received frequent messages, ostensibly from the caregiver, that either provided answers to the puzzle or told the care receiver what to do next; (2) *intrusive/supportive condition,* in which the care receiver received frequent messages that communicated encouragement and emotional support (e.g., "good job," "hard one"); (3) *nonintrusive/supportive condition,* in which the care receiver received two encouraging and emotionally supportive messages during the course of the game (e.g., "good luck, "good job"); and (4) *control condition,* in which the care receiver received no messages during the game. The two intrusive conditions were designed to reflect the absence of the noninterfering, "sit back and wait" aspect of secure base caregiving. After the game, care receivers reported their perceptions of partner support, their mood, and their state self-esteem. Puzzle performance was assessed, and responses to the caregivers' messages were also coded for those who responded. The general pattern of results follow (see Feeney, 2003, for specific details).

Results examining condition differences in perceptions of support (path c) revealed that care receivers in the intrusive/controlling condition viewed their partners' messages as more frustrating and insensitive than did care receivers in the intrusive/supportive condition, who viewed their partners' messages as more frustrating and insensitive than did care receivers in the nonintrusive/supportive condition. Moreover, care receivers in both the intrusive/supportive and nonintrusive/supportive conditions viewed their partners' messages as more helpful than did those in the intrusive/controlling condition. Although care receivers in both intrusive conditions viewed their partners as being more intrusive and interfering than did care receivers in the nonintrusive/supportive and control conditions, care receivers in all experimental conditions rated their partners as being more helpful and supportive than did care receivers in the control condition. Care receivers in the experimental conditions seem to have given their partners some credit for helpful intent.

With regard to immediate outcomes of manipulated caregiving behavior (and perceptions of manipulated caregiving behavior), results indicated that care receivers who perceived their partners' messages to be supportive (as opposed to intrusive and insensitive) experienced increases in state self-esteem and positive mood after the puzzle activity. In contrast, care receivers who viewed their partners' support as being insensitive, intrusive, and interfering experienced decreases in state self-esteem and positive mood from before to after the activity. Interestingly, care receivers in the intrusive conditions who responded to their partners' instant messages were more rejecting of the support than those care receivers who responded to nonintrusive messages. With regard to performance on the puzzle, care receivers in both intrusive conditions scored lower than care receivers in the control condition. Although this finding probably reflects the fact that participants were interrupted frequently in the intrusive conditions, the poorer performance of participants in the intrusive/controlling condition may also reflect a rejection of their partners' intrusive support (given that participants in this condition were given many of the answers to the puzzle). However, this speculation awaits future investigation, and additional work examining these and related processes is currently underway.

Summary of Evidence for Secure Base Processes

This initial investigation of secure base caregiving processes in adulthood provides some preliminary evidence for the paths depicted in the top portion of Figure 10.1 (paths *j* through *d*). However, there has been no empirical examination of the ways in which secure base caregiving and related outcomes influence the safe haven caregiving process (path *e*). As discussed in the next section, much work lies ahead with regard to further specifying the mechanisms and interpersonal dynamics involved at each stage in this portion of the model.

DIRECTIONS FOR FUTURE WORK

It will be important for future work to continue to isolate and examine various components of the caregiving processes outlined in Figure 10.1 and to expand and refine this model as research continues in this area. We view this model as a simplified depiction of what are likely to be very complex interpersonal processes. Although we have come a long way with regard to understanding safe haven caregiving processes, we have barely broken the surface, and there is much knowledge to be gained regarding many of the specific components of this process. For example, research examining important influences on care-seeking behaviors will be crucial for understanding this process. Because care-receiver behaviors have been strongly associated with caregiving behaviors, the care-seeking component of the process should be isolated and examined in a manner similar to the in-depth examinations of the caregiving component. It also will be important to isolate and examine caregivers' cognitive and emotional responses to specific care-seeking behaviors and the resulting influence on caregiving behavior. Sequential coding of couple interactions, as well as experimental studies in which care-seeking behaviors are manipulated, will be extremely helpful in this regard.

Longitudinal investigations examining the long-term outcomes of safe haven caregiving are also important endeavors for future work. The theoretical model depicted in Figure 10.1 suggests that some important long-term outcomes of safe haven caregiving are likely to be (1) better coping with future problems, (2) better problem resolution and related skills, (3) increases in feelings of security, (4) improved relationship quality and satisfaction, (5) changes over time in perceived benefits of seeking, receiving, and providing support, (6) reduced experience of stress and physiological reactivity in response to stressors and daily hassles, and (7) health benefits including improvements in mental and physical well-being. All of these links must be established in future work.

Because secure base caregiving processes in adult relationships are just beginning to be explored, a great deal of research must be done before we are likely to gain an adequate understanding of these processes. The investigation previously described has provided a first step in gaining an overall understanding of some normative secure base processes, including establishing some immediate outcomes of receiving secure base caregiving. It will be important for future research not only to explore the microdynamics of this interpersonal process but also to explore the long-term benefits of secure base caregiving, many of which are likely to be distinct from those afforded by safe haven caregiving. As described previously, individuals whose partners provide them with a secure base from which to explore the world are likely to (1) engage in a variety of exploratory activities, (2) experience increases in self-esteem, self-efficacy, and self-confidence as they gain more knowledge of the world, (3) learn and discover more than they would otherwise, (4) accept challenges and pursue goals, (5) be more healthy emotionally and physically, (6) be more satisfied with their relationships and have better relationship functioning, and (7) hold positive perceptions regarding the benefit of seeking support from others. Hopefully, the project described here will provide a foundation or springboard for other research on secure base processes in adult relationships. New observational, experimental, and daily-experience methods for examining various components of this process are currently being developed, and much exciting research lies ahead.

It is noteworthy that the discussion of secure base caregiving processes presented here emphasizes explorations of the external world that are likely to have important implications for the inner self in terms of self-esteem, perceptions of self-competency, and so forth. However, effective secure base caregiving in adulthood should include not only the support of a relationship partner's exploration of the physical world but also the support of the partner's exploration of his or her inner, psychological world—for example, the exploration of thoughts, feelings, and emotions related to self-understanding and self-discovery. In fact, Main and her colleagues have described the uninhibited exploration of attachment-related events, thoughts, and emotions as a hallmark of secure attachment (Main, 1995; Main, Kaplan, & Cassidy, 1985). Thus the support of this type of exploration, in particular, may have important implications for the development of secure attachment orientations in adulthood (e.g., Byng-Hall, 1999). Future research is needed to explore the specific determinants and outcomes of the support of internal versus external forms of exploration.

Another important goal for future research will be to examine the ways in which the attachment, caregiving, and exploration systems function together in the context of everyday interactions with one's relationship partner in order to demonstrate that a delicate balance of encouraging autonomy (secure base caregiving) yet accepting dependence when needed (safe haven caregiving) is vital for healthy personal and relationship functioning. Future research will be needed in order to examine the ways in which care receivers balance their exploratory and attachment behaviors and the ways in which caregivers balance safe haven and secure base caregiving behaviors. It will also be important for future research to examine the consequences of an effective balance of safe haven and secure base caregiving in relationships (and the consequences of the lack of balanced caregiving). According to attachment theory (Bowlby, 1988), individuals who receive an adequate balance of both types of caregiving are likely to be cheerful, happy, socially cooperative, and effective citizens who are unlikely to break down in adversity, likely to make stable marriages, and likely to provide their own children with the same favorable conditions for healthy development that they enjoyed. In contrast, individuals without a secure home base and safe haven are likely to be less cheerful, to find life and intimate relationships difficult, to be vulnerable in conditions of adversity, and to have difficulties in marriage and child rearing. These important postulates of attachment theory await future investigation.

CONCLUDING STATEMENT

In conclusion, the purpose of this chapter was to review some of the exciting work that is being done on caregiving processes in adult relationships and to lay a foundation for the development of future work in this area. Although we have found some important pieces of the caregiving puzzle, many others are awaiting our discovery. We are fortunate to have a rich and dynamic theory of adult attachment and caregiving processes to light the way. We are grateful to Bowlby for his pioneering work in this area, and to all of our colleagues who have contributed to extending attachment theory to the study of adult relationships.

ACKNOWLEDGMENTS

Preparation of this chapter was supported by National Institute of Mental Health Grant No. MH–066119 to Brooke Feeney and National Science Foundation Grant No. SBR–0096506 to Nancy Collins.

REFERENCES

Allen, J. P., McElhaney, K. B., Land, D. J., Kuperminc, G. P., Moore, C. W., O'Beirne-Kelly, H., & Kilmer, S. L. (2003). A secure base in adolescence: Markers of attachment security in the mother–adolescent relationship. *Child Development, 74,* 292–307.

Ainsworth, M. D. S., Blehar, M. C., Waters, E., & Wall, S. (1978). *Patterns of attachment: A psychological study of the Strange Situation.* Hillsdale, NJ: Erlbaum.

Barbee, A. P. (1990). Interactive coping: The cheering-up process in close relationships. In S. Duck (Ed.), *Social support in relationships* (pp. 47–65). Newbury Park, CA: Sage.

Bowlby, J. (1973). *Attachment and loss: Separation, anxiety and anger.* New York: Basic Books.

Bowlby, J. (1982). *Attachment and loss: Vol. 1. Attachment.* New York: Basic Books. (Original work published 1969)

Bowlby, J. (1988). *A secure base.* New York: Basic Books.

Bretherton, I. (1987). New perspectives on attachment relations: Security, communication, and internal working models. In J. D. Osofsky (Ed.), *Handbook of infant development* (2nd ed., pp. 1061–1100). New York: Wiley.

Byng-Hall, J. (1999). Family and couple therapy: Toward greater security. In J. Cassidy & P. R. Shaver (Eds.), *Handbook of attachment: Theory, research, and clinical applications* (pp. 625–645). New York: Guilford Press.

Carnelley, K., & Ruscher, J. (2000). Adult attachment and exploratory behavior in leisure. *Journal of Social Behavior and Personality, 15,* 153–165.

Carnelley, K. B., Pietromonaco, P. R., & Jaffe, K. (1996). Attachment, caregiving, and relationship functioning in couples: Effects of self and partner. *Personal Relationships, 3,* 257–278.

Carpenter, E. M., & Kirkpatrick, L. A. (1996). Attachment style and presence of a romantic partner as moderators of psychophysiological responses to a stressful laboratory situation. *Personal Relationships, 3,* 351–367.

Cassidy, J. (2001). Truth, lies, and intimacy: An attachment perspective. *Attachment and Human Development, 3,* 121–155.

Collins, N. L., & Feeney, B. C. (2000). A safe haven: An attachment theory perspective on support-seeking and caregiving in intimate relationships. *Journal of Personality and Social Psychology, 78,* 1053–1073.

Collins, N. L., & Feeney, B. C. (2003). *Attachment processes in daily interaction: Feeling supported and feeling secure.* Unpublished manuscript, University of California, Santa Barbara.

Collins, N. L., & Feeney, B. C. (in press). Working models of attachment shape perceptions of social support: Evidence from experimental and observational studies. *Journal of Personality and Social Psychology.*

Collins, N. L., Ford, M. B., Guichard, A., & Feeney, B. C. (2003). *Responding to need in intimate relationships: The role of attachment anxiety.* Unpublished manuscript, University of California, Santa Barbara.

Crowell, J., Treboux, D., Gao, Y., Fyffe, C., Pan, H., & Waters, E. (2002). Assessing secure base behavior in adulthood: Development of a measure, links to adult attachment representations, and relations to couples' communication and reports of relationships. *Developmental Psychology, 38,* 679–693.

Cutrona, C. E. (1996). Social support as a determinant of marital quality: The interplay of negative and supportive behaviors. In G. R. Pierce, B. R. Sarason, & I. G. Sarason (Eds.), *Handbook of social support and the family* (pp. 173–194). New York: Plenum Press.

Emmons, R. A., & King, L. A. (1988). Conflict among personal strivings: Immediate and long-term implications for psychological and physical well-being. *Journal of Personality and Social Psychology, 54,* 1040–1048.

Feeney, B. C. (2003). *A secure base: Responsive support of goal strivings and exploration in adult intimate relationships.* Manuscript submitted for publication.

Feeney, B. C., & Collins, N. L. (2001). Predictors of caregiving in adult intimate relationships: An attachment theoretical perspective. *Journal of Personality and Social Psychology, 80,* 972–994.

Feeney, B. C., & Collins, N. L. (2003). Motivations for caregiving in adult intimate relationships: Influences on caregiving behavior and relationship functioning. *Personality and Social Psychology Bulletin, 29,* 950–968.

Feeney, B. C., & Kirkpatrick, L. A. (1996). The effects of adult attachment and presence of romantic partners on physiological responses to stress. *Journal of Personality and Social Psychology, 70,* 255–270.

Feeney, J. A. (1996). Attachment, caregiving, and marital satisfaction. *Personal Relationships, 3,* 401–416.

Florian, V., Mikulincer, M., & Bucholtz, I. (1995). Effects of adult attachment style on the perception and search for social support. *Journal of Psychology, 129,* 665–676.

George, C., & Solomon, J. (1989). Internal working models of caregiving and security of attachment at age six. *Infant Mental Health Journal, 10,* 222–237.

George, C., & Solomon, J. (1996). Representational models of relationships: Links between caregiving and attachment. *Infant Mental Health Journal, 17,* 198–216.

George, C., & Solomon, J. (1999a). Attachment and caregiving: The caregiving behavioral system. In J. Cassidy & P. R. Shaver (Eds.), *Handbook of attachment: Theory, research, and clinical applications* (pp. 649–670). New York: Guilford Press.

George, C., & Solomon, J. (1999b). The development of caregiving: A comparison of attachment theory and psychoanalytic approaches to mothering. *Psychoanalytic Inquiry, 19,* 618–646.

Hazan, C., & Shaver, P. R. (1990). Love and work: An attachment-theoretical perspective. *Journal of Personality and Social Psychology, 59,* 270–280.

Kunce, L. J., & Shaver, P. R. (1994). An attachment-theoretical approach to caregiving in romantic relationships. In K. Bartholomew & D. Perlman (Eds.), *Advances in personal relationships: Vol. 5. Attachment processes in adulthood* (pp. 205–237). London: Kingsley.

Main, M. (1995). Attachment: Overview, with implications for clinical work. In S. Goldberg, R. Muir, & J. Kerr (Eds.), *Attachment theory: Social, developmental, and clinical perspectives* (pp. 407–474). Hillsdale, NJ: Analytic Press.

Main, M., Kaplan, N., & Cassidy, J. (1985). Security in infancy, childhood, and adulthood: A move to the level of representation. In I. Bretherton & E. Waters (Eds.), Growing points of attachment theory and research. *Monographs of the Society for Research in Child Development, 50*(1–2, Serial No. 209), 66–104.

Marvin, R., Cooper, G., Hoffman, K., & Powell, B. (2002). The Circle of Security Project: Attachment-based intervention with caregiver–pre-school child dyads. *Attachment and Human Development, 4,* 107–124.

Mikulincer, M., & Florian, V. (1995). Appraisal of and coping with a real-life stressful situation: The contribution of attachment styles. *Personality and Social Psychology Bulletin, 21,* 406–414.

Mikulincer, M., Florian, V., & Weller, A. (1993). Attachment styles, coping strategies, and posttraumatic psychological distress: The impact of the Gulf War in Israel. *Journal of Personality and Social Psychology, 64,* 817–826.

Ognibene, T. C., & Collins, N. L. (1998). Adult attachment styles, perceived social support, and coping strategies. *Journal of Social and Personal Relationships, 15,* 323–345.

Reis, H. T., & Shaver, P. (1988). Intimacy as an interpersonal process. In S. Duck & D. F. Hay (Eds.), *Handbook of personal relationships: Theory, research, and interventions* (pp. 367–389). Chichester, UK: Wiley.

Simpson, J. A., Rholes, W. S., & Nelligan, J. S. (1992). Support seeking and support giving within couples in an anxiety-provoking situation: The role of attachment styles. *Journal of Personality and Social Psychology, 62,* 434–446.

Solomon, J., & George, C. (1996). Defining the caregiving system: Toward a theory of caregiving. *Infant Mental Health Journal, 17,* 183–197.

Waters, E., & Cummings, E. M. (2000). A secure base from which to explore close relationships. *Child Development, 71,* 164–172.

Westmaas, J. L., & Silver, R. C. (2001). The role of attachment in responses to victims of life crises. *Journal of Personality and Social Psychology, 80,* 425–438.

CHAPTER 11

Adult Attachment and Relationship Functioning under Stressful Conditions

Understanding Partners' Responses to Conflict and Challenge

JUDITH A. FEENEY

"During one period my partner and I were facing difficulties at work, and they started to affect our relationship. We became temperamental and picked on minor things and blew them up into arguments. But we realized what was happening, and we talked about the situation and worked out ways of supporting each other."

"In stressful times, such as financial problems, a relationship doesn't warrant communication. I have to work out problems myself, because part of me wants to keep things private and personal. I like to keep my problems to myself until I've worked them out. I don't attend to my partner much if my mind's on these things."

Although many studies of adult attachment have tested general hypotheses about attachment and relationship functioning, there are compelling reasons for focusing on stressful situations. In infancy, the attachment system maintains a balance between exploratory behavior and proximity-seeking behavior, taking account of dangers in the environment and the accessibility of attachment figures (Bowlby, 1984). Infants perceive separation from attachment figures as a threat to well-being and resist it by such behaviors as crying and clinging. Thus attachment behavior is activated by conditions of apparent threat. Bowlby (1984) proposed that these conditions fall into three types: conditions of the child (e.g., hunger, illness), conditions of the environment (e.g., alarming events, presence of unfamiliar people), and conditions of the attachment relationship (e.g., the caregiver's absence or discouraging of proximity).

Some of these specific conditions (such as the presence of unfamiliar people) may activate attachment behavior only in the helpless infant, but Bowlby's broad typology is applicable to adult behavior. Based on this typology, attachment researchers have begun to study individual differences in adults' responses to pain and illness, stressful environmental conditions, and conditions that threaten or challenge the attachment bond. This chapter focuses on the third set of conditions (stressful events *within the relationship*), which are of particular relevance to relationship researchers. Two main categories of relationship stressors are discussed: conflictual and challenging situations. The theme of this chapter is that individual differences in attachment behavior are relatively pronounced in these situations. As illustrated by the preceding quotes from research participants (a secure and an insecure male, respectively), individuals with different attachment orientations may respond quite differently to stress, and these responses are likely to affect relationship processes and outcomes.

The link between attachment and stress is consistent with attachment theorists' emphasis on affect regulation. Caregivers' reactions to the child's affective signals are thought to provide a critical context in which the child learns how to deal with negative feelings and achieve "felt security" (Sroufe & Waters, 1977). If caregivers are available and responsive, distress can be regulated by turning to them for comfort, but if they are unavailable, unresponsive, or unpredictable, alternative strategies develop. Over time, the varying strategies are incorporated into rules that guide responses to stressful situations. Hence, different attachment styles are associated with different rules. In terms of infant attachment styles, secure attachment is associated with rules that allow acknowledgment of distress and active support seeking, avoidant attachment with rules that restrict expression of distress and support seeking, and anxious–ambivalent attachment with rules that encourage heightened awareness and expression of distress (Kobak & Sceery, 1988). Because researchers have used a range of approaches to assess adults' attachment orientations, this chapter refers variously to these three styles, to the four-group model of secure, preoccupied, dismissing, and fearful attachment (Bartholomew, 1990), and to the main dimensions underlying these styles: discomfort with closeness (or avoidance) and relationship anxiety.

DEALING WITH CONFLICT AND RELATIONAL TRANSGRESSIONS

Conflict is an inevitable consequence of the interdependence that characterizes couple bonds, and responses to conflict are a major predictor of relationship outcomes (Christensen & Walczynski, 1997). Furthermore, conflict-centered interactions are of particular interest to attachment researchers, because such interactions may cause concern about the partner's availability and hence activate the attachment system (Kobak & Duemmler, 1994). The first half of this chapter focuses on attachment-related differences in responses to conflict and relational transgressions. It presents a series of studies from my research laboratory, together with other key findings in the area, and illustrates the increasing sophistication of research questions.

General Responses to Conflict

Several studies of adult attachment have examined questionnaire-based reports of general conflict behavior. For example, Pistole (1989) used Hazan and Shaver's (1987) three-group measure of attachment style and Rahim's (1983) Organizational Conflict Inventory. She found that secure individuals were more likely to use an integrating (problem-solving) strategy than those who were insecure. Anxious–ambivalent individuals reported little use of compromise but were more likely to oblige the partner's wishes than were avoidant individuals. These findings support the view that secure individuals use more constructive strategies in dealing with conflict; that is, strategies that reflect their concern both for their own interests and for maintaining the relationship. More recently, studies by Gaines and colleagues (1997) assessed the association between attachment security and reported responses to accommodative dilemmas—that is, situations in which a partner engages in negative behavior. As predicted, secure attachment was inversely related to the destructive responses of exit (actively harming the relationship) and neglect (passively allowing the situation to deteriorate).

One of the early studies conducted in our own laboratory also examined reports of general conflict behavior (Feeney, Noller, & Callan, 1994). Although this research ignored the implications of different types of conflict (discussed later), it employed multiple methods, couple data, and a longitudinal design, and addressed the complex relations among attachment, conflict behavior, and marital satisfaction. Couples filled out interaction diaries 6 months after marriage, assessing the quality of their day-to-day interactions in terms of recognition, disclosure, involvement, satisfaction, conflict, and domination. They also attended assessment sessions after 12 months and 21 months of marriage. At these sessions, couples completed questionnaire measures of attachment (discomfort with closeness and relationship anxiety) and conflict behavior (mutuality, coercion, destructive process such as demand–withdraw, and postconflict distress). Finally, they discussed two issues causing conflict in their relationships and provided reports of their own influence strategies; these were coded to yield scores on positivity (reason and support), negativity (manipulation and threat), and conflict avoidance (physical and emotional retreat).

Effects of Individuals' Own Attachment Characteristics

For husbands only, discomfort with closeness was related to diary reports of less involvement, recognition, disclosure, and satisfaction and to questionnaire reports of less mutuality (mutual negotiation). Links between relationship anxiety and conflict behavior were even more widespread, although they were somewhat stronger for wives. Relationship anxiety was linked to diary ratings of low involvement, disclosure, and satisfaction and of high conflict and domination; to questionnaire reports of low levels of mutuality and high levels of coercion, destructive process, and postconflict distress; and to reported use of negative influence strategies. In addition, wives' relationship anxiety predicted their *later* reports of destructive process and postconflict distress, even when earlier conflict scores were controlled. These concurrent and predictive links suggest that anxiety about attachment issues drives a range of destructive conflict behaviors, which may contribute to relationship breakdown and hence exacerbate insecurity.

Effects of the Partner's Attachment Characteristics

Of course, conflict behavior can be influenced by the attachment characteristics of the *partner*, as well as those of the reporter. Recognizing the dyadic nature of attachment bonds, researchers are paying increasing attention to these "partner effects." For example, Kobak and Hazan (1991) reported that when husbands were more securely attached, both husbands and wives showed less rejection and more validation during discussion of a conflict issue. In our study of newlyweds (Feeney et al., 1994), the most consistent partner effects involved husbands' discomfort with closeness and wives' relationship anxiety. When husbands were high in discomfort, wives reported less involvement, recognition, and satisfaction in their day-to-day interactions. Conversely, when wives were high in relationship anxiety, husbands reported more domination and less involvement in day-to-day interactions and more coercion and destructive process in response to conflict.

In the same study, we also investigated possible *interactive* effects of partners' attachment characteristics; that is, does the effect of one person's discomfort or anxiety depend on the partner's attachment profile? The most consistent effect involved husbands' and wives' relationship anxiety, which interacted to predict women's reports of several conflict behaviors, both concurrently and longitudinally. Interestingly, this effect varied in form. For example, wives' reports of conflict avoidance were highest when both spouses were anxious about the relationship (Figure 11.1a), suggesting that their avoidance was driven by the insecurities of both partners. However, anxious wives with husbands low in anxiety reported more coercion than those with anxious husbands (Figure 11.1b). This finding suggests that anxious wives may perceive their nonanxious husbands as unable or unwilling to understand their concerns; this situation may lead to escalating coercion or to *misperceptions* of partners' intentions as coercive. Similarly, a recent study of marital conflict showed complex effects of partners' anxiety levels: Couples with two anxious spouses reported the most conflict, but couples in which only the wife was anxious reported slightly less conflict than those in which both spouses were low in anxiety (Gallo & Smith, 2001). Perhaps anxious wives strive hard to retain their partners and nonanxious husbands take this into account in responding to their needs and concerns.

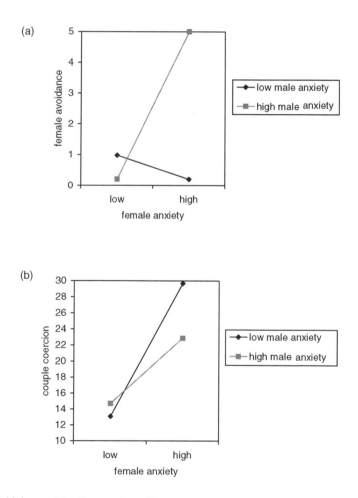

FIGURE 11.1 a and b. Interactive effects of partners' levels of relationship anxiety on females' reports of conflict avoidance and couple coercion.

Attachment, Conflict, and Marital Satisfaction

Relations among attachment, conflict, and marital satisfaction were assessed both in the sample of newlyweds and in a larger sample representing all stages of the marital life cycle (Feeney, 1994). In both studies, we were interested in whether the robust link between security and marital satisfaction was mediated by conflict behavior; that is, can secure individuals' greater satisfaction be explained by their adaptive responses to conflict? This mediation effect was supported in the broad sample (but not in the sample of newlyweds): Relations between attachment and satisfaction became nonsignificant (for wives) or reduced to trends (for husbands) when conflict behavior was controlled. Subsequent studies suggest that secure individuals' greater satisfaction also reflects, in part, their ability to reveal and elicit personal thoughts and feelings (Feeney, 1999a; Keelan, Dion, & Dion, 1998). Together, these findings suggest that insecure individuals may be helped by interventions that promote constructive patterns of negotiation.

Conflict over Closeness and Distance

Although the studies cited previously point to links between attachment security and general reports of conflict behavior, conflicts over closeness and distance are especially relevant to attachment processes. Closeness–distance (or autonomy–connection) is a fundamental relationship dilemma: Relationships cannot survive unless partners give up some autonomy in order to forge a connection, but too much connection stifles the individual entities and may destroy the relationship (Baxter & Montgomery, 1997). Hence, partners must juggle contrasting desires for separateness and closeness, autonomy and commitment. Attachment theory is directly relevant to this issue: Conflicts about closeness and distance may activate the attachment system and are more likely to be intractable if partners differ markedly in attachment orientations (Pistole, 1994). In our laboratory, the implications of attachment for conflicts over closeness and distance have been explored in a study of long-term dating couples (Feeney, 1998, 1999b). This study, discussed next, combined qualitative and quantitative methods.

Open-Ended Reports of Closeness–Distance Conflicts

In the qualitative component, participants were asked to talk about their current relationships, and the talks were tape-recorded and transcribed for content analysis. Content was coded as relevant to the closeness–distance theme if it included explicit mention of "closeness" or "distance" or comment on such issues as the amount of time partners spent together or apart. Several findings supported the salience of this theme and the relevance of attachment security. First, almost all participants (92%) made some reference to the theme. Second, in terms of word count, just over one-third of the content was devoted to discussing these issues. Third, references to this theme often involved strong language: Some participants reported feeling "smothered" and "pressured" by partners' needs for intimacy, whereas others reported feeling "neglected" and "miserable" in the face of partners' needs for distance. Fourth, ongoing conflicts over closeness and distance were reported more frequently when the male was high in discomfort with closeness or the female was high in relationship anxiety.

Struggles over closeness and distance can generate considerable stress and confusion, as evident in these comments from a preoccupied female:

> "Sometimes things just go from bad to worse, because he wants to spend more time with his friends. This causes a lot of problems that we're still trying to resolve. I think maybe he thinks they're resolved, but I'm not sure if I want to continue the relationship—because I'm not sure I've got to know him well enough, because we don't spend enough time together. And—and it's fine if he would prefer to spend time with his friends, but it's letting the situation between us get worse, and I just—it's just—a lot of the time I just try not to think about it—I just don't know."

Struggles over closeness and distance can also maintain, or even exacerbate, an individual's sense of insecurity. For example, another preoccupied woman discussed her concerns about her partner's "cool" and distant behavior and noted that her attempts to discuss these issues met with a guarded response that further increased her anxieties. Her dismissing partner acknowledged that his desire to take occasional "breaks" from the relationship was difficult for her:

> "It's important to have a break in your relationship every now and again; that way, you get to realize whether you really love the person or not, and whether you really want to stay with them. She finds this idea a bit tough."

Given that this man saw the breaks as "testing" the relationship, it is not surprising that his partner found these times difficult. In these accounts, we see that each partner's attitudes and behavior set the stage for subsequent interaction. The interactive cycles that form in this way may involve pursuer–distancer struggles, especially if partners are insecure and have very different preferences for closeness and distance

(Byng-Hall, 1999). Another preoccupied female described this kind of cycle:

> "He used to buy me things all the time and make me feel so special. But when I became more deeply involved, he eased back. I didn't like that, so I eased back too. The moment I did that, it became intense again. But as soon as I start becoming interested, he doesn't show the same keenness."

Her dismissing partner was aware of their differing approaches to intimacy, describing his own relationship style as "stony" and his partner's as "overly emotional." Such rigid patterns can create considerable distress. In fact, Roberts and Noller (1998) found that physical aggression in cohabiting and married couples was linked to the combination of a perpetrator high in relationship anxiety and a partner uncomfortable with closeness. It seems that these couples find it very difficult to deal with stress and conflict, given their contrasting interpersonal goals and styles.

Studying Closeness–Distance Conflicts in the Laboratory

In the study just discussed (Feeney, 1998), dating couples also took part in three interactions involving explicit conflicts of interest. Immediately before one scene (the "leisure scene"), each partner was separately primed to push for a different leisure activity, to be undertaken in a time previously declared as shared couple time. In the remaining scenes, one partner was instructed to act in a cold and distant manner toward the other, who was instructed to try to reestablish closeness. The roles of the man and woman were reversed in the two (counterbalanced) interactions. Responses to partner's distancing were of primary interest; however, the leisure scene enabled a comparison of core relational conflict (i.e., closeness–distance) and more concrete (issue-based) conflict. This distinction is important because core relational conflict is more likely to threaten the relationship and, hence, to activate attachment behavior.

Independent observers rated participants' responses to conflict: Verbal behavior was defined using summary measures of reason, affiliation, and coercion, and nonverbal behavior was assessed using summary measures of touch and avoidance (which tap the extent of involvement with the partner and the situation). The original report of this study (Feeney, 1998) discussed own and partner attachment effects, but the discussion here also includes reanalyses examining interactive effects.

In the leisure scene, the number of significant relations between attachment and conflict behavior did not exceed that expected by chance. In contrast, responses to partner distancing showed many effects, summarized in Table 11.1. These effects again attest to the link between security

TABLE 11.1. Summary of Significant Attachment Effects in Response to Partner's Distancing

Dependent variable	Summary of attachment-related effects
Verbal behavior	
Reason	Females' use of reason was related negatively to their discomfort.
Affiliation	Males' use of affiliation was related negatively to females' discomfort and females' anxiety.
Coercion	Males' use of coercion was related positively to their anxiety.
	Females' use of coercion was highest when both partners were highly anxious.
Nonverbal behavior	
Touch	Males' use of touch was related negatively to their discomfort.
	Females' use of touch was related negatively to their anxiety and was highest when the male was anxious but the female was not.
Avoidance	Males' avoidance was related positively to their discomfort.
	Females' avoidance was related positively to their anxiety, and was highest when both partners were highly anxious.

Note. "Discomfort" refers to discomfort with closeness; "anxiety" refers to relationship anxiety.

and constructive responses to conflict. In terms of nonverbal behavior, males high in discomfort with closeness and females high in relationship anxiety showed less active involvement. Verbal behavior showed effects of both own and partner's attachment characteristics; for example, females high in discomfort with closeness used less reason, and their partners were less affiliative. Females' conflict behavior also showed interactive effects of partners' anxiety levels, but as in our study of newlyweds, this effect varied in form. Females' coercion was highest when both partners were anxious. However, their use of touch was highest when their partners were anxious but they themselves were not, suggesting that women low in anxiety were aware of their partners' insecurities and tried to be supportive.

The fact that attachment-related effects emerged in the partner-distant scene, but not the leisure scene, supports the claim that attachment behavior is activated by perceptions of threat to the relationship. Similarly, in another laboratory study of conflict in dating couples, attachment-related effects (linking ambivalence with distress, hostility, and anxiety and avoidance with lower quality interactions) were stronger for couples who were asked to discuss major, rather than minor, conflicts (Simpson, Rholes, & Phillips, 1996).

Interestingly, the studies reported so far (Feeney, 1998; Feeney et al., 1994) suggest that interactive effects of partners' attachment characteristics are more evident in *women's* responses to conflict. Perhaps women are somewhat more sensitive to relational dynamics, including differences in partners' concerns and anxieties. In line with this claim, Sumer's (2000) study of interpersonal schemas in marriage suggests that secure women may be more effective than secure men in buffering the effects of partners' insecurity.

Relational Transgressions

Conflict between romantic partners can arise from simple differences of opinion or from differing preferences for closeness and distance. Such instances of conflict do not necessarily involve a sense that the partner has transgressed (behaved in a negative or rule-violating way), although even the most innocent differences may be interpreted this way by distressed or insecure spouses. In contrast, the next section of this chapter focuses on partner behaviors that are generally regarded as transgressions. Insecure individuals may find these behaviors particularly stressful, given that they tend to see them as intentional and as caused by internal, stable, and global factors (Gallo & Smith, 2001; Mikulincer, 1998).

Reactivity to Negative Spouse Behavior

A recent study of marriage (Feeney, 2002) examined responses to negative spouse behavior. Given attachment-related differences in attributional patterns (noted previously), negative partner behavior is likely to confirm or exacerbate insecure individuals' doubts about the partner's love and the viability of the relationship. Hence it was hypothesized that insecure individuals would be particularly "reactive" to negative spouse behavior when evaluating their marriages. In other words, the link between marital satisfaction and perceptions of recent negative spouse behavior was expected to be stronger for insecure spouses.

In this study, couples completed categorical and continuous measures of attachment. On each of two successive days, they also completed a checklist of negative spouse behaviors (e.g., "refused to listen to my feelings") and rated their overall satisfaction with the marriage. Reactivity coefficients were formed by correlating negative spouse behavior and satisfaction, averaged across the 2 days. Results were generally as expected: Dismissing and preoccupied husbands were more reactive ($r = -.63$ and $-.61$, respectively) than secure husbands ($r = -.25$), and dismissing and fearful wives ($r = -.63$ and $-.65$, respectively) were more reactive than secure wives ($r = -.30$). Analyses using the attachment scales supported these results, though for husbands only: The link between satisfaction and negative behavior was significant only for those high in discomfort with closeness or relationship anxiety. Overall, these findings suggest that insecure persons' global relationship evaluations are influenced quite strongly by recent negative events. Unfortunately, over time, the tendency to monitor and ruminate over transgressions is likely to erode relationship satisfaction.

Dealing with Hurt Feelings

Psychological hurt is emerging as an important topic for relationship researchers. "Hurt" is regarded as a highly negative emotion (Shaver, Schwartz, Kirson, & O'Connor, 1987), and hurt feelings tend to be particularly strong when the offender is a romantic partner (Leary, Springer, Negel, Ansell, & Evans, 1998). Hence, given that attachment styles reflect learned ways of dealing with negative affect, we would expect attachment-related differences in responses to partners' hurtful behavior. The relevance of attachment theory also fits with Leary and colleagues' (1998) argument that hurt feelings arise when the partner does not seem to value the relationship as much as the offended partner would like. Insecure individuals often interpret ambiguous partner behavior as negative in intention and as jeopardizing the relationship (Collins, 1996).

Hurt is a relational phenomenon, and the outcomes of hurtful events undoubtedly depend on the thoughts, feelings, and behaviors of both partners. For the present discussion, however, let us focus on the victim's perspective. The attachment orientation of the victim is likely to affect an entire chain of events: initial emotions and cognitions, evaluations of offender remorse, behavioral responses, and ongoing experiences of mistrust and self-doubt. Analyses from our studies of hurt feelings support this proposition. This research program began with a retrospective study in which victims gave open-ended and structured accounts of an experience of being hurt by a romantic partner. The open-ended accounts contained references to a range of negative emotions (e.g., anger, sadness, fear), as well as strong metaphorical terms (e.g., "torn apart," "crushed"). Several accounts pointed to the extreme distress that such experiences can elicit. For example, one (preoccupied) participant reported:

> "I didn't eat for a week. I drank alcohol. I was totally at the bottom of my life. I didn't know what to do—complete depression. I cannot accurately describe in words how I felt. Words cannot express the depth of my emotions."

Quantitative analyses from this study (Feeney, in press) involved using structural equations modeling to predict the long-term effects of hurtful events, in terms of victims' ongoing self-doubts and ongoing problems in victim–offender relationships. (Although the retrospective method raises questions about the directionality of links between hurt feelings and the attachment dimensions of avoidance and anxiety, the data are nevertheless useful for demonstrating attachment-related differences in perceptions of hurtful events.) Victims' reports of ongoing self-doubts were predicted by relationship anxiety. This association involved a direct effect, together with indirect effects via initial emotional distress and negative self-perceptions. In other words, the ongoing self-doubts reported by anxious individuals reflect, in part, their initial tendency to be very distressed by partners' transgressions and to see themselves as foolish and undesirable. These results fit with attachment theory: For the anxious individual, hurtful partner behavior confirms existing views of the self as unworthy.

Reports of ongoing relationship problems were predicted by avoidance. This association again involved a direct effect, together with indirect effects through victim behavior and perceived offender remorse. It is important to note the direction of these effects (see Figure 11.2). Overall, avoidance was linked to greater relationship problems. The direct path may reflect avoidant persons' overlearned tendency to downplay attachment needs, particularly in times of stress (Fraley & Shaver, 1997); this tendency may give rise to conflict avoidance and failure to resolve issues. The indirect path through perceived remorse was in the same direction; avoidant victims saw offenders as lacking remorse, and this perception was linked to relationship problems. The path through victim behavior, however, was in the reverse direction: Avoidant victims were *less* likely to

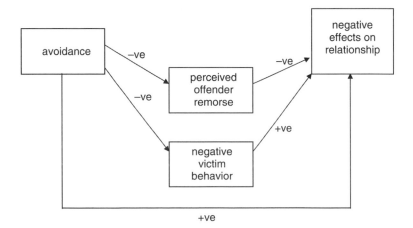

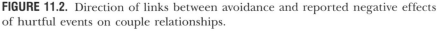

FIGURE 11.2. Direction of links between avoidance and reported negative effects of hurtful events on couple relationships.
+ve, positive association; –ve, negative association.

respond with anger, sarcasm, or rumination, thus reducing relationship problems. This finding suggests that the controlled interpersonal style associated with avoidance may prevent some conflicts from escalating (although, as just noted, issues may resurface in the future). This paradoxical effect of avoidance (i.e., reducing the overall negative effect) highlights the complexity of attachment processes.

DEALING WITH CHALLENGING SITUATIONS

The second half of this chapter focuses on the effects of stressful events that are faced at some time by most couples and that raise issues about the way partners relate to each other. These events are not inherently conflict laden. They are stressful, however, because they require substantial readjustment to patterns of couple interaction. Three kinds of challenging events are considered: separation from partners, caregiving, and new parenthood.

Separation from Partners

The Strange Situation (Ainsworth, Blehar, Waters, & Wall, 1978), which is widely used to assess infant attachment style, involves a series of comings and goings on the part of the parent (usually the mother) and a friendly stranger. These episodes are designed to be mildly stressful, permitting observation of separation and reunion behavior. Of course, adults seldom see short absences from their romantic partners as highly stressful. However, longer absences are likely to raise issues about the benefits and future course of the relationship. In a review paper, Vormbrock (1993) argued that attachment theory provides a useful perspective on separations and reunions between intimate partners. In support of this claim, she noted that spouses react in very similar ways to various types of separation (e.g., wartime, job related) and that the reactions follow stages similar to those seen in children who are separated from their caregivers.

Vormbrock's theoretical analysis of adults' separation behavior focused on universal patterns of response, rather than individual differences. However, studies of responses to "separation reminders" suggest that individuals with different attachment styles differ in the degree of stress associated with thoughts of separation and in the strategies used to deal with such stress. For example, Mikulincer, Florian, Birnbaum, and Malishkewitz (2002) conducted studies in which respondents were asked to imagine being separated from a relationship partner. For individuals high in relationship anxiety, this manipulation led to heightened accessibility of death-related thoughts, suggesting that these individuals experience separation as quite catastrophic. Using a somewhat different experimental procedure, Fraley and Shaver (1997) asked participants to imagine vividly a breakup with their long-term partner and then to stop thinking about it. For individuals high in dismissing avoidance, these instructions led to a decrease in the accessibility of abandonment-related thoughts, together with declines in physiological arousal. These results suggest that dismissing adults have learned to deal with attachment-related concerns by focusing their attention away from the thoughts that activate them.

In our study of long-term dating couples discussed earlier (Feeney, 1998), we obtained reports of actual separation experiences by asking each participant to talk about a time when he or she had been separated from his or her current partner. Some participants described a single separation episode (from 2 weeks to 12 months in length); others described periods of repeated separation in which partners saw each other occasionally. (Importantly, attachment security was not confounded with length or type of separation.) Again, the accounts were tape-recorded and transcribed. Content coding focused on two main issues: strategies used to cope with the partner's absence and effects on the couple relationship. (Other analyses, beyond the scope of this chapter, linked relationship anxiety to extreme emotional distress in response to separation.)

Coping Strategies

Coping strategies were first defined using the broad categories of problem-focused coping (directed at managing the problem), emotion-focused coping (dealing with emotional distress), and support seeking (using resources of the social network). The first two of these categories were further subdivided. Problem-focused coping was divided into maintaining contact with the partner, pursuing personal or couple goals, and confrontive coping (openly discussing the situation with the partner). Emotion-focused coping was divided into positive reappraisal, minimizing, and escape/avoidance (e.g., using drugs). Finally, because coping is a process that typically requires a combination of strategies, the number of strategies used by each participant (e.g., confrontive, support seeking) was tallied.

Links between attachment dimensions and coping strategies are summarized in Table 11.2. All three broad strategies were related to attachment. Males high in discomfort and the partners of anxious males reported more emotion-focused coping, and anxious males reported less problem-focused coping. Males high in discomfort and females high in anxiety reported less support seeking. In terms of the finer subdivisions, males high in discomfort reported less confrontive coping (which represents the most direct attempt to manage the problem) and more escape/avoidance (a very maladaptive approach). Hence, attachment security was linked most strongly to strategies that are clearly constructive or destruc-

TABLE 11.2. Summary of Significant Attachment Effects in Coping with Separation

Coping variable	Example	Attachment-related effects
Problem-focused coping	"I made good use of the time—I kept in touch with him but also made time to catch up with things and work on my own goals."	Males' problem-focused coping was related negatively to own anxiety.
Confrontive coping	"We wrote a lot to each other, and told how we felt, and promised each other that we would be there, and worked out ways of keeping the relationship alive."	Males' confrontive coping was related negatively to own discomfort.
Emotion-focused coping	"I would get very upset but work at hiding it from him. I would make wishes for the future, but wonder whether he wanted to be with me."	Males' emotion-focused coping was related positively to own discomfort; females' emotion-focused coping was related positively to males' anxiety.
Escape/avoidance	"I got drunk a lot; I got stoned a lot. I tried to wipe out so I didn't have to think about what might be happening."	Males' escape/avoidance was related positively to own discomfort.
Support seeking	"I socialized with my friends, talked to them on the phone, told them about what was happening."	Support seeking was related negatively to own discomfort (males) and own anxiety (females).
Diversity of strategies used	n/a	For both genders, diversity was related negatively to own anxiety.

Note. "Discomfort" refers to discomfort with closeness; "anxiety" refers to relationship anxiety.

tive. Finally, for both genders, the number of different strategies was inversely related to their own anxiety.

In summary, secure attachment was linked with constructive patterns of coping: problem-focused coping, support seeking, and more diverse strategies. This finding is consistent with attachment principles and with research linking security to various aspects of the support process, including support seeking, enacted support, and perceived support (Bartholomew, Cobb, & Poole, 1997). Another study of separation dynamics in romantic couples has supported the role of adult attachment (Fraley & Shaver, 1998), although the results were most clear-cut for women. In this innovative study of airport separations, women's self-reported relationship anxiety was associated with observers' ratings of their separation distress. In addition, more avoidant women tended to withdraw from their partners when separation was imminent, whereas avoidance was not linked to withdrawal in nonseparating couples. Hence, attachment-related differences were again more pronounced under stressful conditions.

Effects on the Couple Relationship

In the study by Feeney (1998), reports of the effects of separation were coded dichotomously: Separation was seen either as bringing the partners closer or as creating ongoing problems. Males who reported ongoing problems were higher in discomfort than those who did not, and females who reported ongoing problems were more anxious than those who did not. These findings are important, given that perceptions of relationship problems are likely to predict how the relationship ultimately fares. We were also interested in whether partners had actively renegotiated the relationship on reunion; that is, whether they had discussed what each wanted from the relationship and how much time they could devote to it. Insecure females (those high in discomfort or anxiety) were less likely to report renegotiation. This result may help explain why anxious females reported ongoing problems: They may be reluctant to discuss their concerns and fears with their partners.

The benefits of secure attachment for the reunion process are supported by a study of reunion dynamics following men's deployment on military operations (Cafferty, Davis, Medway, O'Hearn, & Chappell, 1994). Four months after reunion, the men and their wives completed questionnaires assessing attachment, marital satisfaction, conflict, and affect during reunion. For both husbands and wives, secure attachment was related to higher marital satisfaction and less postreunion conflict; preoccupied respondents reported particularly low levels of satisfaction and particularly high levels of conflict. Links between secure attachment and more positive affect during reunion were confined to men, perhaps because their separation experience was more stressful.

Caregiving

Unlike infant–caregiver bonds, adult attachments are characterized (ideally, at least) by mutual caregiving. In other words, each partner is sometimes the giver and sometimes the recipient of care, depending on needs and resources. In fact, Shaver, Hazan, and Bradshaw (1988) argued that attachment and caregiving are behavioral systems that are integrated (along with sexual mating) in romantic love. Given the theoretical arguments linking attachment and caregiving, it is not surprising that several studies have addressed this issue. Most of these studies have assessed general caregiving style or partners' responses to stressful situations in the laboratory.

General Caregiving Style

Kunce and Shaver (1994) conducted a program of research assessing the links between attachment styles and caregiving behavior. Using data derived from interviews and open-ended questionnaires, these researchers developed scales tapping the major dimensions of caregiving in adult relationships: proximity (versus distance), sensitivity (versus insensitivity), cooperation (versus control), and compulsive caregiving. In a student sample, these scales differentiated attachment groups as defined by a four-group measure. As expected, secure respondents reported high proximity and sensitivity, whereas dismissing respondents reported low proximity and sensitivity; both these groups reported a lack of compulsive caregiving. Consistent with their need for the approval of others, preoccupied and fearful respondents reported high compulsive caregiving but low sensitivity. Similarly, in Carnelley, Pietromonaco, and Jaffe's (1996) studies of dating and married couples, individuals who were more securely attached reported giving their partners more beneficial care (i.e., care that involved greater reciprocity and engagement and less neglect). Furthermore, one's own attachment security, partner's attachment security, and partner's provision of beneficial care all contributed to the prediction of relationship satisfaction.

Partners' Responses to Stressful Situations in the Laboratory

In a very different approach to the study of attachment and caregiving, Simpson, Rholes, and Nelligan (1992) had dating couples come to the laboratory and told the female member of each couple that she would soon experience a set of stressful experimental procedures. Observers then rated the extent to which females turned to their partners for comfort and support and the extent to which their partners' behavior was caring and supportive. The central finding of this study was that support seeking and support giving were jointly influenced by attachment security and by coders' assessments of females' anxiety. Specifically, when females seemed very anxious about the situation, female avoidance was associated with physical and emotional retreat from partners, and male avoidance was associated with low levels of support giving. In other words, more avoidant individuals tended to behave in a rather cold and distant manner, but only under higher levels of stress. More recently, Collins and Feeney (2000) observed couples as they discussed a personal concern nominated by one partner. Their results indicated that more avoidant support seekers used indirect (potentially ineffective) means, such as hinting, to show negative affect; further, caregivers who were anxious about their relationships provided lower levels of support.

Spousal Caregiving

In contrast to these studies, the study described next (Feeney & Hohaus, 2001) focused on very challenging situations involving spousal care. Caring for a disabled or distressed spouse may be an inherent part of the marriage contract, but spouses vary in their willingness to care and their ability to respond appropriately to the partner's needs. Our study had two phases. First, spouses gave semistructured accounts of times in their marriages when they had *most* needed to give their partners extra care and support. Second, they completed questionnaires tapping attachment, caregiving style, strength of attachment to spouse, anticipated caregiving burden, and willingness to provide spousal care in the future.

When asked about the time they had most needed to give extra care, spouses identified a range of stressful situations, including spouse's illness, loss of employment and other work stress, death in the family, and severe financial difficulties. Content coding focused on experiences of caregiving (type of care given, caregiver's coping strategies), current evaluations of caregiving (perceived effects on the relationship, feelings about one's own caregiving), and emotional tone of the accounts (negative in tone or accepting of the dependent spouse's needs and feelings).

As shown in Table 11.3, these variables were related to spouses' attachment dimensions. For example, husbands high in discomfort used less support seeking as caregivers and were less likely to be given "complete" care (tangible *and* emotional) as care receivers. Anxious wives used less problem-focused coping and more escape/avoidance as caregivers, and were also less likely to receive "complete" care. Insecurity in self or partner was associated with caregivers' reports of negative effects on the couple relationship and of dissatisfaction with their caregiving efforts. Finally, insecurity (especially relationship anxiety) in self or partner was linked to caregivers' use of negative tone, as reflected in such comments as "he never stopped moaning—what a tragedy queen!" and "She was tedious—bursting into tears for no reason." This important finding shows that insecurity is manifest not only in subjective reports of stressful events but also in judges' ratings of the *tone* of discourse. It seems likely that the negative tone adopted by anxious spouses is played out in actual caregiving interactions, where it may foster hostility and damage the relationship.

The questionnaire phase of this study tested a theoretical model of willingness to provide spousal care in the future. This issue is timely, given the increasing proportion of seniors in Western societies and the limited resources available from public sector and community sources.

TABLE 11.3. Summary of Significant Attachment Effects for Reports of Spousal Caregiving

Dependent variable	Attachment-related effects
Type of care given: practical, emotional, or both	
Husbands giving complete care	Low wife anxiety
Wives giving complete care	Low husband discomfort
Caregivers' coping strategies (coded yes/no)	
Husbands using support seeking	Low husband discomfort
Wives using problem-focused coping	Low wife anxiety
Wives using escape/avoidance	High wife anxiety
Effect on relationship: closer, no effect, or problems	
Husbands reporting increased closeness	Low husband discomfort
Husbands reporting relationship problems	High wife anxiety
Wives reporting increased closeness	Low wife discomfort
Wives reporting relationship problems	High husband anxiety
Caregivers' feelings about care: positive, mixed, or negative	
Wives reporting negative feelings	High wife discomfort
	High husband anxiety
Emotional tone of accounts (negative or not)	
Husbands using negative tone	High husband anxiety
	High wife anxiety
Wives using negative tone	High wife anxiety
	High wife discomfort

Note. "Discomfort" refers to discomfort with closeness; "anxiety" refers to relationship anxiety.

Willingness to care for a dependent spouse was assessed by asking participants to consider a range of disabling conditions and to rate the extent to which they would be willing to care for the spouse should each condition arise. A complete discussion of the results is beyond the scope of this chapter, but for both genders, willingness to provide care was related negatively to own and partner's discomfort and anxiety. These effects generally involved complex paths through caregiving style, strength of attachment, and anticipated burden. The attachment dimension with the most predictive power was discomfort with closeness, especially in predicting wives' willingness to care: The negative association between wives' discomfort and willingness to care involved a direct effect, plus indirect effects through less responsive caregiving, lower attachment strength, and greater anticipated burden.

Overall, findings from this study suggest that the caregiving process is affected by the attachment concerns of both caregiver and care receiver. Caregivers who are uncomfortable with closeness are less responsive to the spouse's needs; those who are anxious tend to feel unappreciated and may have difficulty in setting aside their own needs and concerns. In addition, it seems that the negative attitudes and behaviors of wives high in anxiety and husbands high in discomfort result in their *receiving* less adequate care. Other recent findings from studies of challenging situations support the relevance of both partners' attachment characteristics. For example, in a reanalysis of data from the study by Simpson and colleagues (1992), Campbell, Simpson, Kashy, and Rholes (2001) found that ambivalent (anxious) men and women were rated as hostile and critical; avoidant people (especially avoidant men who reported little dependence on the current partner) both displayed *and* elicited negative behaviors, such as criticism and irritation.

Transition to Parenthood

The transition to parenthood is one of the most precipitous changes that most couples face, and it has implications for the behavioral systems of attachment, caregiving, and sexuality. The marital bond has to accommodate a new and highly dependent family member, additional family tasks are created, and parents have to deal with a range of lifestyle changes and physical and emotional demands. These stresses are likely to prove particularly difficult for insecure individuals, who have less confidence in their own resources and in the couple bond. In a recent study of these issues (Alexander, Feeney, Hohaus, & Noller, 2001; Feeney, Alexander, Noller, & Hohaus, 2003), we recruited married couples who were expecting their first child, together with a comparison sample of childless couples. Couples completed a set of questionnaires on three occasions (for transition couples, the assessments occurred during pregnancy and at 6 weeks and 6 months postbirth) and were interviewed on the first two of these occasions. This report focuses on two aspects of the study: coping strategies (transition group only) and depression (both groups).

Coping with Parenthood

Based on questionnaire reports completed when the babies were about 6 weeks old, each spouse received scores on the major coping strategies of problem-focused coping, emotion-focused coping, and support seeking. This discussion is restricted to emotion-focused coping, which yielded the strongest links with attachment dimensions.

For both genders, higher initial levels of relationship anxiety predicted more emotion-focused coping, although the nature of the effects was gender specific. Husbands' anxiety increased their emotion-focused coping through perceptions of low self-esteem (an internal coping resource) and high parenting strain. Wives' anxiety increased their emotion-focused coping directly, an effect which may reflect overlearned tendencics to monitor situations for negative cues and to focus on distress. However, anxiety also had a weak *negative* effect on wives' emotion-focused coping, through perceptions of less availability of support from family and friends. This paradoxical result may reflect the pressing demands of parenthood: If mothers who are anxious about relationships see little possibility of support from others, they may feel compelled to set aside their own concerns and address the tasks at hand. As with the findings for hurt feelings, these findings illustrate the complex effects of insecurity.

Depression

In this study, we assessed a wide range of variables that may predict wives' depression (measured at time 2). Using the initial questionnaire reports of husbands and wives, we assessed the role of four broad variables: adjustment difficulties (depression and general anxiety), perceived levels of support available from family and friends, marital satisfaction, and attachment security. For the transition group, we also investigated the role of experiences of pregnancy and birth, assessed during the interviews (e.g., reactions to learning of the pregnancy, difficulty of labor).

Of these sets of variables, only the attachment dimensions predicted depression among new mothers. Specifically, wives who were more anxious about relationships at the start of the study reported more depression postbirth. Interestingly, this effect was not reduced when we controlled for initial scores on depression, general anxiety, and marital satisfaction—these results suggest that the link between relationship anxiety and depression is probably causal, rather than simply reflecting overlap among such constructs as insecurity, adjustment problems, and relationship distress. In contrast, in the comparison group, wives' depression at time 2 was predicted strongly by earlier depression, with no additional effect of earlier attachment security. Hence, it seems that in the relatively stressful context of new parenthood, relationship anxiety may predispose women to postbirth depression by raising issues about the partner's commitment and the future of the couple bond. The scope of this problem is highlighted by the finding that wives' postbirth depression predicted subsequent decreases in husbands' marital satisfaction and increases in wives' discomfort with closeness and husbands' relationship anxiety. The latter results fit with attachment theorists' claim that attachment security (and associated models of self and others) can be modified by powerful relationship events (e.g., Shaver, Collins, & Clark, 1996).

In summary, our analyses of coping strategies and depression point to the negative effects of relationship anxiety on adjustment to new parenthood. Another recent study of this topic (Rholes, Simpson, Campbell, & Grich, 2001) supports this conclusion. In this longitudinal study, highly ambivalent (anxious) women reported declines in spousal support and marital satisfaction across the transition period, particularly if they perceived their husbands as providing insufficient support.

GENERAL DISCUSSION AND CONCLUSIONS

Attachment theory offers a useful perspective on relationship functioning under stressful conditions: It helps explain the origins of constructive and destructive responses to stress and generates testable predictions about the strength of attachment-related differences under varying degrees of stress. The studies discussed in this chapter support the view that stress activates the attachment system. Links between attachment security and conflict behavior are stronger when conflict threatens the relationship; this finding suggests that such conflict activates individuals' internal working models. There is also evidence that relationship anxiety is more likely to trigger depression in the (stressful) context of new parenthood and that the tendency for avoidance to predict physical and emotional withdrawal increases under stress. More direct evidence that stressors activate the attachment system is provided by priming studies that focus on responses to threat words (e.g., Mikulincer et al., 2002).

Although research suggests that insecure people are generally more threatened by challenging and conflictual situations, responses to stress often relate differentially to the two major attachment dimensions in ways consistent with theoretical discussions of attachment-related goals and needs. Discomfort with closeness is linked to less support seeking and support giving, both within the couple relationship and in the broader social network. Discomfort also predicts communication difficulties, especially in terms of disclosing personal thoughts and feelings, responding to partners' needs, and adopting reconciliatory approaches to conflict. Relationship anxiety, on the other hand, predicts extreme distress in response to relational stressors, reliance on emotion-focused coping (which may prove ineffective in dealing with these stressors), coercive responses to conflict, and the tendency to minimize or belittle partners' needs.

It is also worth noting the apparent gender differences in the implications of attachment dimensions for responses to stress. Generally speaking, males' discomfort with closeness and females' relationship anxiety seem to be the most consistent predictors of maladaptive responses to stress. For example, males' discomfort with closeness has been related to lack of support seeking and to perceptions of less involvement and mutual negotiation in conflict situations; females' relationship anxiety has been linked to high levels of conflict and coercion and to maladaptive coping behavior. Other researchers have noted the negative effects of males' discomfort with intimacy and females' relationship anxiety, proposing explanations that focus on the effects of sex-role stereotypes about intimacy and dependence (e.g., Kirkpatrick & Davis, 1994). For instance, males who are uncomfortable with intimacy may make less active efforts to maintain relationships with absent partners, especially given that males are not usually seen as the maintainers of relationships. Moreover, females who worry a lot about their relationships may respond to separation with anxiety and jealousy, fueling relationship problems.

Overall, then, the studies reported in this chapter point to attachment-related differences in perceptions of stressful events and in coping behavior. Similarly, based on studies of such diverse stressors as personal failure and war-related events, Mikulincer and Florian (1998) concluded that security is a resource that actively facilitates adjustment: Secure individuals appraise the world in relatively positive ways, have a sense of mastery that nevertheless admits faults and failure, and are open to acquiring new skills and information. Despite the use of a range of research methods and designs, we are still some way from fully understanding how the attachment characteristics of men and women shape their responses to different stressors. Further, the study of stressful events confronts researchers with important practical and ethical issues: Can stress be manipulated in appropriate ways in laboratory contexts? How can we access couples facing important real-life stressors without adding to the demands they face? Given these difficult issues, researchers will need to continue their creative approaches to this area of study.

REFERENCES

Ainsworth, M. D. S., Blehar, M. C., Waters, E., & Wall, S. (1978). *Patterns of attachment: A study of the Strange Situation.* Hillsdale, NJ: Erlbaum.

Alexander, R. P., Feeney, J. A., Hohaus, L., & Noller, P. (2001). Attachment style and coping resources as predictors of coping strategies in the transition to parenthood. *Personal Relationships, 8,* 137–152.

Bartholomew, K. (1990). Avoidance of intimacy: An attachment perspective. *Journal of Social and Personal Relationships, 7,* 147–178.

Bartholomew, K., Cobb, R. J., & Poole, J. A. (1997). Adult attachment patterns and social support processes. In G. R. Pierce, B. Lakey, I. G. Sarason, & B. R. Sarason (Eds.), *Sourcebook of social support and personality* (pp. 359–378). New York: Plenum Press.

Baxter, L. A., & Montgomery, B. M. (1997). Rethinking communication in personal relationships from a dialectical perspective. In S. Duck (Ed.), *Handbook of personal relationships* (pp. 325–349). New York: Wiley.

Bowlby, J. (1984). *Attachment and loss: Vol. 1. Attachment* (2nd ed.). Harmondsworth, UK: Penguin.

Byng-Hall, J. (1999). Family and couple therapy: Toward greater security. In J. Cassidy & P. R. Shaver (Eds.), *Handbook of attachment: Theory, research, and clinical applications* (pp. 625–645). New York: Guilford Press.

Cafferty, T. P., Davis, K. E., Medway, F. J., O'Hearn, R. E., & Chappell, K. D. (1994). Reunion dynamics among couples separated during Operation Desert Storm: An attachment theory analysis. In K. Bartholomew & D. Perlman (Eds.), *Advances in personal relationships: Vol. 5. Attachment processes in adulthood* (pp. 309–330). London: Kingsley.

Campbell, L., Simpson, J. A., Kashy, D. A., & Rholes, W. S. (2001). Attachment orientations, dependence, and behavior in a stressful situation: An application of the Actor–Partner Interdependence model. *Journal of Social and Personal Relationships, 18,* 821–843.

Carnelley, K. B., Pietromonaco, P. R., & Jaffe, K. (1996). Attachment, caregiving, and relationship functioning in couples: Effects of self and partner. *Personal Relationships, 3,* 257–278.

Christensen, A., & Walczynski, P. T. (1997). Conflict and satisfaction in couples. In R. J. Sternberg & M. Hojjat (Eds.), *Satisfaction in close relationships* (pp. 249–274). New York: Guilford Press.

Collins, N. L. (1996). Working models of attachment: Implications for explanation, emotion, and behavior. *Journal of Personality and Social Psychology, 71,* 810–832.

Collins, N. L., & Feeney, B. C. (2000). A safe haven: An attachment theory perspective on support seeking and caregiving in intimate relationships. *Journal of Personality and Social Psychology, 78,* 1053–1073.

Feeney, J. A. (1994). Attachment style, communication patterns and satisfaction across the life cycle of marriage. *Personal Relationships, 1,* 333–348.

Feeney, J. A. (1998). Adult attachment and relationship-centered anxiety: Responses to physical and emotional distancing. In J. A. Simpson & W. S. Rholes (Eds.), *Attachment theory and close relationships* (pp. 189–218). New York: Guilford Press.

Feeney, J. A. (1999a). Adult attachment, emotional control and marital satisfaction. *Personal Relationships, 6,* 169–185.

Feeney, J. A. (1999b). Issues of closeness and distance in dating relationships: Effects of sex and attachment style. *Journal of Social and Personal Relationships, 16,* 571–590.

Feeney, J. A. (2002). Attachment, marital interaction and relationship satisfaction: A diary study. *Personal Relationships, 9,* 39–55.

Feeney, J. A. (in press). Hurt feelings in couple relationships: Towards integrative models of the negative effects of hurtful events. *Journal of Social and Personal Relationships.*

Feeney, J. A., Alexander, R., Noller, P., & Hohaus, L. (2003). Attachment insecurity, depression, and the transition to parenthood. *Personal Relationships, 10,* 475–493.

Feeney, J. A., & Hohaus, L. (2001). Attachment and spousal caregiving. *Personal Relationships, 8,* 21–39.

Feeney, J. A., Noller, P., & Callan, V. J. (1994). Attachment style, communication and satisfaction in the early years of marriage. In K. Bartholomew & D. Perlman (Eds.), *Advances in personal relationships: Vol. 5. Attachment processes in adulthood* (pp. 269–308). London: Kingsley.

Fraley, R. C., & Shaver, P. R. (1997). Adult attachment and the suppression of unwanted thoughts. *Journal of Personality and Social Psychology, 73,* 1080–1091.

Fraley, R. C., & Shaver, P. R. (1998). Airport separations: A naturalistic study of adult attachment dynamics in separating couples. *Journal of Personality and Social Psychology, 75,* 1198–1212.

Gaines, S. O., Jr., Reis, H. T., Summers, S., Rusbult, C. E., Cox, C. L., Wexler, M. O., et al. (1997). Impact of attachment style on reactions to accommodative dilemmas in close relationships. *Personal Relationships, 4,* 93–113.

Gallo, L. C., & Smith, T. W. (2001). Attachment style in marriage: Adjustment and responses to interaction. *Journal of Social and Personal Relationships, 18,* 263–289.

Hazan, C., & Shaver, P. R. (1987). Romantic love conceptualized as an attachment process. *Journal of Personality and Social Psychology, 52,* 511–524.

Keelan, J. P. R., Dion, K. K., & Dion, K. L. (1998). Attachment style and relationship satisfaction: Test of a self-disclosure explanation. *Canadian Journal of Behavioural Science, 30,* 24–35.

Kirkpatrick, L. A., & Davis, K. E. (1994). Attachment style, gender, and relationship stability: A longitudinal analysis. *Journal of Personality and Social Psychology, 66,* 502–512.

Kobak, R. R., & Duemmler, S. (1994). Attachment and conversation: Toward a discourse analysis of adolescent and adult security. In K. Bartholomew & D. Perlman (Eds.), *Advances in personal relationships: Vol. 5. Attachment processes in adulthood* (pp. 121–149). London: Kingsley.

Kobak, R. R., & Hazan, C. (1991). Attachment in marriage: Effects of security and accuracy of working models. *Journal of Personality and Social Psychology, 60,* 861–869.

Kobak, R. R., & Sceery, A. (1988). Attachment in late adolescence: Working models, affect regulation, and representations of self and others. *Child Development, 59,* 135–146.

Kunce, L. J., & Shaver, P. R. (1994). An attachment-theoretical approach to caregiving in romantic relationships. In K. Bartholomew & D. Perlman (Eds.), *Advances in personal relationships: Vol. 5. Attachment processes in adulthood* (pp. 205–237). London: Kingsley.

Leary, M. R., Springer, C., Negel, L., Ansell, E., & Evans, K. (1998). The causes, phenomenology, and consequences of hurt feelings. *Journal of Personality and Social Psychology, 74,* 1225–1237.

Mikulincer, M. (1998). Adult attachment style and individual differences in functional versus dysfunctional experiences of anger. *Journal of Personality and Social Psychology, 74,* 513–524.

Mikulincer, M., & Florian, V. (1998). The relationship between adult attachment styles and emotional and cognitive reactions to stressful events. In J. A. Simpson & W. S. Rholes (Eds.), *Attachment theory and close relationships* (pp. 143–165). New York: Guilford Press.

Mikulincer, M., Florian, V., Birnbaum, G., & Malishkewitz, S. (2002). The death-anxiety buffer function of close relationships: Exploring the effects of separation reminders on death-thought accessibility. *Personality and Social Psychology Bulletin, 28,* 287–299.

Pistole, M. C. (1989). Attachment in adult romantic relationships: Style of conflict resolution and relationship satisfaction. *Journal of Social and Personal Relationships, 6,* 505–510.

Pistole, M. C. (1994). Adult attachment styles: Some thoughts on closeness–distance struggles. *Family Process, 33,* 147–159.

Rahim, M. A. (1983). A measure of styles of handling interpersonal conflict. *Academy of Management Journal, 26,* 368–376.

Roberts, N., & Noller, P. (1998). The associations between adult attachment and couple violence: The role of communication patterns and relationship satisfaction. In J. A. Simpson & W. S. Rholes (Eds.), *Attachment theory and close relationships* (pp. 317–350). New York: Guilford Press.

Rholes, W. S., Simpson, J. A., Campbell, L., & Grich, J. (2001). Adult attachment and the transition to parenthood. *Journal of Personality and Social Psychology, 81,* 421–435.

Shaver, P. R., Collins, N., & Clark, C. L. (1996). Attachment styles and internal working models of self and relationship partners. In G. J. O. Fletcher & J. Fitness (Eds.), *Knowledge structures in close relationships: A social psychological approach* (pp. 25–61). Mahwah: NJ: Erlbaum.

Shaver, P. R., Hazan, C., & Bradshaw, D. (1988). Love as attachment: The integration of three behavioral systems. In R. J. Sternberg & M. L. Barnes (Eds.), *The psychology of love* (pp. 68–99). New Haven, CT: Yale University Press.

Shaver, P., Schwartz, J., Kirson, D., & O'Connor, C. (1987). Emotion knowledge: Further exploration of a prototype approach. *Journal of Personality and Social Psychology, 52,* 1061–1086.

Simpson, J. A., Rholes, W. S., & Nelligan, J. S. (1992). Support seeking and support giving within couples in an anxiety-provoking situation: The role of attachment styles. *Journal of Personality and Social Psychology, 62,* 434–446.

Simpson, J. A., Rholes, W. S., & Phillips, D. (1996). Conflict in close relationships: An attachment perspective. *Journal of Personality and Social Psychology, 71,* 899–914.

Sroufe, L. A., & Waters, E. (1977). Attachment as an organizational construct. *Child Development, 48,* 1184–1199.

Sumer, N. (2000, June). *The interplay between attachment mental models and interpersonal schemas among married couples.* Paper presented at 2nd Joint Conference of International Society for the Study of Personal Relationships and International Network of Personal Relationships, Brisbane, Australia.

Vormbrock, J. K. (1993). Attachment theory as applied to wartime and job-related marital separation. *Psychological Bulletin, 114,* 122–144.

PART V

CLINICAL AND APPLIED ISSUES

Therapy, Psychopathology, and Well-Being

CHAPTER 12

Attachment Theory

A Guide for Healing Couple Relationships

SUSAN M. JOHNSON

Until very recently, couple and family therapists intervened in the multidimensional, complex drama of distressed family relationships without the benefit of a cogent theory of family relatedness and nurturance or a theory of adult love (Mackay, 1996; Roberts, 1992). The field has relied on conceptualizations of dysfunction, such as the idea that dysfunction arises from a lack of boundaries and "enmeshment," or from a lack of communication skills, or from an unconscious compulsion to reenact past relationships with parents. In addressing distressed adult relationships, in particular, therapists have had no coherent, integrative, research-supported map to rely on when formulating problems, delineating treatment goals, or focusing moment-to-moment change processes in therapy sessions. One potential resource has been exchange theory. This theory focuses on the cognitive evaluation of profit and loss in a relationship and how this evaluation affects satisfaction. This perspective centers the therapy process on helping partners to negotiate more skillfully. However, it does not take into account the powerful emotions at play in close relationships and seems, focusing as it does on concepts such as cost and profit, to be more appropriate for business relationships than intimate bonds.

I believe that, for the first time in the history of couple and family therapy, attachment theory offers a rich theoretical map (Johnson, 2003a; Johnson & Whiffen, 1999) that provides a broad explanatory perspective on close relationships and has enough depth and specificity to guide the process of healing those relationships (Johnson & Whiffen, 2003). This chapter focuses on attachment theory as a basis for effective interventions for relationship distress in adult partnerships and for healing particularly problematic injuries in such partnerships. At present, the emotionally focused model of couple therapy (EFT; Greenberg & Johnson, 1988; Johnson, 1996) is the approach that most directly relies on attachment theory to understand and repair close relationships (Johnson, 1986, 2003b).

The EFT model is also one of the few empirically supported couple interventions (Johnson, Hunsley, Greenberg, & Schindler, 1999), and it demonstrates the most positive treatment outcomes in terms of significant improvement (90% in the most rigorous studies) and rates of recovery (70–73% in the most rigorous studies) and also shows evidence of stability of results across time even with at-risk populations (Clothier, Manion, Gordon Walker, & Johnson, 2002; Johnson, 2002). The studies on EFT have been relatively rigorous. For example, they have used control groups, monitored the implementation of interventions, and recorded dropout rates, which are generally low. Treatment is brief; studies have used 10 to 12 sessions. However, it is important to note that therapists in studies usually have expert training and ongoing clinical supervision. In everyday clinical practice, 15–20 sessions is more common. Research on predictors of success in therapy and the process of change has also been conducted. The best predictors of success seem to be the task element of the therapeutic alliance—that is, how relevant partners perceive the tasks set out by the therapist to be—and the female client's belief that her partner still cares for her. Engagement in therapy appears to be more important than initial distress level in terms of predicting success. Research on the process of change has found that the completion of key change events in therapy leads to recovery from relationship distress and that specific therapist interventions, such as the heightening of attachment-oriented emotions, predicts this completion (Bradley & Furrow, in press; Johnson & Greenberg, 1988). A recent article also reviews the field of couple therapy and places EFT in the context of other interventions (Johnson, 2003c).

It is perhaps worth noting, right from the beginning, one of the key reasons that attachment theory appears to be so suited as a guide to clinical intervention in couple and family therapy. Attachment is a systemic theory (Erdman & Caffery, 2002; Johnson & Best, 2002). It integrates a focus on how interactions with significant others construct models of self and other and default modes of affect regulation with a focus on how these models and modes then affect habitual ways of engaging others. Bowlby described his theory as a control systems theory and focused on feedback loops and homeostatic or self-regulatory patterns of interaction (Bowlby, 1969). He viewed these patterns as being linked to and organized by inner states of security or anxiety. Both traditional systems and attachment theories view dysfunction in terms of loss of flexibility and rigid, constricted ways of processing information and responding. Both are essentially nonpathologizing. Bowlby (1979), for example, views negative models of attachment that define others as untrustworthy and the self as unlovable as "perfectly reasonable constructions" (p. 23). He stresses that both are adaptive in particular contexts. Attachment theory, systemic as it is, does what a couple therapist needs a guiding theory to do: It links dancer and dance, self and system, into a "holistic evolving picture" (Johnson & Best, 2002, p. 168; see also Johnson, 2003b).

Attachment theory informs the couple therapist of the critical organizing or "leading elements" (Bertalanffy, 1968) and defining events in a close relationship. It then offers therapists specific goals, tasks, and pathways to significant change. These critical or leading elements consist of the following:

- Powerful attachment-oriented emotions, such as fear and rage.
- Habitual ways of regulating these emotions and engaging with one's partner in repeating self-reinforcing patterns of interaction.
- Expectations or cognitive models that arise from these interactions.

This attachment perspective is consonant with recent research into the nature of marital distress (Gottman, Coan, Carrere, & Swanson, 1998; Pasch & Bradbury, 1998), which stresses the power of emotional engagement and responsiveness to define the quality of close relationships and the negative impact of patterns such as demand–withdraw that limit responsiveness. Recent research also stresses the importance of reaching for and offering soothing and comfort as a predictor of positive relatedness. This parallels Bowlby's (1969) observation that mutual accessibility and emotional responsiveness are the key features of a secure bond. Attachment theory also fits with the experience of distressed partners and with how they express that experience. For example, critical, angry wives, when given hope and safety, will very often disclose desperation and loss in the face of their partners' unavailability and unresponsiveness, whereas their more defended, distancing partners describe how they shut down to protect the relationship and prevent fights, all the while tortured by fears of inadequacy and loss. Change events in EFT such as "softenings," in which a previously hostile spouse risks asking for contact and comfort, are also obvious examples of bonding events and are associated with dramatic changes in relationship definition (Johnson & Greenberg, 1988). The unusually low dropout rate in EFT also indcates how powerfully an attachment framework speaks to clients and makes sense of their experience.

On a more general level, a sizable body of research on the relevance of this theory to the quality of adult relationships now exists (Cassidy & Shaver, 1999; Shaver & Hazan, 1993). A more secure attachment style has been found to predict such positive aspects of relationship functioning as greater interdependence, commitment, trust, and satisfaction in couples (e.g., Kirkpatrick & Davis, 1994; Simpson, 1990); higher levels of support seeking and providing (Simpson, Rholes, & Nelligan, 1992); greater intimacy and less withdrawal and verbal aggression (Senchak & Leonard, 1992); more sensitive and appropriate caregiving behaviors (Kunce & Shaver, 1994); and less jealousy (Hazan & Shaver, 1987). A secure style also appears to promote a more complex, articulated, positive, and coherent sense of self (Mikulincer, 1995). This last finding supports Bowlby's belief that an autonomous sense of self is positively associated with a secure sense of connectedness and the ability to depend on attachment figures, rather than being in opposition to it. Both Bowlby (1988) and feminist writers (Jordan, Kaplan, Miller, Stiver, & Surrey, 1991) have noted the pathologization of dependency in Western cultures. This kind of finding also offers an explanatory framework as to why attachment-oriented interventions such as EFT seem to affect "intrapsychic" problems such as depression and posttraumatic stress disorder (Dessaulles, Johnson, & Denton, 2003; Johnson, 2002).

It is important to note that a couple therapist deals with each partner's general orientation to attachment; for example, a partner might say, "I don't trust my husband very much, but then I have never trusted anyone very much. I have never really thought of asking for comfort from anyone." For this kind of client, secure attachment is foreign territory, and she will need more support as she begins to deal with attachment needs and fears. However, the goal of therapy is to repair a specific attachment relationship, so the focus is on each partner's relationship-specific attachment "style" or strategy and how the general dimensions of insecurity, namely anxiety and avoidance, play out and are confirmed in a specific couple's relationship. The couple therapist is more likely to focus on a partner's habitual forms of engagement with his or her spouse rather than on the partner's general attachment style—that is, on emotional and behavioral regulation rather than on general abstract models of self and other (Fraley & Shaver, 2000). Collins and Allard (2001) suggest that, because working models are complex and because most people have more than one model of attachment, the word "style" be reserved for models that are general, abstract, and chronic. However, when summarizing recent studies of how interactions are evaluated by romantic partners, they also stress that generally insecure models negatively bias perceptions of a partner's behavior, regardless of the quality of their current relationship. In clinical experience using EFT with survivors of childhood abuse and their partners, it is clear that the chronic negative attachment style of these survivors often requires a longer therapy process and many repetitions of positive bonding events to shape a more secure attachment bond, even with relatively responsive partners (Johnson, 2002).

It is a question for future research whether a corrective, security-enhancing experience that changes attachment responses and working models in a specific relationship will, over time, also change general models of attachment toward security. There is evidence that one's own or a partner's responses in key life transitions in which attachment needs come to the fore, such as the transition to parenthood, can shift an individual's attachment style. Disconfirming experiences, in therapy or in everyday life, have the potential to change a person's general attachment style (Simpson, Rholes, Campbell, & Wilson, 2003).

WHAT DOES ATTACHMENT THEORY TEACH THE COUPLE THERAPIST?

1. According to attachment theory, seeking and maintaining contact with significant others is an innate, primary motivating principle in human beings across the lifespan. Dependency is seen as an innate part of being human rather than as a childhood trait that we outgrow. According to attachment theory, there are no such things as complete independence from others or overdependence (Bretherton & Munholland, 1999). There is only effective or ineffective dependence. Secure dependence fosters autonomy and self-confidence. Health means maintaining a felt sense of interdependence, rather than being self-sufficient and separate from others. An EFT therapist will validate people's need for secure connection and respect the power of the emotions associated with this innate need, the fear of rejection and abandonment, the rage of desperation, the sadness of loss, and the shame that accompanies the fear of being unworthy of love and care.

2. Secure attachment offers a safe haven and a secure base. The *safe haven* that contact with attachment figures offers is an innate survival mechanism. The presence of an attachment figure, which usually means parents, children, spouses, and lovers, provides comfort and security and buffers against stress and uncertainty, whereas the perceived inaccessibility of such figures creates distress (Mikulincer, Florian, & Weller, 1993). Proximity to a loved one normatively tranquilizes the nervous system (Schore, 1994) and provides a natural antidote to anxiety and vulnerability. Secure attachment also provides a *secure base* from which individuals can explore their universe and learn to reflect on themselves, their behavior, and their mental states (Fonagy & Target, 1997; Mikulincer, 1997). It promotes the confidence necessary to risk, to learn, and to continually update models of self, others, and the world so that adjustment to new contexts is facilitated.

These concepts encourage the couple therapist to focus on fostering safety in the therapy session and on the gradual shaping of a felt sense of safe connection between partners. A sense of connection with a loved one is a primary built-in emotional regulation device. Bowlby believed that isolation and loss of connection is inherently traumatizing. He stated that when someone is confident that a loved one will be there when needed, "a person will be much less prone to either intense or chronic fear than will an individual who has no such confidence" (1973, p. 406). Attachment to key others is then our "primary protection against feelings of helplessness and meaninglessness" (McFarlane & van der Kolk, 1996). Attachment theory thus also helps the therapist understand how lack of safety and fears that attachment figures will be unresponsive narrow down distressed partners' responses and prevent the use of skills and insights that are often accessible to them in other relationships. It also helps us grasp and articulate relationship-defining attachment injuries in close relationships (Johnson, Makinen, & Millikin, 2001). These are situations in which partners fail to provide a safe haven and secure base at times of urgent need.

3. According to attachment theory, the building blocks of secure bonds are emotional accessibility and responsiveness. Separation distress results from the appraisal that an attachment figure is inaccessible. If there is no engagement, no emotional responsiveness, the message from the attachment figure reads as, "Your signals do not matter, and there is no connection between us." Emotion is central to attachment, and this theory provides a guide for understanding and normalizing many of the extreme emotions that accompany distressed relationships. It is worth noting that in many research studies relationship distress is associated with a pattern in which one spouse displays emotion to which the other spouse does not respond (Johnson & Bradbury, 1999). Emotions tell us and communicate to others what our motivations and needs are; they are the music of the attachment dance (Johnson, 1996). As Bowlby suggests, "the psychology and psychopathology of emotion is . . . in large part the psychology and psychopathology of affectional bonds" (1979, p. 130). This perspective not only focuses the therapist on emotions and how they are processed and communicated but also helps the therapist to evoke and shape emotions, such as the longing for reassurance to cue new interactional responses and to help couples take new risks with each other. New corrective emotional experiences of mutual accessibility and responsiveness are then also seen as necessary to significantly change the nature of a specific attachment bond. Attachment theory can also help the therapist understand a partner's general model of attachment relationships and extreme responses infused with attachment emotions, such as compulsive sexuality and extreme sexual demands of the spouse. Hazan and Zeifman (1994) suggest that sex is a key way of expressing attachment needs in adult relationships.

4. The process of separation distress is predictable and offers a framework that makes sense of research findings on marital distress—for example, the findings that a cycle of angry accusation and emotional demands followed by defensive distance from the other partner is an extremely accurate predictor of divorce (Gottman, 1994). Attachment theory states that if behavior that seeks comfort from an attachment figure

fails to evoke a comforting response, a prototypical process of angry protest, clinging, depression, and despair occurs, culminating eventually in detachment. Depression is a natural response to loss of connection. Bowlby viewed the expression of anger in close relationships as often being an attempt to make contact with an inaccessible attachment figure. He distinguished between the anger of hope and the anger of despair, which becomes desperate and coercive. In secure relationships, protest at inaccessibility is recognized and accepted (Holmes, 1996). Using attachment theory as a guide, a therapist can understand the plotline underlying the drama of distress and so understands what is necessary to change that plotline.

5. Attachment theory tells us that the number of ways human beings have to deal with the unresponsiveness of attachment figures, and so the stances partners can take in the drama of relationship distress, is limited. There are only so many ways of coping with a negative response to the question, "Can I depend on you when I need you?" Attachment responses seem to be organized along two dimensions, anxiety and avoidance (Fraley & Waller, 1998). When the need for connection is frustrated, the attachment system may become hyperactivated or go into overdrive. Attachment behaviors become heightened and intense as anxious clinging, pursuit, and even aggressive attempts to obtain a response from the loved one escalate. Alternately, the second strategy, especially when hope for responsiveness has been lost, is to deactivate the attachment system and suppress attachment needs by focusing on tasks and avoiding distressing attempts at emotional engagement with attachment figures. These two basic strategies, anxious–preoccupied clinging and detached avoidance, can develop into habitual styles of engagement with intimate others.

A third insecure strategy has also been identified. This is essentially a combination of seeking closeness and then fearfully avoiding closeness when it is offered. This strategy is usually referred to as "disorganized" in the child literature and "fearful–avoidant" in the adult literature (Bartholomew & Horowitz, 1991). It is associated with chaotic and traumatic attachment relationships in which others are, at one time, the source of and solution to fear (Alexander, 1993; Johnson, 2002).

These three strategies are "self maintaining patterns of social interaction and emotion regulation strategies" (Shaver & Clarke, 1994, p. 119), but they will also play out differently depending on the attachment characteristics of a particular partner and the way in which the strategies affect satisfaction in a specific relationship. Individuals whose partners characteristically use one of the three insecure strategies mentioned before report lower satisfaction. Couples in which neither partner relies on an insecure strategy report better adjustment than couples in which either or both partners use insecure strategies (Feeney, 1994; Lussier, Sabourin, & Turgeon, 1997).

Knowledge of attachment strategies and how they play out focuses the change process in couple therapy. In key change events in EFT (Johnson 1996), the therapist actively helps avoidant spouses to reengage and deal with the attachment insecurities that block emotional engagement. The therapist also helps anxious spouses deal with their anxiety in a way that leads to the clear communication of needs in a manner that pulls the other spouse toward them and facilitates responsiveness. In general, attachment theory helps the EFT therapist adapt interventions to individual differences—to the strategies (or attachment style) of each partner (Johnson & Whiffen, 1999). Anxious partners are helped in every session to differentiate their emotions and articulate the attachment vulnerabilities and needs underlying their angry criticism of their partners. The therapist has to support avoidant partners in staying in contact with and developing their emotions, so that they can access attachment needs and fears and block exits into rationalizations and instrumental issues. Fearful–avoidant partners have to be particularly encouraged to ask for comfort in the face of their belief that they are not entitled to or worthy of such caring.

6. Attachment involves representational models of self and others. These models of self and others, distilled out of thousands of interactions, become expectations and biases that are carried forward into present interactions and new relationships. They are not one-dimensional cognitive schemas. They are procedural scripts for how to create relatedness. A person may have more than one model, but one will usually be more accessible and dominant in a given context. These models involve goals, beliefs, and strategies, and they are heavily infused with emotion. Models arise in couple therapy sessions and often are associated with problems that accompany relationship distress, such as depression. A secure attachment style is characterized by a working model of self that is worthy of love and care and that is confident and competent, and, indeed, research has found secure attachment to be associated with greater self-efficacy (Mikulincer, 1995). Secure people, who believe others will be responsive when needed, also tend to have working models of others as dependable and worthy of trust. The concept of working models helps the therapist to move to the level of key representations of self and others and to focus on shifting these representations if necessary. For example, partners who are filled with shame and believe themselves to be unlovable can, if supported, disclose their fears about themselves in a way that evokes disconfirming responses from the other partner. When key interactions with loved ones change, our sense of who we are can also often begin to change.

The question posed at the beginning of this section is what attachment theory has to teach the couple therapist. It tells the therapist what the goal of an effective couple therapy should be in concrete interactional terms. Attachment strategies were first specifically identified in experimental separations and reunions between mothers and infants (Ainsworth, Blehar, Waters, & Wall, 1978). Some infants were able to modulate their distress on separation because they had confidence in the connection with the mother (they did not expect to be abandoned or rejected). They were then able to give clear, unambiguous signals and so evoke reassuring contact with the mother when she returned. They were able to take in and use this contact to regulate distress; then, confident of the mother's responsiveness if she was needed, they were able to return to exploration and play. These infants were viewed as securely attached. This is also what an emotionally focused therapist is able to see in sessions with partners who are ready to terminate therapy. Adult partners can regulate and express attachment needs and fears, ask for connection in an open manner, offer and receive soothing, and, as a result of better affect regulation and communication about attachment needs, can solve problems more efficiently. In fact, the first study of EFT (Johnson & Greenberg, 1985) showed that those who received EFT were as able to display improved problem-solving as those who had received problem-solving training interventions.

In summary, attachment theory tells the therapist what to target in couple sessions; namely, emotional communication patterns that maintain separation distress and insecurity, such as accusing–distancing. These must be deescalated. Attachment needs and fears must be brought to the fore in a way that fosters the reengagement of distancing partners and the "softening" of attacking partners so that mutual soothing and emotional connection are possible. Insights, communication skill sequences, and new negotiated contracts will not, if the couple is in significant distress, be enough to ensure these relationship-transforming events. Attachment theory directs the therapist to a specific process focus on the ongoing construction of emotion and on attachment needs and attachment anxieties and fears, and it further suggests that these must be addressed in a context of a therapeutic relationship that offers a safe haven and a secure base. In short, attachment theory clarifies the essential nature of the drama of marital distress and offers the therapist a guide as to how to address this distress and help it to heal. A description of key change events in EFT, a therapy that operationalizes the precepts outlined previously, now follows.

SNAPSHOTS OF CHANGE

The EFT process of change moves through three stages: the deescalation of negative interactional cycles (Stage 1), the creation of key bonding events that create more secure attachment (Stage 2), and the consolidation of these changes into the couple's everyday life (Stage 3). What are some of the key points in this change process, as seen through an attachment lens? What does the EFT journey toward a more secure attachment look like?

Toward Deescalation

In Stage 1 of EFT, negative patterns such as attack–withdraw are clarified and deescalated, and the partners begin to see how their cycle of interaction isolates both of them and fuels their attachment hurts and fears. In a couple who had immigrated to Canada a few years previously and in which the man had then become depressed, the wife states, "You were always distant, but now it's like you can pick me up for a moment and then put me down and shut me out. I am alone. Nothing I do makes any difference. I get enraged. I can't do this anymore." First, her spouse denies that there are "real problems" in the relationship and focuses on pragmatic issues such as her stress at work. As the therapist explores his emotional responses, however, he begins to encapsulate his view of the relationship as, "There is no point in talking. If I try, we fight and suddenly the whole house is on fire. I can't do this closeness thing. I'm not good at it—never come up to the mark. So I just try to keep things calm. Then, when I can't, I kind of numb out." The therapist hears themes of isolation and abandonment, helplessness and failure, and sees the familiar cycle of angry protest by the wife and avoidance by the husband. The therapist puts each person's responses in the context of the perceived availability and responsiveness of the other partner. The wife's anger is framed in terms of her fighting to get close to him, and his avoidance is framed as an attempt to calm himself and the relationship down and so preserve it. An attachment frame validates and gives meaning to each partner's feelings and needs. Both partners become clear about the cycle that holds their relationship hostage and come to see this cycle, which constantly confirms their worst fears, as the problem. They then begin to access and share marginalized feelings, such as her grief and fear, which she usually does not show to him, and his longing to be accepted and fear of her rejection. They are able to step aside from and modify their negative cycle and to create more safety and hope between them. The task is now to create positive bonding interactions that provide an antidote to this negative cycle.

Change Event: Withdrawer Reengagement

In Stage 2 of EFT, the therapist helps the more withdrawn spouse articulate his position and its attachment significance. With the therapist's support, this man is able to stay connected with his present emotional experience and articulate his fears and his needs. The key moments in his reengagement are exemplified as follows:

"I just feel that I can never be enough. I feel pathetic—inadequate. Like a whiney wimp. So, I frantically try to turn down the volume between her and me. If I can't, I just give up—I guess I shut down. So then she thinks that I am gone—that I don't care."

"It's bloody scary, that's what it is. Like right now, I can't breathe. [He turns to his wife.] I can't win with you—your words drown me out. It's hopeless—I give up." [He weeps.] The therapist helps him express these feelings directly to his spouse and helps her hear and respond to them. Once he has owned and congruently expressed these emotions and had them accepted by his spouse, he can begin to touch his longings and feel entitled to his partner's caring. He says:

"I want you to give me a break. You must stop evaluating and interrogating me—so I can breathe. I don't want to shut down. I want to feel like you respect me—close and safe like I did in the first years of our relationship."

Change Event: Blamer Softening

In Stage 2, the second change event involves the blaming spouse risking being soft and vulnerable and asking for her attachment needs to be met. As the husband in this couple reengages and reaches for his wife, she first talks about protecting herself. She says, "Well, now you are here, are you? After I've wept and wept and killed myself trying to get you to open up. How do I know you won't just shut me out again?"

As the therapist helps the wife clarify her fear and sense of loss, she says, "I don't know if I can—like—put myself in his hands again. I'll be out there, on a limb then, vulnerable as hell. It's terrifying—it's almost easier to give up and just let him go." The therapist validates her doubts and encourages her to confide in her husband directly and to help him understand her anguish. As she begins to reach for him and finds him responsive, she suddenly becomes cold and bitter. She articulates an attachment injury in which she had "given up" and withdrawn during his depression and he had turned briefly to another woman. As she expresses her grief and rage about this, the therapist helps the husband take responsibility for how he hurt her and elaborate on how this liaison occurred. He then comforts and reassures her, and the therapist helps the couple return to the softening process.

The wife begins to access and give shape to her "desperation" to "pin him down" so she can feel less lost and alone. When the husband continues to be accessible and responsive, she allows herself to express her grief and abandonment. She is able to share how devastated she is by the rift between them and her longings for reassurance. She says quietly, with downcast eyes, "I need him to show me that he really wants this relationship—to set my mind at ease." When the therapist asks her to look at and directly address her husband with these words, she says, "No, I can't. I can't—it's too much." The therapist then asks her husband to help her. He takes her hands and says, "Come and let me hold you. I can do it now. I have let you down—but now I can do it. I want us to be close. I want you to risk it and let me in. We can learn together. [She weeps.] Can I hold you?" She nods and they embrace.

The therapist reflects the process of this session and heightens the attachment significance of each partner's responses. After this session and throughout the consolidation phase of therapy, the communication between the partners is clear and open, and they can soothe and comfort each other. Each can ask for and give support and reassurance. Each expresses a sense of felt security and commitment to the relationship. The couple said that they now saw each other "in a different light." They were able to construct a joint narrative of how the relationship had become distressed and how they had healed it together. They reported that they were now able to deal with the emotions that arose between them in a way that brought them together rather than pushed them apart.

There are times when the process described here becomes derailed in an impasse in which one spouse refuses to trust or risk with the other. This began to happen, in a minor way, in the preceding case, when the wife brought up the husband's affair during the softening process. Attachment theory helps to clarify these impasses and offers a guide to EFT therapists as to how to heal specific relationship traumas or injuries that block the creation of transforming bonding events. Let us now consider the nature and resolution of attachment injuries.

ATTACHMENT INJURIES: IMPASSES IN RESHAPING ATTACHMENT

There is a growing body of work on forgiveness in the literature on intimate relationships (Enright & Fitzgibbons, 2000; Worthington & DiBlasio, 1990), but there is also little understanding in the literature of the specific nature of the kinds of negative events that call for forgiveness or the process of interpersonal forgiveness that allows for the restoration of trust and closeness. This area offers an excellent example of how attachment theory can make sense of specific relationship-defining events and patterns and so guide the process of intervention. Attachment injuries can be defined as relationship traumas (Johnson, 2002; Johnson et al., 2001) of abandonment and betrayal at key moments of need which, if unable to be healed, block relationship renewal and the restoration of trust. Injured partners describe how these injuries are easily evoked in the manner of traumatic flashbacks and how they become hypervigilant to possible hurts or reminders of these injuries. They also speak of numbing themselves in the manner described in classic examples of posttraumatic stress disorders. These events illustrate the "indelible imprint" (Herman, 1992, p. 35) of traumatic experience.

These injuries became apparent when couples are able to create deescalation in their distressed relationships but change events in Stage 2 of EFT (withdrawer reengagement and blamer softening) are blocked by a partner's refusal to risk emotional engagement with the other. A past injury in which attachment needs were not met and expectations of being able to rely on the partner were shattered then emerges in the session in an alive and emotionally charged way. These incidents are often difficult for the therapist to understand and to address, until they are placed in an attachment frame. This frame suggests that isolation and separation from an attachment figure at increased moments of vulnerability evoke traumatic helplessness and so disproportionally influence the quality of an attachment relationship (Simpson & Rholes, 1994). It is the attachment significance of such events that is crucial, rather than the specific content of the events. If this significance is missed, partners can be seen as obdurate or resistant or even as personality disordered or as rejecting the relationship.

So in therapy, Matthew and Helen describe their relationship as relatively happy until Matthew became involved in environmental issues and the founding of a wildlife protection plan in his community. This couple had three children, and at first the family had all taken part in this activism. However, as demands on Matthew's time increased, Helen began to feel deprived of support and companionship. They began to get stuck in a pattern of Helen complaining and becoming angry while Matthew defended his commitment to "the cause" and withdrew more and more from his wife, taking on an increasingly consuming role in the cause. Their relationship, however, remained stable until Helen's mother died, and Helen then had "no one to turn to—no one to hold me. I was so alone—I finally got so upset—I had to tell Matt he should go." This couple was able to address the negative patterns of interaction in their relationship and construct a plan to limit the time Matthew donated to "the cause" so that he could be more involved with his wife and family. Matthew became more open and emotionally accessible and confided that, as his wife expressed disappointment in him, the positive feedback he got from colleagues in the cause became more and more important and compelling, and he had turned to it as an escape. He then was able to state his desire to again be close to his wife and his longing for and fear of losing her. Helen did become less angry and would begin to be more open and vulnerable to her spouse, but then she would return again and again to the events around her mother's death. As the couple tried to talk about this issue, Helen would become overwhelmed with grief and despair, and Matthew would retreat and become distant and intellectual. He would then reiterate that he had already apologized for being "distracted by other commitments" at the time of her mother's death. This couple had reduced their relationship distress but, as we now understand it, unless this kind of attachment injury is healed, the creation of positive bonding interactions and the accompanying mutual emotional accessibility and responsiveness that leads to stable recovery and more secure attachment is impossible.

HEALING ATTACHMENT INJURIES

When a therapist can use a coherent theory of relatedness to focus the intervention process, he or she is better able to describe, predict, and explain the steps involved in change as it evolves in a session and to construct change events more deliberately. A recent study of softening change events suggests, for example, that heightening emotional responses and reframing them in terms of attachment, before structuring the sharing of attachment needs and fears, results in successful softening events that then are associated with recovery from distress (Bradley & Furrow, in press; Johnson & Greenberg, 1988). This process of delineating the key steps in the change event that concerns the healing of an attachment injury is currently underway, and key interventions associated with successful completion of this healing process are beginning to be understood better.

From the observations of cases and the construction of a rational outline of the change process, the process of resolution of attachment injuries appears to be as follows (Johnson, 2002, in press):

Step 1

As the EFT therapist begins to encourage a spouse to risk connecting with his or her partner, this spouse becomes flooded by emotion from an incident in which he or she felt abandoned and helpless, experiencing a violation of trust that damaged his or her belief in the relationship as a secure bond. The spouse relates this incident in an alive, highly emotional manner reminiscent of a traumatic flashback. The partner tends to stay emotionally distant and to discount or minimize the incident and the injured partner's pain.

Step 2

With the therapist's help, the injured spouse explores the injury and begins to articulate its specific emotional impact and its attachment significance. New emotions frequently emerge at this point. Anger often evolves into clear expressions of helplessness, fear, and shame. The therapist attunes to the injured partner's emotion and acts as a surrogate processor, helping this partner express and organize this overwhelming negative emotion and the meaning it has for the person, his or her stance in the relationship, and the cycles that characterize the relationship. So Helen told Matthew of how alone, "naked and abandoned," she felt at her mother's funeral when he sat at the back of the church rather than with her.

Step 3

The other partner, supported by the therapist, begins to be able to hear the significance of the injurious event and to understand it in attachment terms; that is, as a reflection of how crucial his or her comfort and reassurance is to the injured spouse. This partner then is able to explicitly acknowledge and emotionally connect with the injured partner's pain and suffering. He or she elaborates on how the event evolved in a manner that makes his or her response more predictable and understandable to the injured partner. In the case of Matthew and Helen, Matthew was able to express how his sense of having already let Helen down during her mother's illness and his fear of her rage at his involvement with "the cause" (which she termed "his mistress") all prompted him to stay distant and even to believe that she was "calmer and better if he wasn't around her."

Step 4

The injured partner then tentatively moves toward a more integrated and complete articulation of the injury and expresses the loss involved in it and his or her fears concerning the change in the bond with the partner. The injured partner begins to allow the other to witness his or her vulnerability. The therapist helps the injured partner to "make sense of" his or her emotional experience and to integrate this experience into his or her sense of self and the relationship. Helen is able to weep and to tell Matthew directly about how much she needed and missed his comfort and reassurance in the dark days after her mother's death and about her fears that she had lost him, too.

Step 5

The other spouse then becomes more emotionally engaged and is able to acknowledge explicit responsibility for his or her part in the attachment injury and to express empathy, regret, and/or remorse in a congruent and emotionally compelling manner that the injured spouse finds comforting and reassuring. The message conveyed by this is, as Helen put it when Matthew wept for the pain he had caused her, "He does see my pain—it does impact him. He cares—he wanted to be there for me—so many things got in the way."

Step 6

The injured spouse then risks asking for the comfort and caring from the partner that were unavailable at the time of the injurious event. This is done, as in softening events, in a way that pulls the partner toward him or her. Helen weeps for her mother and her own loss of the "safe place" with Matthew and asks to be held. He holds and soothes her.

Step 7

The other spouse is now able to respond in a caring manner that appears to act as an antidote to the traumatic experience of the attachment injury. The partners are calm and able to reflect on the event and to construct together a new narrative of this event. In general, healing from trauma involves the ability to construct an integrated narrative of the traumatic event together with its meaning and its consequences, the ability to process and integrate the emotion associated with the event, and the ability to risk emotional engagement with others that offers corrective experiences of efficacy and belonging (Harvey, 1996).

Once the attachment injury is resolved, the therapist can more effectively foster the continued growth of trust and the beginning of general positive cycles of bonding and connection.

FROM A SCIENCE OF RELATIONSHIPS
TO A SCIENCE OF HEALING RELATIONSHIPS

A revolution is occurring in the field of couple therapy (Johnson, 2002, 2003c). This revolution appears to reflect what has been termed the "greening of relationship science" (Berscheid, 1999, p. 260). The increasing application of attachment theory as an explanatory framework for the patterns of marital distress outlined in observational studies is a key part of this relationship science. The coherent map of adult relatedness offered by attachment theory and research addresses the critical goals that have been identified in reviews of the couple therapy field (Johnson & Lebow, 2000; Pinsof & Wynne, 1995). It addresses the need for conceptual coherence by providing clear links between models of adult love and pragmatic "if this . . . then that" interventions. It addresses the need for both theory and practice to become more empirically based. It addresses the need to bridge the gap between research and practice, to delineate the therapist and client behaviors leading to important moments of change (Beutler, Williams, & Wakefield, 1993), and so to constantly refine interventions. It also extends the relevance of couple therapy to problems previously treated as individual intrapsychic issues (such as depression or posttraumatic stress disorders), as the significance of a safe haven and secure base in terms of individual functioning, growth, and resilience is becoming clearer and clearer (Anderson, Beach, & Kaslow, 1999; Uchino, Cacioppo, & Kiecolt-Glaser, 1996). Gurman (2001) also points out that for any change, however it has occurred, to endure, it must be supported in a person's natural environment. The most important part of this environment is most often a person's attachment relationships, and there is evidence that involving attachment figures as adjuncts, even in primarily individually oriented interventions, enhances the effectiveness of treatment (Barlow, O'Brien, & Last, 1984; Cerny, Barlow, Craske, & Himadi, 1987).

John Bowlby believed that love was the crowning achievement of human evolution and that the need for secure attachment was the script underlying the oldest and most universal of dramas, the drama of couple and family relationship distress. Knowledge of this script is contributing to the development of couple therapy into a sophisticated and mature discipline that offers healing for close relationships and a crucial arena for the positive definition of self. As has been previously noted (Johnson 2003a), a map that outlines the nature of a terrain makes the difference between a "glorious adventure or getting lost in the woods and reaching a dead end" (p. 104). Couple therapy is now advancing on the path of a glorious adventure in which the prize is improved and restored relationships with the people we love the most.

REFERENCES

Ainsworth, M. D. S., Blehar, M. C., Waters, E., & Wall, S. (1978). *Patterns of attachment: A study of the Strange Situation.* Hillsdale, NJ: Erlbaum.

Alexander, P. C. (1993). Application of attachment theory to the study of sexual abuse. *Journal of Consulting and Clinical Psychology, 60,* 185–195.

Anderson, P., Beach, S. R., & Kaslow, N. J. (1999). Marital discord and depression: The potential of attachment theory to guide integrative clinical intervention. In T. Joiner & J. C. Coyne (Eds.), *The interactional nature of depression* (pp. 271–298). Washington, DC: APA Press.

Barlow, D. H., O'Brien, G. T., & Last, C. G. (1984). The treatment of agoraphobia. *Behavior Therapy, 15,* 41–58.

Bartholomew, K., & Horowitz, L. M. (1991). Attachment styles among young adults: A test of a four-category model. *Journal of Personality and Social Psychology, 61,* 226–244.

Berscheid, E. (1999). The greening of relationship science. *American Psychologist, 54,* 260–266.

Bertalanffy, L. von. (1968). *General system theory.* New York: Braziller.

Beutler, L. E., Williams, R. E., & Wakefield, P. J. (1993). Obstacles to disseminating applied psychological science. *Applied and Preventative Psychology, 2,* 53–58.

Bowlby, J. (1969). *Attachment and loss: Vol. 1. Attachment.* New York: Basic Books.

Bowlby, J. (1973). *Attachment and loss: Vol. 2. Separation: Anxiety and anger.* New York: Basic Books.

Bowlby, J. (1979). *The making and breaking of affectional bonds.* London: Tavistock.

Bowlby, J. (1988). *A secure base: Clincal applications of attachment theory.* New York: Basic Books.

Bradley, B., & Furrow, J. (in press). Therapist interventions in change events in emotionally focused couples therapy. *Journal of Marital and Family Therapy.*

Bretherton, I., & Munholland, K. A. (1999). Internal working models in attachment relationships. In J. Cassidy & P. Shaver (Eds.), *Handbook of attachment: Theory, research, and clinical applications* (pp. 89–111). New York: Guilford Press.

Cassidy, J., & Shaver, P. R. (Eds.). (1999). *Handbook of attachment: Theory, research and clinical applications.* New York: Guilford Press.

Cerny, J. A., Barlow, D. H., Craske, M. D., & Himadi, W. G. (1987). Couples treatment of agoraphobia: A two-year follow-up. *Behavior Therapy, 18,* 401–415.

Clothier, P., Manion, I., Gordon Walker, J., & Johnson, S.M. (2002). Emotionally focused interventions for couples with chronically ill children: A two-year follow-up. *Journal of Marital and Family Therapy, 28,* 391–399.

Collins, N. L., & Allard, L. M. (2001). Cognitive representations of attachment: The content and function of working models. In G. J. O. Fletcher & M. S. Clark (Eds.), *Blackwell handbook of social psychology: Vol. 2. Interpersonal processes* (pp. 60–85). Oxford, UK: Blackwell.

Dessaulles, A., Johnson, S. M., & Denton, W. (2003). The treatment of clinical depression in the context of marital distress: Outcome for emotionally focused interventions. *American Journal of Family Therapy, 31,* 345–353.

Enright, R. D., & Fitzgibbons, R. P. (2000). *Helping clients forgive.* Washington, DC: APA Press.

Erdman, P., & Caffery, T. (2002). *Attachment and family systems: Conceptual, empirical and therapeutic relatedness.* New York: Springer.

Feeney, J. A. (1994). Attachment style, communication patterns, and satisfaction across the life cycle of marriage. *Personal Relationships, 1,* 333–348.

Fonagy, P., & Target, M. (1997). Attachment and reflective function: Their role in self-organization. *Development and Psychopathology, 9,* 679–700.

Fraley, R. C., & Shaver, P. (2000). Adult romantic attachment: Theoretical developments, emerging controversies, and unanswered questions. *Review of General Psychology, 4,* 132–154.

Fraley, R. C., & Waller, N. G. (1998). Adult attachment patterns: A test of the typological model. In J. A. Simpson & W. S., Rholes (Eds.), *Attachment theory and close relationships* (pp. 77–114). New York: Guilford Press.

Gottman, J. (1994). *What predicts divorce?* Hillsdale, NJ: Erlbaum.

Gottman, J., Coan, J., Carrere, S., & Swanson, C. (1998). Predicting marital happiness and stability from newlywed interactions. *Journal of Marriage and the Family, 60,* 5–22.

Greenberg, L. S., & Johnson, S. M. (1988). *Emotionally focused therapy for couples.* New York: Guilford Press.

Gurman, A. (2001). Brief therapy and family and couple therapy: An essential redundancy. *Clinical Psychology: Science and Practice, 8,* 51–65.

Harvey, M. (1996). An ecological view of psychological trauma and trauma recovery. *Journal of Traumatic Stress, 9,* 3–23.

Hazan, C., & Shaver, P. (1987). Romantic love conceptualized as an attachment process. *Journal of Personality and Social Psychology, 52,* 511–524.

Hazan, C., & Zeifman, D. (1994). Sex and the psychological tether. In K. Bartholomew & D. Perlman (Eds.), *Advances in personal relationships: Vol. 5. Attachment processes in adulthood* (pp. 151–177). London: Kingsley.

Herman, J. L. (1992). *Trauma and recovery.* New York: Basic Books.

Holmes, J. (1996). *Attachment, intimacy and autonomy: Using attachment theory in adult psychotherapy.* Northdale, NJ: Aronson.

Johnson, M. D., & Bradbury, T. N. (1999). Marital satisfaction and topographical assessment of marital interaction: A longitudinal analysis of newlywed couples. *Personal Relationships, 6,* 19–40.

Johnson, S. M. (1986). Bonds or bargains: Relationship paradigms and their significance for marital therapy. *Journal of Marital and Family Therapy, 12,* 259–267.

Johnson, S. M. (1996). *Creating connection: The practice of emotionally focused marital therapy.* New York: Brunner/Mazel.

Johnson, S. M. (2002). *Emotionally focused couple therapy with trauma survivors: Strengthening attachment bonds.* New York: Guilford Press.

Johnson, S. M. (2003a). Attachment theory: A guide for couples therapy. In S. M. Johnson & V. E. Whiffen (Eds.), *Attachment processes in couple and family therapy* (pp. 103–123). New York: Guilford Press.

Johnson, S. M. (2003b). Introduction to attachment: A therapist's guide to primary attachments and their renewal. In S. M. Johnson & V. E. Whiffen (Eds.), *Attachment processes in couple and family therapy* (pp. 3–17). New York: Guilford Press.

Johnson, S. M. (2003c). The revolution in couple therapy: A practitioner-scientist perspective. *Journal of Marital and Family Therapy, 29,* 365–384.

Johnson, S. M. (in press). Emotion and the repair of close relationships. In W. Pinsof & T. Patterson (Eds.), *Family psychology: The art of the science.* New York: Oxford University Press.

Johnson, S. M., & Best, M. (2002). A systematic approach to restructuring adult attachment: The EFT model of couples therapy. In P. Erdman & T. Caffery (Eds.), *Attachment and family systems: Conceptual, empirical and therapeutic relatedness* (pp. 165–189). New York: Brunner-Routledge.

Johnson, S. M., & Greenberg, L. S. (1988). Relating process to outcome in marital therapy. *Journal of Marital and Family Therapy, 14,* 175–183.

Johnson, S. M., & Greenberg, L. S. (1985). The differential effects of experiential and problem solving interventions in resolving marital conflict. *Journal of Consulting and Clinical Psychology, 53,* 175–184.

Johnson, S. M., Hunsley, J., Greenberg, L., & Schindler, D. (1999). Emotionally focused couples therapy: Status and challenges. *Clinical Psychology: Science and Practice, 6,* 67–79.

Johnson, S. M., & Lebow, J. (2000). The coming of age of couple therapy: A decade review. *Journal of Marital and Family Therapy, 26,* 9–24.

Johnson, S. M., Makinen, J., & Millikin, J. (2001). Attachment injuries in couple relationships: A new perspective on impasses in couples therapy. *Journal of Marital and Family Therapy, 27,* 145–155.

Johnson, S. M., & Whiffen, V. (1999). Made to measure: Attachment styles in couples therapy. *Clinical Psychology: Science and Practice, 6,* 366–381.

Johnson, S. M., & Whiffen, V. E. (Eds.). (2003). *Attachment processes in couple and family therapy.* New York: Guilford Press.

Jordan, J., Kaplan, A., Miller, J., Stiver, I., & Surrey, J. (1991). *Women's growth in connection: Writings from the Stone Center.* New York: Guilford Press.

Kirkpatrick, L. E., & Davis, K. E. (1994). Attachment style, gender, and relationship stability: A longitudinal analysis. *Journal of Personality and Social Psychology, 66,* 502–512.

Kunce, L. J., & Shaver, P. R. (1994). An attachment-theoretical approach to caregiving in romantic relationships. In K Bartholomew & D. Perlman (Eds.), *Advances in personal relationships: Vol. 5. Attachment processes in adulthood* (pp. 205–237). London: Kingsley.

Lussier, Y., Sabourin, S., & Turgeon, C. (1997). Coping strategies as moderators of the relationship between attachment and marital adjustment. *Journal of Social and Personal Relationships, 14,* 777–791.

Mackay, S. K. (1996). Nurturance: A neglected dimension in family therapy with adolescents. *Journal of Marital and Family Therapy, 22,* 489–508.

McFarlane, A. C., & van der Kolk, B. A. (1996). Trauma and its challenge to society. In B. A. van der Kolk, A. C. McFarlane, & L. Weisaeth (Eds.), *Traumatic stress: The effects of overwhelming experience on mind, body, and society* (pp. 24–45). New York: Guilford Press.

Mikulincer, M. (1995). Attachment style and the mental representation of the self. *Journal of Personality and Social Psychology, 69,* 1203–1215.

Mikulincer, M. (1997). Adult attachment style and information processing: Individual differences in curiosity and cognitive closure. *Journal of Personality and Social Psychology, 72,* 1217–1230.

Mikulincer, M., Florian, V., & Weller, A. (1993). Attachment styles, coping strategies, and posttraumatic psychological distress: The impact of the Gulf War in Israel. *Journal of Personality and Social Psychology, 64,* 817–826.

Pasch, L. A., & Bradbury, T. N. (1998). Social support, conflict and the development of marital dysfunction. *Journal of Consulting and Clinical Psychology, 66,* 219–230.

Pinsof, W., & Wynne, L. (1995). The efficacy of marital and family therapy: An empirical overview, conclusions, and recommendations. *Journal of Marital and Family Therapy, 21,* 585–613.

Roberts, T. W. (1992). Sexual attraction and romantic love: Forgotten variables in marital therapy. *Journal of Marital and Family Therapy, 18,* 357–364.

Schore, A. N. (1994). *Affect regulation and the organization of self.* Hillsdale, NJ: Erlbaum.

Senchak, M., & Leonard, K. (1992). Attachment styles and marital adjustment among newlywed couples. *Journal of Social and Personal Relationships, 9,* 51–64.

Shaver, P., & Clarke, C. (1994). The psychodynamics of adult romantic attachment. In J. M. Masling & R. F. Borstein (Eds.), *Empirical perspectives on object relations theory* (pp. 105–156). Washington, DC: American Psychological Association.

Shaver, P., & Hazan, C. (1993). Adult romantic attachment: Theory and evidence. In D. Perlman & W. Jones (Eds.), *Advances in personal relationships* (Vol. 4, pp.29–70). London: Kingsley.

Simpson, J. A. (1990). The influence of attachment styles on romantic relationships. *Journal of Personality and Social Psychology, 59*(5), 971–980.

Simpson, J., & Rholes, W. (1994). Stress and secure base relationships in adulthood. In K. Bartholomew & D. Perlman (Eds.), *Advances in personal relationships: Vol. 5. Attachment processes in adulthood* (pp. 181–204). London: Kingsley.

Simpson, J. A., Rholes, W. S., Campbell, L., & Wilson, C. L. (2003). Changes in attachment orientations across the transition to parenthood. *Journal of Experimental Social Psychology, 39,* 317–331.

Simpson, J., Rholes, W., & Nelligan, J. (1992). Support seeking and support giving within couples in an anxiety-provoking situation: The role of attachment styles. *Journal of Personality and Social Psychology, 62,* 434–446.

Uchino, B. N., Cacioppo, J. T., & Kiecolt-Glaser, J. K. (1996). The relationship between social support and physiological processes: A review with emphasis on underlying mechanisms and implications for health. *Psychological Bulletin, 119,* 488–531.

Worthington, E. L., & DiBlasio, F.A. (1990). Promoting mutual forgiveness within the fractured relationship. *Psychotherapy, 27,* 219–223.

CHAPTER 13

Attachment-Related Trauma and Posttraumatic Stress Disorder
Implications for Adult Adaptation

ROGER KOBAK
JUDE CASSIDY
YAIR ZIR

From early in his writing, Bowlby conceptualized attachment as a behavioral system that is activated by appraisals of danger and accompanying feelings of fear. From this perspective, the attachment system plays a major role in how individuals cope with frightening experience. In this chapter, we consider a set of extreme and distinct frightening experiences that we term "attachment-related trauma." These traumas result from frightening experiences that co-occur with a perceived threat to the availability of an attachment figure. The importance of perceived threats to the availability of an attachment figure has often been neglected in the clinical literature on trauma. In addition to expanding our understanding of traumatic events, attachment theory and research provide an account of how individuals cope with and resolve traumatic experiences. Attachment research can also shed light on the posttraumatic cognitive and emotional processes that interfere with the resolution of trauma. Unresolved traumatic experience may have important consequences for stress regulation and management of adult attachment and caregiving relationships. In the clinical literature, unresolved trauma has been extensively studied among individuals who develop posttraumatic stress disorder (PTSD). We propose that consideration of the attachment literature related to unresolved trauma in combination with clinical research on PTSD can lead to further specification of the mechanisms through which unresolved traumatic experience may impair child and adult adaptation.

In the first part of this chapter, we define attachment-related trauma. Attachment-related traumas share a common feature of a fear-provoking threat to the self that is accompanied by a perceived threat to the availability of the attachment figure. Four types of attachment-related traumas are considered: disruptions in which an attachment figure is perceived as unavailable as the result of a substantial unplanned separation; parental abuse when the attachment figure is the source of danger; attachment injuries that occur when an individual feels abandoned by an attachment figure at a time of crisis; and loss of an attachment figure through death. These events can have lasting influence if they undermine the individual's confidence in self and attachment figures. The influence of these two kinds of threat appraisal changes with development. In infancy and childhood, a threat to the availability of the attachment figure is also likely to be perceived as a threat to the self. By adolescence and adulthood, individuals are better able to distinguish threats to the attachment figure's availability from perceived threats to the self.

Next, we consider the processes that interfere with the resolution of attachment-related trauma. We describe Main and Goldwyn's (1998) "unresolved loss and trauma" classification in the Adult Attachment Interview (AAI) and review the clinical research on PTSD. We then identify common mechanisms, including failure to reappraise traumatic memories, dissociative breakdowns in organized coping, and stress reactivity, as factors common to unresolved status and PTSD. Despite the similarities of these two approaches, consideration of attachment theory and research can extend clinical research in several important ways. Our notion of attachment-related trauma expands the range of events that should be viewed as possible traumas, particularly traumas experienced in childhood and adolescence. In addition, attachment theory provides an account of the interpersonal context that may either facilitate or impede an individual's ability to resolve a traumatic event. We conclude by identifying factors that should facilitate the resolution of attachment-related traumas.

A DEVELOPMENTAL VIEW OF ATTACHMENT-RELATED TRAUMA: PERCEIVED THREATS TO THE AVAILABILITY OF AN ATTACHMENT FIGURE

The fourth edition of the *Diagnostic and Statistical Manual of Mental Disorders* (American Psychiatric Association [APA], 2000) provides two criteria for a traumatic event: (1) "a threat to life or physical integrity" that (2) is accompanied by "intense fear, helplessness, or horror" (p. 463). Much of the research on trauma has focused on situations involving threats to the individual or to the individual's survival. The DSM definition is concerned exclusively with the experience of trauma in adulthood. As a result, there has been less consideration of the nature of trauma experience early in life or of how trauma experience changes with development. A developmental approach can inform our understanding of adult experiences of trauma and its effects by considering the role that the attachment system plays in either mitigating or exacerbating an individual's experience of a frightening event. We believe that examination of attachment relationships and processes can inform our understanding of traumatic experience in important ways.

Attachment researchers have focused extensively on the role that the attachment figure plays in providing a haven of safety during times of distress. Observations of infants and young children provide ample evidence that the presence of an attachment figure is likely to make a frightening experience less traumatic by virtue of the safety derived from the attachment figure (Bowlby, 1973). Although the specific situations that elicit fear and activate attachment change with development, the extreme fear associated with trauma is likely to activate the attachment system across the lifespan. For instance, an individual of any age who faces a natural disaster would most likely seek contact with an attachment figure. Available and responsive attachment figures can reduce the sense of fear and provide an important alliance that facilitates coping with the perceived threat. As a result, when the individual maintains a confident expectation of an attachment figure's availability, he or she is less likely to experience the "intense fear, helplessness, or horror" that constitutes a traumatic experience.

Just as the presence of an attachment figure provides safety and reduces fear, so can a perceived threat to an attachment figure's availability itself be the source of intense fear and anxiety. The second volume of Bowlby's (1973) attachment trilogy provides a comprehensive review of evidence indicating that both children and adults respond with intense fear if they perceive a threat to the availability of attachment figures.

Events that constitute a threat to the availability of an attachment figure change dramatically from infancy through adulthood. In infancy, a brief separation can cause considerable distress when accompanied by fear-eliciting stimuli such as a strange environment and a stranger. The young infant lacks the cognitive and linguistic abilities to understand the separation or to plan a reunion, and, as a result, even a brief separation is appraised as a threat to the availability of the attachment figure. These threats to the availability of the attachment figure may elicit intense fear and intensify efforts to ensure the continued availability of an attachment figure.

The complex of cognitive, linguistic, and regulatory changes that occur during childhood fundamentally transform the way the child appraises the availability of attachment figures. Separations now can be planned in ways that ensure the continued availability of the attachment figure, if needed. The child's growing competencies also make it increasingly possible to manage for long period of times without proximity to the attachment figure. As a result, daily stresses are increasingly managed more autonomously and are guided by internal representations that an attachment figure is available if needed. This confidence often suffices for managing daily challenges (Kobak, 1999). Yet despite the older child's and adult's ability to be guided by confident expectations of the availability of an attachment figure and of their own abilities, extreme events that are appraised as threats to an attachment figure's availability continue to elicit intense fear and anxiety. In adolescence and adulthood, threats to the availability of the attachment figure increasingly involve more extreme threats, such as death of the attachment figure or abandonment (Johnson, 2002).

Consideration of the attachment system broadens our definition of what may be experienced as a traumatic event. From this perspective, traumatic experience may result from two broad types of appraisal. The first type of appraisal focuses on serious threats to the individual's well-being or survival. This type of appraisal readily activates the attachment system and orients thoughts and behavior toward seeking safety and protection from an attachment figure. A wide variety of situations, such as accidents, illnesses, natural disasters, robbery, physical assault, or fires, may be appraised as threatening by both children and adults (see Norris, 1992). The second type of traumatic appraisal involves threat of loss of or abandonment by an attachment figure. For an infant, even relatively minor separations may be appraised as such a threat. In older children and adults, threats of abandonment by or loss of an attachment figure may result from conflict with, rejection by, or death of an attachment figure.

Four Types of Attachment-Related Trauma

Attachment-related trauma occurs when a frightening experience is accompanied by or results from the appraisal of loss, rejection, or abandonment by an attachment figure. Because children's survival is often dependent on their parents' availability and protection, it is not uncommon for appraised threats of rejection, abandonment, and loss to be simultaneously perceived as a threat to survival. By adulthood, threats to the availability of an attachment figure do not necessarily signal threats to survival, and, as a result, many adult traumas may be the product of compound fear situations in which a threat to the self is combined with a perceived threat of loss or abandonment by an attachment figure.

Four major types of attachment-related trauma are described here: (1) attachment disruptions, (2) physical or sexual abuse by a parent, (3) loss of an attachment figure through death, and (4) attachment injuries.

Attachment Disruptions

Attachment disruptions are an extreme form of separation that differ from normal daily separations in important ways. First, the separation is prolonged and often involves little communication with the attachment figure. Second, the separation is unanticipated and occurs without a joint plan for reuniting with the attachment figure. The way in which the child appraises and evaluates the disruption will be influenced both by developmental level and by experience. Infants and young children may be particularly vulnerable to prolonged separation, as they lack the ability to form joint plans or represent the attachment figure during the absence. Older children are more capable of managing long separations from parents as long as the separations are accompanied by planning and continued communication. It is likely that attachment-related experience is particularly relevant to the appraisal of separations. For instance, parents who threaten to abandon or send the child away may increase the likelihood that the child will appraise physical separation as abandonment. Similarly, when divorce or marital separations are accompanied by high levels of conflict or disagreements about child rearing, the child will be more likely to appraise a separation as an abandonment (Grych & Fincham, 1993).

In a sample of 9- to 11-year-old boys, Kobak, Little, Race, and Acosta (2001) examined the effects of attachment disruptions on psychopathology and functioning at school. Disruptions were classified on a 4-point scale ranging from maintaining a continuous relationship to complete abandonment or loss of the attachment figure. Boys who had been placed in classrooms for severely emotionally disturbed children had much higher rates of attachment disruptions with their biological mothers. Across all the boys, higher levels of attachment disruptions were associated with higher teacher ratings of dissociative symptoms and more dependency on ratings of the teacher–student relationship.

Physical and Sexual Abuse by an Attachment Figure

Physical or sexual assault is nearly always likely to be an experience in which the individual is intensely frightened and helpless. This type of trauma is inflicted by other human beings and is likely to shake an individual's confidence in others. When the perpetrator of abuse is also an attachment figure, the child faces an inescapable dilemma. Two factors make abuse especially complex. First, as Main and Hesse (1990) have pointed out, abuse creates a unique attachment-related trauma in which the attachment figure becomes a source of alarm. When the child's haven of safety also becomes a source of danger, the child is faced with a dilemma that has no solution. Abuse creates a further problem for the child insofar as it is frequently a chronic aspect of the parent–child relationship. The child is thus faced with an ongoing source of trauma.

A central contribution of attachment research in infancy and early childhood has been to identify traumatic experience in early periods of development that may not be accessible to adult memory or recall. The disorganized pattern identified in infancy is thought to be associated with children adapting to a caregiver who is frightened or frightening (Main & Hesse, 1990). This disorganization pattern may well reflect the infant's early experience of trauma in the context of the parent–child relationship. At this point, relatively little is known about how traumatic experiences that occur early in life are later recalled or processed by adults.

Loss of an Attachment Figure

The loss of an attachment figure through death may or may not be a frightening experience (Bonanno & Kaltman, 1999). Fear is more likely if the loss is sudden, making it impossible to prepare for the absence of the attachment figure. Under more favorable circumstances, coping with the anticipated death of an attachment figure and with the subsequent bereavement occurs gradually over an extended period of time. Bowlby (1980) provides an extensive description of the process of anticipating and mourning the loss of an attachment figure in the third volume of his attachment trilogy.

Fear usually accompanies the threat of loss rather than actual loss. Thus initial news of events involving perceived danger to the life of the attachment figure can produce extreme fear even if the events do not necessarily result in the death of the attachment figure. Although the threat of loss is ultimately an appraisal process that is likely to differ across individuals, several contextual factors are likely to make the threat of loss particularly traumatic. There is evidence that violent death (e. g., from homicide, suicide, or accidents) is more likely to produce intense fear and difficulties following the loss in comparison with losses that occur through natural causes (Zisook, Chentsova-Dutton, & Schuchter, 1998). Bowlby (1973) emphasized how children's exposure to violence or suicide threats could be particularly frightening to children.

Although children are not attachment figures to parents, perceived threats to children's survival are likely to produce intense fear in a parent and thereby activate the parental caregiving system. Studies of bereaved adults have failed to clarify whether the loss of a child is more or less traumatic than the loss of a conjugal partner (Bonanno & Kaltman, 1999). Factors that influence postloss symptoms include the age of the parent and the degree of forewarning of the child's death (Lehman, Wortman, & Williams, 1987). Another study found that the reproductive age of the child affected parents' ability to cope with the loss of a child, with the loss of a child in the 15- to 25-year age range producing the most difficulties in postloss adjustment (Crawford, Salter, & Jang, 1989).

Attachment Injuries

Drawing on her clinical work with distressed couples, Johnson has suggested a fourth type of attachment-related trauma (Johnson, 2002; Johnson, Makinen, & Millikin, 2001). She describes compound fear situations in which an adult, when faced with a life-threatening situation, feels abandoned by his or her attachment figure. Attachment injuries are "wounds arising from abandonment by a present attachment figure in a situation of urgent need" (Johnson, 2002, p. 15). These events are traumatic in that they elicit intense fear associated with the isolation and abandonment. In addition, these events fundamentally shake the adult's confidence in the partner's availability and responsiveness.

The intense fear and sense of betrayal that accompany an attachment injury create a nodal event whichthat may fundamentally alter an individual's expectations about the partner's availability. These events often make the work of the couple therapist, particularly efforts to restore confidence in the partner's availability, more difficult. One important implication of the attachment-injuries notion is that these events often need to be addressed in order to overcome impasses in therapy.

If attachment injuries can occur in the context of adult attachment relationships, similar events may have a profound influence on parent–child attachments. In addition to the feelings of abandonment that accompany attachment disruptions and parental abuse, children may be victimized by peers or adults outside the family. If the attachment figure ignores, dismisses, or denies these events when they occur, the child may feel abandoned and isolated at a time of urgent need. Diamond and Stern (2003) has identified these moments as the basis of potential impasses in treatment of adolescent children and their parents.

FAILURE TO RESOLVE TRAUMATIC EVENTS

Epidemiological research in the past decade suggests that exposure to traumatic events is relatively common. Several large-scale studies have found the lifetime prevalence of exposure to traumatic events to be between 39 and 70% (Freedy & Donkervoet, 1995). In one national probability sample of more than 4,000 adult American women, over 35% of the women had experienced at least one of four traumatic "criminal" events: rape, molestations or attempted sexual assault, physical assault, and homicide of a close friend or relative (Resnick, Kilpatrick, Dansky, Saunders, & Best, 1993). Although the majority of trauma survivors manage to successfully cope with the event, failure to cope with trauma can have severe and long-lasting consequences.

Both attachment and clinical researchers have focused attention on trauma survivors who have failed to successfully resolve trauma. For attachment researchers, individuals who show difficulty resolving traumatic experience in the context of the AAI are believed to suffer from unresolved loss and trauma. For clinical researchers, the diagnosis of PTSD results from a cluster of symptoms that typically impair survivors' functioning more than a month after the occurrence of the event. The DSM criteria for the disorder include three distinct symptom clusters: (1) *reexperiencing* the event in the form of intrusive thoughts or nightmares; (2) avoiding reminders of the event and *emotional numbing;* and (3) *hyperarousal,* involving irritability and exaggerated startle response. We believe that these two research literatures—attachment research on unresolved loss and trauma and clinical research on PTSD—share an overlapping set of concerns and can inform each other about the processes involved in failing to resolve traumatic experience.

Unresolved Loss and Trauma in the Adult Attachment Interview

The AAI (George, Kaplan, & Main, 1996) is a semistructured interview that probes attachment-related experiences during childhood, such as memories of feeling loved or unloved, memories of being upset or ill, and memories of separation, rejection, and loss. Participants are asked to provide general descriptions of their relationships with each parent and to integrate specific instances with these more general descriptions. Contained within the AAI is an assessment of attachment-related trauma and the extent to which adults have managed to "resolve" attachment-related trauma.

Based on their AAI narratives, adults are classified into one of three principal groups: *secure/autonomous, dismissing of attachment,* and *preoccupied with attachment* (Main & Goldwyn, 1998). In addition, individuals may receive an *unresolved* classification if they have experienced an attachment-related childhood or adult trauma (i.e., loss or abuse) with which they have been unable to successfully come to terms. Individuals classified as unresolved on the AAI are also assigned an underlying classification of secure, dismissing, or preoccupied (i.e., unresolved/secure, unresolved/dismissing, or unresolved/preoccupied). For example, a person whose AAI revealed a lack of resolution, as well as a reliance on dismissing attachment strategies, would be classified as unresolved/dismissing.

The coding of unresolved status focuses on two of the four major categories of attachment-related trauma described earlier: loss and abuse in the context of an attachment relationship. It is the parts of the interview related to loss (all important losses during the person's life) and abuse (e.g., physical or sexual abuse, bizarre punishments, parental suicide or suicide attempts in the child's presence) that are important for coding lack of resolution. Specifically, a person is classified "unresolved with respect to loss or trauma" if his or her speech shows lapses in the monitoring of *reasoning* (i.e., temporary lack of conventional logic or reality testing when discussing loss or trauma) or lapses in the monitoring of *discourse* (i.e., marked shifts or irregularities in the narrative style used by the speaker when discussing loss or trauma). Lapses in the monitoring of reasoning may indicate intrusions of incompatible belief systems into consciousness, whereas lapses in the monitoring of discourse suggest a shift into a state involving considerable absorption and diminished awareness of the interview situation. Despite the differences between these two types of lapses, both are considered to be examples of lack of resolution.

Lapses in the monitoring of reasoning during discussion of a loss through death can take a number of forms, including (1) indications of disbelief that the person is dead; (2) suggestions that the speaker was somehow responsible for the death, despite evidence to the contrary; (3) indications of confusion between the identity of the dead person and the individual him- or herself; (4) psychologically confused statements; (5) indications that the dead person may be attempting to manipulate the speaker's mind; and (6) disorientation with respect to time and space. An example of a lapse in reasoning was observed by Ainsworth and Eichberg (1991) in an otherwise high-functioning mother. When the woman was asked whether she recalled any loss experiences, she responded, "Yes, there was a little man," and then began to cry. According to the woman, this man had been her caretaker for a few months when she was 8 years old and had given her what little affection she obtained in her early years. One day, he had asked her whether she would marry him when she grew up, and she had replied, "I can't because by then you'll be dead." He died 2 weeks later of a brain hemorrhage. While crying and still describing this event to the interviewer, the woman said, "Strange, how you can kill a person with just one sentence." This single statement placed her interview in the unresolved-attachment category. Another interview offers an example of a belief that the lost person is simultaneously dead and alive: "It's probably better that he is dead because he can get on with being dead and I can get back to my business."

Lapses in the monitoring of discourse when discussing loss also can take a number of different forms, including (1) unusual attention to detail, (2) marked shift in the style or rhythm of the discourse, (3) unfinished sentences, and (4) prolonged silences. This type of lapse is illustrated in the following description of an interview (from Main & Goldwyn, 1998) with a parent of a disorganized infant who had used an ordinary conversational style during the earlier portions of the AAI.

When asked to describe the death of a young cousin, she exhibited a marked changed in discourse register and responded,

> "She was young, she was lovely, she was dearly beloved by all who knew her and who witnessed her as she was torn from us by that most dreaded of diseases, tuberculosis. And then, like a flower torn from the ground at its moment of splendor, she was taken from us in that most terrible moment of her death. The sounds of the weeping, the smell of the flowers, her mother in her black dress cast across her daughter's coffin, I remember it still." (p. 104)

Such a sudden shift to a eulogistic form of speech is typical of the altered state of consciousness conveyed during lapses in the monitoring of discourse.

As we noted earlier, these types of lapses also occur with regard to unresolved trauma. Lapses in monitoring of reason can be seen in the disorganized thinking that is sometimes exhibited in survivors of sexual abuse and physical abuse. Examples of such lapses include stating that an event both happened and did not happen, taking responsibility for one's victimization for implausible reasons (e.g., "I was seductive and caused it"), and fearing having one's mind controlled by the abuser. Lapses in monitoring of discourse include disoriented speech, such as, "I would . . . um . . . get to me . . . didn't really . . . couldn't say." As these examples suggest, lapses in the monitoring of reasoning or discourse sufficient to lead to placement in the unresolved AAI category are often very brief and may appear in conjunction with speech that is otherwise secure, dismissing, or preoccupied. It is also important to note that lapses do not include expressions of continuing pain or regret or mild fearfulness regarding parents' behavior.

Mechanisms Characterizing Both Unresolved Loss/Trauma and PTSD

Both the classification of "unresolved loss or trauma" in the AAI and the clinical diagnosis of PTSD point to an important distinction in how individuals cope with trauma. Whereas some individuals manage to successfully cope with traumatic experience in a manner that allows them to return to normal life, others remain vulnerable to reexperiencing the traumatic event in ways that disrupt normal functioning. We believe that the symptoms that characterize PTSD and the lapses in monitoring discourse and reason that result in AAI "unresolved" status share several common features. These include: (1) failure to integrate memory of a traumatic experience into a coherent autobiographical narrative; (2) avoidance of the painful emotion associated with traumatic memories, perhaps through dissociation; and (3) increased stress reactivity or tendency to experience dysfunctional arousal when exposed to subsequent triggers or stressful events.

Failure to integrate memories of trauma characterizes both individuals with PTSD and those classified as unresolved. For individuals with PTSD, memories of the trauma intrude in unexpected ways on mental life in the form of intrusive images or nightmares. Ehlers and Clark (2000) suggested that data-driven encoding of traumatic experience and the subsequent failure to elaborate trauma memories increases risk for developing PTSD. In these individuals, memories of the event are less integrated into an autobiographical narrative, and, as a result, these memories are less available to higher order search strategies that are under cognitive control. Because these memories are often poorly elaborated and integrated, they tend to be activated less by controlled search strategies and more by sensory cues. This situation results in relatively unpredictable activation of trauma memories. The sensory and relatively unelaborated nature of trauma memories is also evident in the AAI. The excessive level of detail found in the narratives of some participants or the more general lapse in monitoring of discourse or reasoning suggests that the memory of the trauma has not been elaborated or integrated in a way that allows controlled processing of the event in the interview context.

A second feature common to PTSD and AAI unresolved status involves the use of dissociative or avoidant ways of managing the painful emotion that accompanies traumatic memory. Attempts to avoid traumatic memories or to restrict emotion (numbing) are central features of PTSD. In the AAI, the unresolved individual's tendency to become absorbed in memories is manifested in a momentary loss of the interview context. Such absorption or dissociation may reduce painful emotions that are associated with loss or trauma memories. However, these dissociative processes serve to isolate the memory from the kinds of reappraisal that would help an individual to make sense of the event and integrate it into a coherent autobiographical narrative. Halligan, Michael, Clark, and Ehlers (2003) suggested that the failure to integrate and elaborate trauma memories can be traced to encoding processes that are likely to occur shortly after a traumatic event. They noted that this type of failure is similar to the dissociative process of depersonalization. Dissociation that occurs when recalling a traumatic event impedes the cognitive and emotional processing of the event and is likely to maintain a disorganized trauma memory.

A third shared feature of PTSD and AAI unresolved status is increased reactivity to stress. The diagnostic criteria for PTSD identify hyperarousal (as indicated by exaggerated startle response, disturbed sleep, anger outbursts, poor concentration, and hypervigilance) as markers of stress reactivity (American Psychiatric Association, 1994). Individuals with these symptoms tend to be highly reactive to both conditioned cues that trigger traumatic memories and nonconditioned cues involving daily stressful events (van der Kolk, 1996). Instead of responding to daily stressors with the normal coping efforts, individuals with symptoms of hyperarousal may be prone to breakdowns in organized coping strategies that result in momentary loss of organized behavior, characterized by angry outbursts. Individuals classified as unresolved in the AAI may also be reactive to stress. The lapses in monitoring discourse and reason that occur in the interview are focused entirely on sections of the interview in which the individual is recalling emotionally challenging or stressful events. The momentary breakdown in monitoring could be a marker that the individual is having difficulty maintaining an organized discourse strategy at a moment of high stress.

In the AAI, this reactivity to stress is observed in the lapses of metacognitive monitoring observed in the interview. The AAI is a context that is likely to trigger memories of loss or trauma and to test the individual's ability to maintain cognitive control over trauma-related memories. In this sense, the lapses in reasoning and discourse can be viewed as a momentary breakdown of metacognitive strategies for monitoring discourse. The AAI creates a context in which it is possible to observe the types of momentary dissociative processes that both result from and maintain disorganized memories of traumatic experience. A similar breakdown in regulatory functioning, observed in some infants in the Strange Situation, has been classified as "disorganized" attachment behavior (Main & Solomon, 1986). Attachment theory and research also suggest a mechanism that may account for dissociation. At moments of high stress, normal coping and monitoring strategies become vulnerable to breakdown that leads to disorganized behavior or thinking. Such a process may account both for the lapses in discourse and reasoning in the AAI and also the disorganized behaviors shown by infants at moments of high stress in the Strange Situation. The failure or breakdown of coping strategies leaves the individual vulnerable and helpless.

In sum, attachment and PTSD researchers have identified similar characteristics of unresolved trauma. First, both sets of researchers emphasize that failed resolution of trauma is characterized by disorganized or sensory memories that are not integrated into a self-referential autobiography. Second, both sets of researchers suggest that the emotional numbing or dissociative types of symptoms may accompany breakdowns in organized coping. Dissociative symptoms include reduced awareness of one's surroundings, derealization, depersonalization, and emotional numbing. This type of symptom may represent an attempt at coping when other strategies have failed. Third, both sets of researchers have found that individuals with unresolved trauma are vulnerable to stress reactivity and may show marked lapses in organized coping under conditions of stress.

In addition to the difficulties that are common to PTSD and AAI unresolved status, individuals exposed to attachment-related traumas face some unique difficulties. Whereas many adult traumas involve threats to the self, they do not necessarily involve threats to the availability of an attachment figure. These relatively simple traumas allow the individual to use his or her attachment relationships as a source of safety, emotional comfort, and means of coping with traumatic experience. In contrast, attachment-related traumas are inherently more complex and difficult to resolve. Individuals facing attachment-related traumas have usually experienced a major threat to their safety, along with a threat to the availability of their attachment figures. In the case of loss, the threat to availability becomes a reality with which the individual must cope. As a result, attachment-related trauma may be more difficult to resolve for two reasons. First, the level of fear or threat may be compounded. Bowlby (1973) described this as a "compound fear" situation. Second, the individual's ability to use an attachment as a source of safety and comfort may be drastically reduced or eliminated.

The Interpersonal Consequences of Unresolved Trauma

Unresolved trauma may create a variety of interpersonal problems for trauma survivors and family members. The interpersonal effects of unresolved trauma have been most intensively investigated in the parent–infant relationship. Several studies indicate that unresolved loss and trauma reflected in a parent's AAI may predict the infant's inability to establish an organized attachment strategy (for reviews, see Cassidy & Mohr, 2001; van IJzendoorn, Schuengel, & Bakermans-Kranenburg, 1999). The mechanisms through which parental unresolved trauma influences the infant are thought to be the parent's frightened or frightening behavior toward the infant (Main & Hesse, 1990). Main and Hesse (1990) further suggested that the infant is likely to be frightened by unpredictable parental behavior and consequently unable to maintain a consistently organized strategy for maintaining the attachment relationship. This difficulty becomes evident in the momentary disorganized, disoriented, or frightened behavior displayed by the infant during the Strange Situation procedure.

Although the link between unresolved trauma in the AAI and disorganized attachment in infants requires further investigation, several mechanisms associated with AAI unresolved status may increase an infant's likelihood of being alarmed by his or her caregiver. For instance, the stress reactivity and angry outbursts of a parent with unresolved status could lead the child to experience the parent as frightening. Similarly, a parent's dissociative lapses or emotional numbing may result in helpless behavior that leads the child to perceive the parent as frightened. Furthermore, intrusive and poorly integrated memories of traumatic experience may lead to unpredictable shifts in parental behavior and mood that could frighten a young infant or child.

Because living with a parent who has unresolved trauma is likely to result in chronic and cumulative experiences of fear, older children may develop strategies for maintaining a relationship with a parent who is unpredictable, frightening, or frightened. There is longitudinal evidence that disorganized infants develop controlling–caregiving or controlling–hostile strategies that are thought to provide the child with a way of managing a parent who is a source of fear or alarm (Lyons-Ruth, Bronfman, & Atwood, 1999; Main & Cassidy, 1988; Wartner, Grossman, Frommer-Bombik, & Suess, 1994). Much less is known about how unresolved trauma influences adolescent–parent or adult–adult attachment relationships. However, the controlling patterns identified in younger children may persist in adolescent–parent relationships. In addition to examining patterns of interaction in which the child controls the relationship with a parent, concurrent assessment of the parent's states of mind with respect to loss and trauma are needed. Moreover, there is some evidence that the AAI may need to be accompanied by other assessments of traumatic experience and lack of resolution. Investigations of high-risk samples suggest that many adult participants who report sexual abuse in structured interviews fail to report sexual abuse on the AAI (K. Lyons-Ruth, personal communication, August 28, 2002). In addition, the criteria for unresolved status in the AAI may be overly restricted to lapses of metacognitive monitoring without assessing other markers of failure to resolve loss or trauma.

Individuals with unresolved trauma are also at increased risk for major difficulties in adult attachment relationships. For instance, the severity of PTSD symptoms has been linked to relationship distress among male combat veterans (Riggs, Byrne, Weathers, & Litz, 1998). Nearly one-half of women who experience sexual abuse will be revictimized (Follette, Polusny, Bechtle, & Naugle, 1996). The mechanisms that account for the link between PTSD and interpersonal difficulties have not been studied. However, many of the same mechanisms that may link unresolved trauma in the AAI to parent–child attachments may also account for difficulties in adult relationships. Both stress reactivity and emotional numbing are likely to make establishing open communication with an adult partner especially difficult. In more extreme cases, in which past trauma results from interpersonal violence, there is some evidence that survivors may fail to appraise risk in relationships or act to protect themselves (Wilson, Calhoun, & Bernat, 1999).

ATTACHMENT AND THE RESOLUTION OF TRAUMA

The literature on PTSD and AAI unresolved status identify processes that interfere with the resolution of traumatic experience. These processes suggest several challenges to successfully resolving a traumatic experience. One challenge centers on stress regulation or, more specifically, on managing the intense fear and helplessness that accompanies a traumatic event. A second challenge involves coping with the effects that the traumatic event has on core cognitive assumptions about oneself and the world. A third challenge involves integration and reappraisal of the traumatic event in a way that restores positive expectations for oneself and others.

The intense fear and helplessness associated with a trauma and subsequent memory for the event can easily undermine normal ways of coping with stressful experience. Foa's emotional processing model suggests that later PTSD symptoms are more likely to occur in individuals who initially respond with numbing to the trauma situation (Foa & Kozak, 1986; Foa & Riggs, 1993). As a result of numbing, the fear associated with trauma memories remains high, leading to subsequent difficulties in processing or integrating traumatic memories. In contrast, if individuals can tolerate the stress of the traumatic experience, memories of the event gradually become less fear provoking and subject to reappraisal. Trauma researchers suggest that social support usually plays a critical role in helping survivors tolerate the stress of the trauma experience and in predicting better long-term resolution of the event. This literature on social support can be substantially strengthened by the consideration of principal attachment figures from whom survivors are most likely to initially seek comfort and reassurance (Johnson, 2002). In optimal situations, the attachment figure increases safety enough to allow the survivor to tolerate memories of trauma and go through a process of reappraising the traumatic memory, coming to accept the event and integrating the memory into a continuous autobiographical narrative. Thus secure attachment relationships play an integral role in helping trauma survivors manage the intense fear associated with trauma memories.

Survivors' abilities to use attachment relationships as a source of safety and stress regulation may be severely challenged in the case of attachment-related traumas. If the trauma has shaken the individual's confidence in the availability of an attachment figure, he or she faces a second challenge of restoring confident expectations and a secure attachment relationship. In cases involving loss, the individual must reorganize his or her attachment hierarchy, replacing the deceased person with another attachment figure. In cases in which an attachment figure has become a source of threat or alarm, successful resolution is likely to involve establishing a secure relationship with an alternative or secondary attachment figure. Other types of threat may be subject to repair through reappraising the event in a way that restores confidence in the attachment figure's availability. This may require reappraisals of the circumstances surrounding the event and attributions of responsibility for the event. Threats that are attributed to intentional acts by the attachment figure or attributions of personal responsibility to the victim are usually associated with difficulty resolving or integrating the traumatic event. Ultimately, the individual needs to reestablish a secure attachment relationship marked by confident expectations of the attachment figure's availability.

Finally, if the individual can tolerate the negative emotions involved in the traumatic event and has a secure relationship to support exploration, he or she can begin the process of reappraising the traumatic event and integrating it into a coherent autobiographical narrative. This may involve finding meaning or making sense of the traumatic event. Although trauma poses a severe challenge to core beliefs about oneself and the world (Janoff-Bulman, 1992; Parkes & Weiss, 1983), this challenge creates the conditions for cognitive reappraisal and restructuring. One study of recovery from loss focused on the process of meaning making that occurs following a significant loss (Davis, Nolen-Hoeksema, & Larson, 1998). Two aspects of meaning were emphasized: (1) "sense making," or the ability to integrate the experience of loss into a broader set of assumptions of oneself and the world, and (2) finding benefit or positive meaning in the experience. Individuals who were able to make sense of a loss reported less distress immediately following the loss but were as depressed as other respondents at 13 and 18 months after the loss. In contrast, participants who reported finding positive benefit in loss reported less distress at 13 and 18 months.

The integration and reappraisal of traumatic memories can be either facilitated or undermined by the presence or absence of a secure attachment. Listening to intense fear and negative emotions may be extremely challenging for others and may drive away people who would normally be sources of support and comfort (Coyne, 1976; Silver, Boon, & Stones, 1990). Yet, if the attachment figure can provide a secure base for exploring memories of the traumatic experience, the processes of fear reduction, reappraisal, and integration of trauma memories can be enhanced and facilitated. Relatively little is known about how a supportive attachment relationship can provide the basis for reevaluation and reappraisal of traumatic memories.

Ultimately, resolution of traumatic experience can be tested in several ways. The individual needs to be capable of managing stress in adaptive ways, particularly the fear associated with the traumatic experience. Another critical factor centers on reestablishing positive expectancies that one is worthy and that others are available and trustworthy. These expectations are most likely to be manifested in a secure attachment relationship characterized by trust, commitment, and open communication. Finally, if the first two conditions are met, the individual is in a position to reappraise and reevaluate the traumatic experience. This is a gradual process that would lead to the ability to provide an organized, coherent account of the trauma and its effects on oneself and on significant relationships.

SUMMARY AND FUTURE DIRECTIONS

Attachment research has made a significant contribution to understanding traumatic experience of infants and adults. A central contribution of this work has been in identifying how infant vulnerability to forming disorganized attachments results largely from alarming experiences with caregivers (Main & Hesse, 1990). In this chapter, we have focused on traumas that are remembered and reported by older children and adults in both attachment research using the AAI and clinical research on PTSD. The AAI unresolved classification represents a significant methodological advance that has shed light on the failure to resolve traumatic experience. This classification has also shown promise in predicting both infant disorganization and adult psychopathology. Nonetheless, additional work on the effects of trauma is needed in several ways.

The range of events that may be experienced as traumatic needs to be expanded and differentiated. The categories of attachment-related trauma that we have described provide one way of differentiating types of trauma. As we have suggested, the nature of attachment-related trauma is influenced by the developmental status of the child, by contextual factors, and by the expectations for an attachment figure's availability that a child brings to appraising a traumatic event. Some types of trauma may be more difficult to resolve, especially insofar as the availability of an attachment figure is compromised. In many cases, the effects of attachment-related trauma may become a chronic feature of a relationship and may result in long-term patterns of disorganization that are extremely difficult to resolve. It is also likely that early attachment traumas may have more lasting effects than later traumas.

Finally, the mechanisms that account for resolving or failing to resolve traumatic experience need to be further specified and tested. We believe that research on PTSD provides valuable clues to mechanisms, including stress reactivity, dissociative emotion numbing, and hyperarousal, that are associated with difficulties in resolving traumatic experience. Further, each of these mechanisms is likely to profoundly influence current attachment relationships and to compromise an individual's ability to use attachment as a source of safety and eventually a secure base for reappraising traumatic experience. However, attachment quality may moderate the extent to which stress reactivity, dissociative coping, and hyperarousal emerge in the aftermath of a traumatic event. Studies of PTSD can benefit by inclusion of attachment measures, and attachment studies can be informed by consideration of the mechanisms that contribute to the PTSD classification. Both attachment and PTSD mechanisms need to be tested in prospective studies to better understand how adults cope with traumatic experience.

ACKNOWLEDGMENTS

This chapter was supported by National Institute of Mental Health Grant No. RO1-MH59670 to Roger Kobak and by Grant No. MH50773 and MH58907 to Jude Cassidy.

REFERENCES

Ainsworth, M. D. S., & Eichberg, C. (1991). Effects of infant-mother attachment of mothers' unresolved loss of an attachment figure, or other traumatic experience. In C. M. Parkes, J. Stevenson-Hinde, & P. Marris (Eds.), *Attachment across the life cycle* (pp. 160–183). London: Routledge.

American Psychiatric Association. (2000). *Diagnostic and statistical manual of mental disorders* (4th ed., text rev.). Washington, DC: Author.

Bonanno, G., & Kaltman, S. (1999). Toward an integrative perspective on bereavement. *Psychological Bulletin, 125*(6), 760–776.

Bowlby, J. (1973). *Attachment and loss: Vol. 2. Separation: Anxiety and anger.* New York: Basic Books.

Bowlby, J. (1980). *Attachment and loss: Vol. 3. Loss: Sadness and depression.* New York: Basic Books.

Cassidy, J., & Mohr, J. (2001). Unsolvable fear, trauma, and psychopathology: Theory, research, and clinical considerations related to disorganized attachment across the lifespan. *Clinical Science and Practice, 8,* 275–298.

Coyne, J. C. (1976). Depression and the response of others. *Journal of Abnormal Psychology, 85,* 186–193.

Crawford, C. B., Salter, B. E., & Jang, K. L. (1989). Human grief: Is its intensity related to the reproductive value of the deceased? *Ethology and Sociobiology, 10,* 297–307.

Davis, C. G., Nolen-Hoeksema, S. N., & Larson, J. (1998). Making sense of loss and benefiting from the experience: Two construals of meaning. *Journal of Personality and Social Psychology, 75,* 561–574.

Diamond, G. S., & Stern, R. S. (2003). Attachment-based family therapy for depressed adolescents: Repairing attachment failures. In S. M. Johnson & V. E. Whiffen (Eds.), *Attachment processes in couple and family therapy* (pp. 191–212). New York: Guilford Press.

Ehlers, A., & Clark, D. M. (2000). A cognitive model of posttraumatic stress disorder. *Behaviour Research and Therapy, 38,* 319–345.

Foa, E. B., & Kozak, M. J. (1986). Emotional processing of fear: Exposure to corrective information. *Psychological Bulletin, 99,* 20–35.

Foa, E. B., & Riggs, D. S. (1993). Posttraumatic stress disorder in rape victims. In J. Oldham, M. B. Riba, & A. Tasman (Eds.), *American Psychiatric Press review of psychiatry* (Vol. 12, pp. 273–303). Washington, DC: American Psychiatric Press.

Follette, V. M., Polusny, M. A., Bechtle, A. E., & Naugle, A. E. (1996). Cumulative trauma: The impact of child sexual abuse, adult sexual assault, and spouse abuse. *Journal of Traumatic Stress, 9,* 25–35.

Freedy, J. R., & Donkervoet, J. C. (1995). Traumatic stress: An overview of the field. In J. R. Freedy & S. E. Hobfoll (Eds.), *Traumatic stress: From theory to practice* (pp. 3–28). New York: Plenum Press.

George, C., Kaplan, N., & Main, M. (1996). *Adult Attachment Interview protocol* (3rd ed.). Unpublished manuscript, University of California at Berkeley.

Grych, J. H., & Fincham, F. D. (1993). Children's appraisals of marital conflict: Initial investigations of the cognitive-contextual framework. *Child Development, 64,* 215–230.

Halligan, S. L., Michael, T., Clark, D. M., & Ehlers, A. (2003). Posttraumatic stress disorder following assault: The role of cognitive processing, trauma memory, and appraisals. *Journal of Consulting and Clinical Psychology, 71,* 419–431.

Janoff-Bulman, R. (1992). *Shattered assumptions: Towards a new psychology of trauma.* New York: Free Press.

Johnson, S. M. (2002). *Emotionally focused couple therapy with trauma survivors: Strengthening attachment bonds.* New York: Guilford Press.

Johnson, S. M., Makinen, J., & Millikin, J. (2001). Attachment injuries in couple relationships: A new perspective on impasses in couples therapy. *Journal of Marital and Family Therapy, 27,* 145–155.

Kobak, R. (1999). The emotional dynamics of disruptions in attachment relationships: Implications for theory, research and clinical intervention. In J. Cassidy & P. R. Shaver (Eds.), *Handbook of attachment: Theory, research, and clinical applications* (pp. 21–43). New York: Guilford Press.

Kobak, R., Little, M., Race, E., & Acosta, M. (2001). Attachment disruptions in seriously emotionally disturbed children: Implications for treatment. *Attachment and Human Development, 3,* 243–257.

Lehman, D. R., Wortman, C. B., & Williams, A. F. (1987). Long-term effects of losing a spouse or child in a motor vehicle crash. *Journal of Personality and Social Psychology, 52,* 218–231.

Lyons-Ruth, K., Bronfman, E., & Atwood, G. (1999). A relational diathesis model of hostile–helpless states of mind: Expressions in mother–infant interaction. In J. Solomon & C. George (Eds.), *Attachment disorganization* (pp. 33–70). New York: Guilford Press.

Main, M., & Cassidy, J. (1988). Categories of response to reunion with parent at age six: Predictable from infant attachment classifications. *Developmental Psychology, 24,* 415–426.

Main, M., & Goldwyn, R. (1998). *Adult attachment scoring and classification system, Version 6.3.* Unpublished manuscript, University of California at Berkeley.

Main, M., & Hesse, E. (1990). Parents' unresolved traumatic experiences are related to infant disorganized attachment status: Is frightened and/or frightening parental behavior the linking mechanism? In M. T. Greenberg, D. Cicchetti, & E. M. Cummings (Eds.), *Attachment in the preschool years: Theory, research and intervention* (pp. 161–182). Chicago: University of Chicago Press.

Main, M., & Solomon, J. (1986). Discovery of an insecure–disorganized/disoriented attachment pattern: Procedures, findings, and implications for classification of behavior. In T. B. Brazelton & M. Yogman (Eds.), *Affective development in infancy* (pp. 95–124). Norwood, NJ: Ablex.

Norris, F. (1992). Epidemiology of trauma: Frequency and impact of different potentially traumatic events on different demographic groups. *Journal of Consulting and Clinical Psychology, 60,* 409–418.

Parkes, C., & Weiss, R. S. (1983). *Recovery from bereavement.* New York: Basic Books.

Resnick, H. S., Kilpatrick, D. G., Dansky, B. S., Saunders, B. E., & Best, C. L. (1993). Prevalence of civilian trauma and posttraumatic stress disorder in a representative national sample of women. *Journal of Consulting and Clinical Psychology, 61,* 984–991.

Riggs, D. S., Byrne, C. A., Weathers, F. W., & Litz, B. T. (1998). The quality of intimate relationships of male Vietnam veterans: Problems associated with posttraumatic stress disorder. *Journal of Traumatic Stress, 11,* 87–101.

Silver, R. L., Boon, C., & Stones, M. H. (1990). The role of coping in support provision: The self-presentational dilemma of victims of life crises. In B. R. Sarason, I. G. Sarason, & G. R. Pierce (Eds.), *Social support: An interactional view* (pp. 397–426). New York: Wiley.

van der Kolk, B. A. (1996). The complexity of adaptation to trauma: Self-regulation, stimulus discrimination, and characterological development. In B. A. van der Kolk, A. C. McFarlane, & L. Weisaeth (Eds.), *Traumatic stress: The effects of overwhelming experience on mind, body, and society* (pp. 182–212). New York: Guilford Press.

van IJzendoorn, M. H., Schuengel, C., & Bakermans-Kranenburg, M. (1999). Disorganized attachment in early childhood: Meta-analysis of precursors, concomitants, and sequelae. *Development and Psychopathology, 11,* 225–249.

Wartner, U. G., Grossman, K., Frommer-Bombik, E., & Suess, G. (1994). Attachment patterns at age six in south Germany: Predictability from infancy and implications for preschool behavior. *Child Development, 65,* 1014–1027.

Wilson, A. E., Calhoun, K. S., & Bernat, J. A. (1999). Risk recognition and trauma related symptoms among sexually revictimized women. *Journal of Consulting and Clinical Psychology, 67,* 705–710.

Zisook, S., Chentsova-Dutton, Y., & Schuchter, S. R. (1998). PTSD following bereavement. *Annals of Clinical Psychiatry, 10,* 157–163.

CHAPTER 14

Anxious Attachment
and Depressive Symptoms

An Interpersonal Perspective

JEFFRY A. SIMPSON
W. STEVEN RHOLES

John Bowlby (1969, 1973, 1980) proposed that psychological disturbance in adulthood often originates from disturbed relationships with attachment figures, both early in life and across the lifespan. He claimed, for example, that

> when a child's attachment behaviour is responded to tardily and unwillingly and is regarded as a nuisance, he [sic] is likely to become anxiously attached, that is apprehensive lest his caregiver be missing or unhelpful when he needs her [sic] and therefore reluctant to leave her side, unwillingly and anxiously obedient, and unconcerned about the troubles of others. Should his caregivers . . . actively reject him, he is likely to develop a pattern of behavior in which avoidance of them competes with his desire for proximity and care and in which angry behavior is apt to become prominent. (1988, p. 82)

According to attachment theory, inadequate or unpredictable care from attachment figures forms the foundation of insecure working models, wherein the self is viewed at some level as being unworthy of love and support and relationship partners are viewed as unable or unwilling to meet one's basic emotional needs. People who develop insecure models tend to have difficult and unhappy relationships in adulthood (Feeney, 1999), and they are more vulnerable to a variety of clinical problems and disorders (Dozier, Stovall, & Albus, 1999; van IJzendoorn & Bakermans-Kranenburg, 1996).

One of Bowlby's central aims in developing attachment theory was to explain why some people are particularly susceptible to depression and depressive symptoms (Bowlby, 1980, 1988). Within the past decade, a growing body of theoretical and empirical work has begun to clarify some of the interpersonal origins of depression (Ingram, 2003). Informed by attachment theory and other recent interpersonal models of depression, we introduce in this chapter a diathesis–stress process model that has organized much of our research concerning how and why the anxious–ambivalent attachment orientation is associated with greater depressive symptomatology (see also Rholes & Simpson, 2004). Although depressive symptoms are more prevalent in both anxiously and avoidantly attached people, the processes through which each attachment orientation is related to depressive symptoms is likely to be quite different. This chapter focuses on attachment ambivalence, primarily because mounting evidence indicates that attachment ambivalence may be more strongly and more closely tied to depressive symptoms than is avoidance. Most of the chapter is organized around a new process model that proposes that, when highly anxious–ambivalent individuals encounter stressful life events, they might display perceptual and behavioral reactions that precipitate, sustain, or perhaps exacerbate depressive symptoms. After discussing features of attachment theory that are most relevant to depression, we review the model, along with several recent studies that provide preliminary support for different pathways in the model. Besides offering a detailed description of processes that might generate and sustain depressive symptoms, the model also accentuates some novel pathways to depression and introduces two new theoretical concepts: dysfunctional relationship attitudes and relationship deprivation.

ADULT ATTACHMENT ORIENTATIONS

Structured on the premise that patterns of attachment established early in life could affect attachment orientations in adulthood, two independent lines of adult attachment research were launched in the 1980s. Both lines sought to establish whether Ainsworth, Blehar, Waters, and Wall's (1978) concept of attachment patterns in children might describe attachment organization in adults. In the first attempt to measure adult attachment orientations, Main, Kaplan, and Cassidy (1985) developed a standardized interview that inquired about childhood experiences with and perceptions of attachment figures (the Adult Attachment Interview, AAI; Main & Goldwyn, 1994). The AAI measures adults' "state of mind" with regard to various important attachment issues. Individuals who respond to the AAI in ways indicating that they cannot or have not come to terms with what they view as adverse early experiences with their attachment figures are classified as being "preoccupied" with relationships. Those who answer the AAI by trying to suppress their attachment system to avoid thinking about or remembering difficult childhood experiences with their attachment figures are classified as "dismissive" of relationships. Persons classified as "secure" (free/autonomous) respond to the AAI in a less defensive manner than dismissive individuals, and they discuss difficult attachment issues from their childhoods more directly and openly than preoccupied people.

Almost concurrently with Main and colleagues' work, Hazan and Shaver (1987) developed a brief self-report measure of attachment orientations. This measure, which inquires about romantic relationships in adulthood instead of perceptions of early parent–child interactions and events, categorized respondents into one of three exclusive attachment categories that paralleled Ainsworth and colleagues' (1978) secure, avoidant, and anxious–ambivalent patterns of infant–caregiver attachment. Recent research has confirmed that two orthogonal dimensions actually underlie Hazan and Shaver's three categories (Griffin & Bartholomew, 1994; Simpson, Rholes, & Phillips, 1996), and these dimensions have become the focus of most contemporary research on adult romantic attachment (Brennan, Clark, & Shaver, 1998). The first dimension, commonly labeled *avoidance*, measures the degree to which individuals desire limited intimacy with, and strive to remain psychologically and emotionally independent from, their romantic partners. The second dimension, typically labeled *anxiety* or *ambivalence*, indexes the degree to which people worry that their romantic partners cannot be relied on to provide care and emotional support. The model that we describe here focuses on attachment anxiety–ambivalence as measured by self-report scales, most of which are based on Hazen and Shaver's original three-category attachment measure.

ADULT ATTACHMENT AND DEPRESSION

Adult attachment measures—both the AAI and the self-report romantic scales—correlate with many problematic conditions, including depression, eating disorders, alcohol abuse, domestic violence, and assorted personality disturbances (Brennan & Shaver, 1998; Dozier et al., 1999; van IJzendoorn & Bakermans-Kranenburg, 1996). Given its prevalence and close theoretical connections with interpersonal processes, depression and depressive symptoms have been granted proportionally more attention by attachment researchers. Several studies of psychiatric patients have shown that unipolar depression is more common in people classified as preoccupied (Cole-Detke & Kobak, 1996; Fonagy et al., 1996; Rosenstein & Horowitz, 1996) and dismissive (Patrick, Hobson, Castle, Howard, & Maughan, 1994) on the AAI. Research investigating adult romantic attachment orientations (styles) has also established clear links between avoidant and, particularly, anxious–ambivalent attachment and depressive symptoms. In a representative U.S. sample of adults, for instance, Mickelson, Kessler, and Shaver (1997) found that, relative to secure people, those who reported being more avoidant or more anxious–ambivalent scored higher on a measure tapping DSM-III major depressive episodes. Administering the Brief Symptom Index (Derogatis & Melisaratos, 1983) to a large community sample, Cooper, Shaver, and Collins (1998) confirmed that anxiously attached individuals experience the highest levels of depressive symptoms, secure individuals report the lowest levels, and avoidant individuals fall in between. Similar effects have been found for young women making the somewhat stressful transition from high school to adult life (Burge et al., 1997; Hammen et al., 1995). In marriages, anxiously attached individuals are more likely to report depressive symptoms, especially if their marital adjustment scores are lower (Scott & Cordova, 2002). Viewed together, these studies reveal that people who are insecurely attached to their parents or their romantic partners—particularly preoccupied (as measured by the AAI) or anxious–ambivalent (from self-reports) individuals—are at greater risk for experiencing unipolar depression as well as more temporary depressive symptoms.

In recent years, there has been burgeoning interest in understanding the interpersonal processes through which depressive symptoms might be instigated, maintained, or exacerbated (see Hammen, 1995). Two types of interpersonal dysfunction were initially believed to trigger or worsen depressive symptoms (Arieti & Bemporad, 1980). One form, known as the *dependent type,* originates from perceiving oneself as being extremely dependent on support from others and worrying that sufficient support might not be available. A second form, termed the *evaluative type,* stems from perceiving that significant others will accept a person only if certain conditions of worth are met.

Informed by this perspective, Hammen (1995) developed an integrative cognitive–interpersonal model of depression whereby susceptibility to depression is presumed to be governed by three factors: (1) biological and/or socialization experiences in the family of origin, (2) exposure to highly stressful current events or environments, and (3) dysfunctional perceptions of self and/or significant others, all of which increase the probability of engaging in maladaptive interpersonal behaviors (see also Hammen, 2000). What makes Hammen's model appealing is its breadth, its recognition that early life events may affect the onset and maintenance of depressive symptoms in adulthood, and the ease with which concepts and principles central to attachment theory fit with different components of the model.

Few attachment scholars have proposed models outlining the specific interpersonal processes that might render highly ambivalent people so vulnerable to depressive symptoms. To fill this conceptual gap, we have developed a preliminary process model. Portions of our model and the research that has tested it have been guided by a diathesis–stress approach that incorporates certain elements contained in Hammen's (1995) model, particularly those that involve dysfunctional perceptions and maladaptive interpersonal behaviors. Our model, however, focuses more directly on attachment-relevant constructs, processes, and issues per se.

AN INTERPERSONAL MODEL OF AMBIVALENCE
AND DEPRESSIVE SYMPTOMS

Attachment theory maintains that working models (schemas) comprise at least four components: (1) beliefs and expectations about partners and relationships, (2) rules that link particular beliefs and expectations to behaviors, (3) habitual emotional reactions to attachment-related events, and (4) episodic memories of attachment experiences (Bowlby, 1980; Collins & Allard, 2001). Two of the cardinal beliefs that anchor anxious working models are the sense that one is unworthy of care and support and that others cannot be relied on to provide care and support. These negative beliefs presumably generate negative expectations about what one is likely to experience in close relationships. In tandem, these beliefs and expectations function as negative perceptual filters, systematically biasing the partner and relationship perceptions of highly anxious–ambivalent persons (Bowlby, 1973, 1980).

These beliefs and expectations should motivate highly anxious persons to take steps to prevent their partners from ignoring and eventually leaving them, especially in stressful situations that activate their attachment systems (Cassidy & Berlin, 1994). To guard against the prospect of relationship loss, highly anxious individuals become hypervigilant in relationship-threatening situations (Simpson, Ickes, & Grich, 1999), leading them to enact suspicious, controlling, and/or clingy behaviors and to make exaggerated and persistent demands concerning their need for support. Characteristically anxious emotions include fear about abandonment and anger directed at partners who do not meet their exaggerated desires for care, attention, and emotional support. Many of the episodic memories associated with anxious working models should confirm and strengthen the negative beliefs and expectations that highly anxious individuals have about themselves and their partners. Salient memories are likely to involve specific past experiences of either rejection or neglect or role-reversal experiences in which individuals had to provide inappropriate emotional care and support to someone who should have served as an older and wiser attachment figure.

Model Constructs

Our model, which is shown in Figure 14.1, contains several constructs. From the outset, we draw a clear distinction between "baseline" and "activated" levels of attachment ambivalence, concepts that are analogous to trait-versus-state forms of anxiousness. The baseline attachment ambivalence level reflects the degree to which an individual possesses the central, defining features of anxious working models. Individuals vary in the strength and confidence with which they endorse beliefs or harbor expectations that epitomize anxious models; in the strength of the connections between beliefs, expectations, and behavioral rules; in the intensity of the habitual emotional reactions evoked in response to critical attachment events; and in the number and type of episodic memories housed within their anxious models. Together, these variations produce individual differences in baseline attachment ambivalence levels, which are indirectly assessed by self-report attachment-style scales.

The activation-level construct refers to the current cognitive accessibility of anxious working models. We assume that the greater the accessibility, the more likely ongoing perceptions, emotions, and behavior will be influenced by anxious working models. Thus, when anxious models are highly accessible, individuals should be more likely to perceive the social environment, to react emotionally, and to behave in ways that are prototypical of highly anxious people. When accessibility is low, however, individuals should be less prone to perceive, feel, and behave in a characteristically anxious manner.

The level of activation should be contingent on specific situational factors. Bowlby (1969) proposed that attachment behaviors in young children, such as searching for or signaling an attachment figure, are typically elicited by hunger, fear, fatigue, illness, or separation from attachment figures (i.e., by felt insecurity; Sroufe & Waters, 1977). Similar vulnerabilities also appear to activate attachment working models in adults (Shaver & Mikulincer, 2002). In addition, situations that are directly relevant to (or associated with) the central components of working models (such as relationship or self-related beliefs and expectations, characteristic behaviors and affect, episodic memories) should also trigger working models. For example, one central feature of anxious working models is the staunch expectation that attachment figures might eventually leave. For persons who possess these models, any situation that accentuates the possibility of abandonment (e.g., a serious relationship conflict) ought to increase the activation of anxious models, even if they do not produce conscious feelings of greater vulnerability. According to our model, therefore, working models can be activated in two ways: through exposure to strong, situationally induced feelings of vulnerability (felt insecurity) and through exposure to common events that trigger the core concerns underlying specific working models.

Direct measures of attachment activation have yet to be developed. Nevertheless, several studies have shown that persons with equivalent baseline levels of attachment ambivalence and avoidance behave differently when they encounter situational factors that should engage their working models. Simpson, Rholes, and Nelligan (1992), for instance, found that highly avoidant women who were more distressed about engaging in an impending anxiety-provoking task were less likely to seek emotional support from their romantic partners than were less distressed highly avoidant women. Conversely, highly secure women who were more distressed were more likely to seek support than highly secure women who were less distressed. In other words, heightened distress appeared to increase the accessibility of avoidant and secure working models, which in turn led women to behave in ways prototypical of either high avoidance (not seeking support) or high security (actively seeking support).

Our model contains two new constructs: dysfunctional relationship attitudes and perceptions of relationship deprivation. Based on observations in therapy sessions, Aaron Beck noted that depressed people tend to place stringent and rigid conditions on their personal happiness (see Beck, Rush, Shaw, & Emery, 1979; Weissman & Beck, 1978). They often agree, for instance, with statements such as "I can be happy only if everyone likes and respects me." Beck referred to these conditions on happiness as "dysfunctional" because they often are very difficult to fulfill and, hence, may unduly limit personal happiness. Extending these ideas, we propose that highly anxious individuals may impose similar conditions on their intimate relationships. One such condition might be that happiness in life cannot be attained without a nearly perfect partner and relationship. To the extent that this condition (attitude) is adopted, it should place tremendous daily pressure on partners and relationships. Highly anxious individuals do, in fact, base more of their personal well-being on their daily perceptions of their partners and relationships, and their relationships tend to suffer more as a result of this (Campbell, Simpson, Boldry, & Kashy, 2003).

Allowing one's general life satisfaction to be heavily dictated by one's relationship should be especially dysfunctional if the conditions that must be satisfied to achieve a "great" relationship are themselves dysfunctional. According to our model, the conditions that people place on their partners and relationships can be either rigid or more flexible, and they can be either easy or difficult to fulfill. Rigid conditions must be fully met at all times in order for a relationship to be considered satisfactory. Flexible conditions can be met only partially or occasionally, with failures to meet them being excused when other conditions are sufficiently met. Conditions on relationship satisfaction that are rigid, unrealistic, or virtually impossible to achieve are dysfunctional in that they impose severe constraints on the attainment of relationship satisfaction. According to our model, the more dysfunctional attitudes an individual holds, the more he or she should view the partner and relationship as disappointing.

Thus we propose that individuals can hold dysfunctional attitudes about partners and relationships at two levels. Higher level dysfunctional attitudes make satisfaction with one's life too heavily contingent on the nature of one's current relationship, whereas lower level dysfunctional attitudes make satisfaction with one's relationship contingent on rigidly held conditions that are unrealistic and difficult to fulfill. The combination of higher level and lower level dysfunctional relationship attitudes should increase the probability that individuals feel something important is missing from their lives. We hypothesize that higher level and lower level dysfunctional relationship attitudes should be more prevalent in persons who manifest higher baseline (state) levels of attachment ambivalence.

A likely consequence of holding dysfunctional relationship attitudes is a sense of relationship deprivation. Relationship deprivation differs from both loneliness and dissatisfaction with one's current relationship. We define it as a sense of being deprived of something one deserves, which occurs when people believe that satisfactory relationships are a mandatory condition for happiness in life, and when their current relationships (or their history of relationships) do not meet their conditions for satisfaction. Individuals who experience strong relationship deprivation may feel as if they have been cheated by life or by their partners. Accompanying feelings and emotions are likely to include frustration, anger, resentment, self-blame, and ultimately a sense of hopelessness.

Model Pathways

We now turn to the pathways that link the constructs in our model. Consistent with Bowlby (1969), we propose that baseline ambivalence levels should be partially determined by experiences (or perceptions of experiences) with parents and peers in attachment-relevant situations throughout social development (see Path A in Figure 14.1). At the same time, we acknowledge that early attachment experiences could have direct effects on depressive symptoms later in adulthood that are not mediated through current baseline levels of ambivalence (Path M). Path B indicates that activation levels should be higher when an individual experiencing an activating situation enters it with a higher baseline level of ambivalence. Path C suggests that the triggering situational factors discussed previously should heighten the activation and the influence of anxious working models.

Paths D, E, F, and G indicate the proposed processes through which anxious working models should operate once they are activated. When

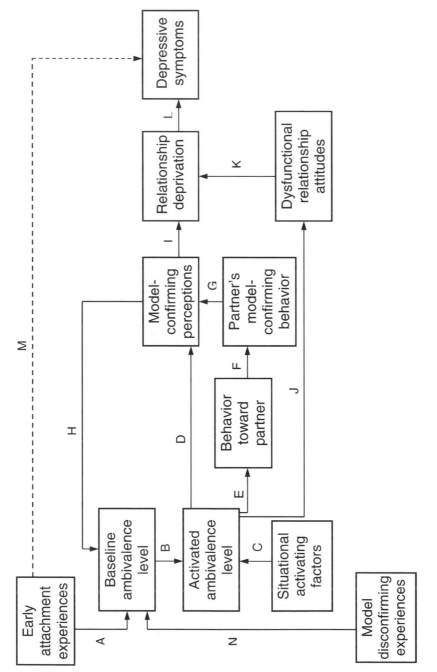

FIGURE 14.1. Interpersonal model of attachment ambivalence and depressive symptoms.

the activation level of anxious working models increases, the likelihood that social perceptions will be processed through the "negative filters" contained in these models should increase. This in turn should increase the likelihood that relationship partners and events will be construed in ways that confirm the pessimistic beliefs and expectations that characterize anxious working models (Path D). Increasing the activation level should also increase the likelihood that behavior—particularly behavior toward relationship partners—will be directed by the beliefs, expectations, and behavioral routines housed in anxious working models (Path E). The consequence of such behavior is likely to be withdrawal, anger, or other forms of behavior by the partner that are consistent with, and thus confirm, the already pessimistic beliefs and expectations contained in these working models (Path G). Over time, model-confirming perceptions may feed back on baseline ambivalence levels (Path H), either sustaining or increasing these levels. Baseline ambivalence levels, however, may be attenuated by major model-disconfirming experiences (Path N).

Path J represents the hypothesized association between activated ambivalence levels and dysfunctional relationship attitudes. Paths I and K indicate that the combination of more negative perceptions of one's partner or relationship and greater dysfunctional attitudes should produce greater feelings of relationship deprivation, which should launch, maintain, or aggravate depressive symptoms (Path L).

We now discuss two large-scale research projects that provide provisional tests of some of the pathways in our model (Figure 14.1). Because the model emphasizes the crucial role that stress and the vulnerability associated with it assume in activating the ambivalent working model, both projects focus on how individuals with different early experiences and/or contemporary attachment orientations cope during major life transitions. We first describe the findings of a project that explored how perceptions of childhood experiences with parents and current romantic partners are linked to depressive symptoms in young adults as they navigate a common life transition—leaving home and starting college. We then describe several sets of findings from another research project that has investigated a different stressful life transition—having a first child.

ATTACHMENT EXPERIENCES WITH PARENTS
AND ADJUSTMENT TO COLLEGE LIFE

Bowlby believed that growing up with "ordinarily affectionate" parents usually produces such strong expectations for emotional support that it becomes "difficult to imagine a world in which support is not available" (Bowlby, 1973, p. 208). Growing up with unsupportive parents, on the other hand, is likely to leave one with "no confidence that a care-taking figure can ever be truly available and dependable" (Bowlby, 1973, p. 208). Paths A and M represent the effects that these early experiences with attachment figures are likely to have on depressive symptoms in adulthood. Path A suggests that adverse experiences in the family of origin launch the formation of anxious working models. It implies that persons who have higher baseline levels of ambivalence in adulthood should have experienced more difficult childhoods than their less anxious counterparts. A substantial body of research shows that patterns of attachment to caregivers in infancy are related to the ways in which caregivers behave toward their children (Ainsworth et al., 1978; van IJzendoorn, 1995). Furthermore, longitudinal research has confirmed that patterns of attachment to caregivers in childhood are correlated with adult attachment orientations assessed by the AAI (Waters, Merrick, Treboux, Crowell, & Albersheim, 2000; Waters, Weinfield, & Hamilton, 2000). Nonetheless, there appears to be a reasonable amount of predictable discontinuity between attachment to caregivers and attachment orientations in adulthood (see Fraley and Brumbaugh, Chapter 4, this volume). This is consistent with Path H in the model, which implies that attachment working models must be periodically reconfirmed by social experience to remain stable over time.

We do not know of any longitudinal studies that relate early experiences to self-reported attachment orientations in adulthood. Some research indicates that memories of experiences with early attachment figures systematically vary with adult romantic attachment orientations. Individuals with anxious–ambivalent romantic attachment styles, for instance, recount having had colder and less caring fathers, less understanding mothers, and poorer parental relationships in general (Hazan & Shaver, 1987). Highly ambivalent people also hold mixed and sometimes conflicting views of their parents from childhood, describing them as inconsistent and punitive but also as more benevolent (Levy, Blatt, & Shaver, 1998). People with more ambivalent attachment styles also remember their fathers as less loving and more neglectful during early childhood (Shaver, Belsky, & Brennan, 2000). Research relevant to Path A, therefore, seems to provide modest support for this segment of the model.

Much less is known about whether early attachment experiences exert a *direct* effect on depressive symptoms later in life (which explains why Path M is depicted with a dashed line in our model). Some recent studies have hinted that insecure attachment to parents (Sund & Wichstrom, 2002) and memories of parental rejection (Crockenberg & Leerkes, 2003) may both directly contribute to the development of depressive symptoms in adulthood. Moreover, Hammen (1995) has conjectured that certain critical events within the family of origin might directly precipitate depressive symptoms years later. Evidence pertaining to Path M from attachment research is provided most directly by the small literature on "earned security." Researchers within the AAI tradition have labeled persons who are categorized as secure on the AAI despite having experienced troubled parenting as "earned secures." Because family experiences and attachment state of mind are at odds with one another, earned secures provide an ideal group with which to study Path M.

Only one such study has examined depression. Pearson, Cohn, Cowan, and Cowan (1994) found that earned secures were as vulnerable to depressive symptoms as persons who had adverse childhoods but who were classified as insecure. Though this might be taken as evidence that earned security is not a valuable concept, the results of this study suggest otherwise. Even though they were equally vulnerable to depression, earned secures and insecures with equivalent family histories differed in their own parenting effectiveness. Earned secures were rated to be more effective parents. With respect to depression, this study reveals that early attachment experiences may exert separate effects on depressive symptoms in adulthood that are not mediated by adult attachment orientations.

To our knowledge, only one study of earned security has measured self-report attachment orientations. Grich (2001) proposed that poor parenting initiates the processes through which anxious working models develop, but that attachment ambivalence and poor parenting are far from isomorphic, owing to experiences outside of the parent–child relationship that may influence attachment orientations. She also proposed that the experience of poor parenting (defined as having memories of one or both parents being unloving, rejecting, or neglecting) should be especially likely to translate into depressive symptoms in adulthood if poor parenting is viewed during adulthood through the negative lens of anxious working models. Grich argues that persons who experienced adverse parental behavior yet still developed a sense of security in adulthood should have found meaning in their difficult childhoods, might have found ways to forgive their parents, or could have otherwise defused the emotional impact of the adverse parenting they received. She also suggests that earned security may counteract the potentially negative residue of having received deficient parenting.

To test this diathesis–stress hypothesis, Grich (2001) asked people who had just entered college to complete the AAI, standard self-report measures of adult romantic attachment orientations, and the College Adjustment Scale (Anton & Reed, 1991), which contains a depressive-symptoms subscale. Trained raters then scored participants' AAI transcripts, focusing on the AAI state-of-experience scales. Participants were assigned scores for "parenting risk" based on the amount of unloving, rejecting, or neglectful behavior that raters inferred the interviewees had experienced.

Consistent with the studies reviewed previously, highly ambivalent individuals (assessed by the self-report romantic attachment scales) were more likely to report depressive symptoms compared with other persons.

In addition, people who had higher parenting-risk scores also reported more depressive symptoms. Providing provisional support for the direct effect implied by Path M in our model, both attachment ambivalence and parenting risk predicted greater depressive symptoms when the other was statistically controlled. A significant interaction involving adult ambivalence and childhood experience also emerged. It revealed that individuals who scored lower in attachment ambivalence reported fewer depressive symptoms, regardless of the quality of their earlier parenting. Similarly, those who were highly ambivalent and experienced good parenting also reported relatively few symptoms. Highly ambivalent individuals who experienced poor parenting, however, reported substantially higher depressive symptoms than all other participants in the study. The impact of perceived early parenting on depressive symptoms, therefore, was moderated by individuals' degree of ambivalence.[1] Grich's (2001) results suggest that how adverse early experiences are construed may determine how damaging they are in adulthood.

THE TRANSITION TO PARENTHOOD

Becoming a parent for the first time is a challenging and stressful event for the vast majority of people. It is commonly associated with declines in marital satisfaction, increases in marital conflict, reductions in companionate activities, and, in some cases, increases in depression (Belsky, Lang, & Rovine, 1985; Belsky & Pensky, 1988; Belsky, Spanier, & Rovine, 1983; Cowan & Cowan, 2000; Cowan, Cowan, Core, & Core, 1978; Cowan et al., 1985; Heinicke, 1995; Levy-Shiff, 1994). These decrements in well-being are not universal, however. Tucker and Aron (1993) have found that variation in personal and marital well-being tends to increase during the transition period, with most new parents experiencing declines but some actually showing improvements.

During the past few years, we have investigated the ways in which self-reported romantic attachment orientations—especially ambivalence—are systematically related to pre- to postnatal changes in marital satisfaction (Rholes, Simpson, Campbell, & Grich, 2001), depressive symptoms (Simpson, Rholes, Campbell, Tran, & Wilson, 2003), and attachment orientations (Simpson, Rholes, Campbell, & Wilson, 2003). These studies, all of which were conducted on the same sample of married couples, are relevant to the concept of activated ambivalence levels and pathways D, E, F, G, and H in Figure 14.1.[2]

The data for this project were collected from 106 couples (both wives and their husbands) at two points during the transition to parenthood: approximately 6 weeks before the birth of their first child and at 6 months postpartum. During the prenatal period, women completed self-report scales that assessed their attachment orientations, their perceptions of the amount of support available from their husbands, their perceptions of the amount of anger their husbands directed toward them, their marital satisfaction, and their depressive symptoms.[3] Husbands completed scales that assessed their attachment orientations, the amount of support they perceived giving to their wives, the amount of anger they perceived directing at their wives, their martial satisfaction, and their depressive symptoms. During the postnatal period, the same information was collected a second time.

Chronic Stress as an Activator of Working Models

Certain situations should enhance the impact that insecure attachment orientations have on relationship-based perceptions, information processing, and behavior (Bowlby, 1969, 1988; Kobak & Duemmler, 1994). The situations that should do so are those that increase the activation level of an individual's working model. Situations that produce feelings of vulnerability—such as those that induce fear, illness, pain, fatigue, or prolonged stress, as well as those that signal the loss of or prolonged separation from attachment figures—should activate attachment needs and working models in nearly all individuals. Under these general activating conditions, attachment orientations (and the working models that underlie them) should have a stronger influence on interpersonal perceptions and behavior than is true of more mundane situations (Mikulincer, Florian, & Weller, 1993; Simpson et al., 1992, 1996). Working models should also be activated by situations that make salient the "core" fears and concerns associated with different forms of attachment insecurity. With respect to attachment ambivalence, serious problems or conflicts with attachment figures are likely to make beliefs and emotions associated with relationship loss or abandonment salient, thereby activating ambivalent working models above their chronically high baseline levels, even if they do not produce strong feelings of vulnerability (Kobak & Duemmler, 1994; Simpson & Rholes, 1994). Because the arrival of a new child often heightens stress and conflict in many relationships and may elicit memories of deficient caregiving by one's own parents (Bowlby, 1988), the transition to parenthood—especially the early postnatal phase—should activate the working models of highly ambivalent people.

The pivotal role that these factors assume in triggering ambivalent working models is represented in Path C of our model (reflecting situational activating factors). We reason that when chronic or acute stress is low, ambivalent working models should remain relatively quiescent (at their baseline ambivalence levels). When stress is high, however, ambivalent models should become more accessible or activated. In general, the stronger the degree of activation, the more influence ambivalent models should exert on attachment-relevant perceptions and behavior. Thus the escalating amount of stress and vulnerability that most people experience between the prenatal and the postnatal periods (stemming from factors such as the lingering effects of childbirth, sleep deprivation, fatigue, the daily demands of child care, and increased relationship conflicts) should activate the working models of highly ambivalent women in particular, causing their attachment and relationship-relevant perceptions and behavior to change correspondingly. Increases in activation levels from the prenatal to the postnatal period should lead to stronger correlations between ambivalence levels, as measured by self-report scales, and perceptions, emotions, and behaviors.

Consistent with this premise, the correlations between women's levels of ambivalence and their perceptions of spousal support, spousal anger, and marital satisfaction in our transition-to-parenthood data were significantly larger during the more taxing postnatal period than during the relatively less stressful prenatal period (Rholes et al., 2001). In combination with other studies that have examined different stressors (e.g., Mikulincer et al., 1993; Simpson et al., 1996), these findings imply that ambivalent working models do affect attachment-relevant thoughts, feelings, and actions more strongly during heightened stress.

Ambivalence and Marital Processes

According to attachment theorists, highly ambivalent individuals should have attachment systems that are easily activated (see Path B) and tend to remain "online" (Bowlby, 1973; Kobak & Duemmler, 1994; Simpson & Rholes, 1994). Moreover, the working models of these individuals should bias their information processing in model-confirming and sustaining ways (Bowlby, 1973; Collins & Allard, 2001). Bowlby (1973, pp. 368–369), in fact, claimed that the cognitive predispositions underlying attachment orientations "determine what is perceived and what ignored, how a new situation is construed, and what plan of action is likely to be constructed to deal with it." Because they perceive having received unpredictable care and support in the past, highly ambivalent persons should anticipate that future attachment figures also might not be supportive in times of need. Accordingly, we hypothesized that highly ambivalent women would perceive less prenatal spousal support than other women. Bowlby also conjectured that working models should lead people to behave in ways that might compel their attachment figures to confirm their worst fears and worries (that is, their "core" concerns). Hence, we also expected that highly ambivalent women might behave in ways that undermine their husbands' motivation or tendency to provide support. We also predicted that the adverse impact of perceiving lower levels of spousal support on measures of marital satisfaction and depressive symptoms would be stronger for highly ambivalent women because, despite their mistrust of attachment figures, they should still crave support and react more negatively to its absence. Finally, we surmised that, even though these effects should be stronger during the more stressful postnatal period, they should also be evident during the somewhat stressful prenatal phase.

Supporting these hypotheses and various paths in our model (Figure 14.1), highly ambivalent women viewed their husbands as less supportive during the prenatal period than did less ambivalent women. These perceptions, of course, could be an accurate reflection of their husbands' behavior (Path G in the model), a result of the perceptual biases of these women (Path D), or both processes. The perceptions of husbands offer some support for the first alternative (Path G). Regardless of their own attachment scores, men married to more ambivalent women perceived offering less support to their wives, especially during the more stressful postnatal period. They also viewed their wives as more immature, more dependent, emotionally weaker, and less emotionally stable than did men married to less ambivalent women.

Other evidence, however, suggests that highly ambivalent women may have perceived lower-than-justified levels of spousal support (Path D). Despite the fact that their husbands reported being less supportive, highly ambivalent women perceived that their husbands were significantly less supportive than even their husbands perceived being, whereas less ambivalent women perceived that their husbands were more supportive than their husbands perceived being. The associations between women's ambivalence and these "over" and "under" perceptions of spousal support remained statistically significant when wives' and husbands' marital satisfaction and other measures of marital quality (e.g., love, the amount of daily conflict) were partialed. In other words, the tendency for highly ambivalent women to perceive less support than their husbands claimed to provide was *not* entirely attributable to differences in the marital quality or functioning of more versus less ambivalent women. This suggests that the low perceptions of spousal support harbored by highly ambivalent women might be partially distorted by their working models.

A recent laboratory study lends credence to this interpretation. Collins and Feeney (2000) gave participants either a clearly supportive message or an ambiguously worded message (ostensibly written by each participant's dating partner) right before participants were about to engage in a moderately stressful task (delivering an impromptu speech). Highly ambivalent people interpreted the ambiguous message as much less supportive than did less ambivalent people. They also perceived their partner's behavior in a subsequent, unrelated task as significantly less supportive than did neutral observers. These findings also indicate that highly ambivalent people are "prepared" to perceive their partners in a less supportive light, providing further evidence for Path D in our model.[4]

In sum, the negatively skewed perceptions of highly ambivalent people may emanate both from perceptual biases driven by their working models *and* from reduced levels of actual support provided by their partners (Paths D and G in the model).

What might discourage the partners of highly ambivalent people from providing greater support? The findings of three recent studies suggest that highly ambivalent women may behave in ways that alienate their partners, particularly when they are upset (see Paths E and F in the model). Rholes, Simpson, and Oriña (1999) led women to believe that they were going to experience a set of "anxiety-provoking" procedures. Before the procedures began, each woman was led to a room where she waited with her nonstressed male dating partner, who was waiting to do a different, mundane task and, therefore, could provide support. After 5 minutes, each woman was told that, due to equipment malfunctions, she would not have to do the anxiety-provoking task. Both the 5-minute "stress" period and the 5-minute "recovery" period (after women had been told that they would not experience the procedures) were unobtrusively videotaped and then rated by trained observers. Highly ambivalent women who displayed greater anxiety and sought more comfort and support from their partners during the "stress" period behaved in a more withdrawn and angry manner toward their partners during the "recovery" period, largely because they viewed the support they had received during the "stress" period as deficient. If this pattern of resentful behavior becomes chronic, it could erode their partners' motivation or willingness to provide support, especially in situations in which highly ambivalent persons truly need comfort and support.

Simpson, Rholes, and Phillips (1996) have also documented that, when highly ambivalent women try to resolve major, relationship-based problems with their romantic partners, they tend to display greater anxiety and more dysfunctional conflict resolution tactics (rated by observers). They also report being more distressed and angrier than other women, and they report significant pre- to postdiscussion declines in feelings of subjective closeness to their partners. Less ambivalent women, by comparison, feel slightly closer to their partners after discussing major relationship problems. These behavioral and perceptual reactions also might alienate the partners of highly ambivalent individuals. Finally, though not focusing on attachment per se, Downey, Freitas, Michaelis, and Khouri (1998) have found that women who are more rejection sensitive (most likely highly ambivalent women) display similar behaviors that eventually elicit rejection from their romantic partners.

Additional processes could also undermine partner support. To the extent that highly ambivalent women perceive their husbands as less supportive than their husbands perceive they really are (Rholes et al., 2001), the feedback that these husbands receive from their wives is likely to be neither self-verifying (Swann, 1990) nor self-enhancing (Murray & Holmes, 1997). Over time, these husbands may come to believe that their ambivalent wives' needs for support are unending and flow from their stable—and perhaps unchangeable—personality traits. This interpretation would explain why the husbands of highly ambivalent women in our transition project viewed their wives as more dependent, weak, immature, and emotionally unstable. Alternately, wives' negative perceptions of spousal support might gradually change how their husbands view themselves (see Drigotas, Rusbult, Wieselquist, & Whitton, 1999). It is possible that a negotiated reality may emerge between highly ambivalent wives and their husbands, whereby husbands eventually accept their wives' views of them as being unsupportive and then behave in a less supportive manner (see Path G).[5]

Path J implies that people who are more ambivalent (1) believe that "great" relationships are essential to happiness in life and (2) impose stringent conditions that must be met before they can be happy with their relationships. The idea that stringent conditions must be met in order for highly ambivalent people to be happy with their relationships suggests that problems in relationships will have a stronger impact on more ambivalent people. The results of our transition study provide support for this hypothesis. Highly ambivalent women who perceived that their husbands were less supportive before childbirth also reported being more dissatisfied with their marriages than did less ambivalent women who also viewed their husbands as equally unsupportive. Furthermore, statistical interactions involving women's prenatal ambivalence and their prenatal perceptions of spousal support confirmed that highly ambivalent women who perceived less prenatal support became significantly more dissatisfied between the prenatal and the postnatal period and perceived that their husbands became significantly less supportive across time. As discussed earlier, one of the "core" concerns of highly ambivalent individuals involves wanting emotional support yet fearing that it will not be available when needed. When support is perceived as low or deficient during a critical life event such as the transition to parenthood, highly ambivalent individuals' worst suspicions and fears about their attachment figures may be implicitly confirmed.[6]

Ambivalence and Depression

According to our model, ambivalence should be linked to depressive symptoms most directly through feelings of relationship deprivation (Path L)—the sense that one's current partner is not fulfilling basic relationship needs that are essential to happiness. Relationship deprivation, in turn, should be affected by model-confirming perceptions (Path I) and dysfunctional relationship attitudes (Path K). As discussed earlier, dysfunctional relationship attitudes exist when individuals believe that they cannot be happy unless their current partners can meet their lofty and rather inflexible relationship expectations. Individuals who are most likely to experience relationship deprivation should: (1) place many stringent relationship-based contingencies on their happiness (e.g., "Without the 'right' kind of relationship, I simply cannot be happy") and (2) be highly critical and judgmental of their partner or relationship. According to our model, dysfunctional relationship attitudes are a specific form of Beck's more general dysfunctional attitudes construct, and they should be associated with depressive symptoms in the same way that general dysfunctional attitudes are.[7]

Highly ambivalent persons meet almost all of the criteria for vulnerability to depressive symptoms. They perceive their partners and relationships more negatively than may be warranted, they view their relationships as not fully meeting their strict contingencies for total happiness (cf. Crocker & Wolfe, 2001), and they endorse many of Beck's dysfunctional general attitudes (Roberts, Gotlib, & Kassel, 1996). Depressive symptoms in highly ambivalent people, therefore, should be more closely yoked to their current perceptions of the partner and relationship. When they perceive their relationships as good (i.e., as currently meeting the conditions necessary for happiness), highly ambivalent persons should experience fewer depressive symptoms—perhaps even fewer than securely attached individuals. However, when they perceive that their relationships are not meeting their stringent standards, highly ambivalent individuals should be more susceptible to depressive symptoms. The relationship perceptions of highly ambivalent persons do, in fact, vacillate more across short periods of time than is true of other people (Campbell et al., 2003; Tidwell, Reis, & Shaver, 1996). This evidence insinuates that depressive symptoms could also be more temporally variable in highly ambivalent people, depending on the degree to which they perceive that their relationship needs and expectations are being met at specific points in time.

When we started our transition-to-parenthood project, validated scales measuring relationship deprivation and dysfunctional relationship attitudes (the two new constructs in our model) had not been developed. Consequently, we were able to test only the connections between women's ambivalence, their perceptions of their husband's support and anger, and their depressive symptoms. As reported in Simpson and colleagues (2003), women who were more ambivalent did report having more prenatal depressive symptoms than other women, and this effect was partially mediated through their perceptions of receiving lower prenatal spousal support. When stress was greater at 6 months postpartum, ambivalence accounted for twice as much variance in women's depressive symptoms as it did during the prenatal period. Moreover, postnatal ambivalence and postnatal perceptions of spousal support interacted, with depressive symptoms being greatest among highly ambivalent women who perceived less postnatal spousal support. Similar to the prenatal period, the main effect of postnatal ambivalence on postnatal depressive symptoms was partially mediated through perceptions of lower postnatal spousal support. Most important, changes in depressive symptoms from the prenatal to the postnatal period exhibited similar patterns. That is, highly ambivalent women became significantly more depressed across the transition than did less ambivalent women, and this was most evident in highly ambivalent women who entered the transition perceiving less spousal support. In addition, the link between prenatal ambivalence and pre- to postnatal increases in depressive symptoms was partially mediated by perceived pre- to postpartum declines in spousal support, just as Bowlby (1988) anticipated.

To summarize, data from the first two published studies of our transition-to-parenthood project (Rholes et al., 2001; Simpson et al., 2003) primarily address issues pertaining to Paths B, C, D, E, F, and G in our model. The findings revealed that highly ambivalent women perceive less spousal support across the transition to parenthood, especially during the more stressful postnatal period. These perceptions of low or deficient support appear to have their origins both in the perceptual biases of these women (to not "see" or acknowledge available support) and in differences in the amount of support their husbands most likely provided. Highly ambivalent women are also more susceptible to declines in marital quality and increases in depressive symptoms across the transition period. Both of these changes are partially mediated through perceived pre- to postpartum declines in spousal support, which highly ambivalent individuals—particularly women—should find especially troubling. Thus the conditions that highly ambivalent people may "require" to be happy—having highly stable and unwaveringly supportive relationships—may be eroded by their perceptual biases, their interpersonal styles of relating, and their partners' behavioral responses to them, particularly when highly ambivalent people are distressed.

Changes in Attachment Orientation

Our model suggests that baseline levels of ambivalence should be established by earlier attachment experiences (Path A) and by feedback from contemporary model-confirming perceptions and events (Path H). One major misconception about attachment theory is the belief that, once formed, attachment orientations remain relatively unchanged across development. This view is incorrect. Bowlby (1973) believed that attachment orientations and the working models that anchor them ought to change when individuals encounter significant model-inconsistent or incongruent life events. Stability and change of attachment orientations most likely occur via dynamic processes that operate in daily experiences (see Fraley and Brumbaugh, Chapter 4, and Davila and Cobb, Chapter 5, this volume). Although early experiences with attachment figures launch the development of attachment orientations (Path A), people who have insecure orientations should not remain insecure simply because of negative childhood memories. Instead, they actively experience and construe their daily social worlds in ways that usually sustain and "justify" their existing levels of insecurity.

The feedback loop near the middle of Figure 14.1 shows how both one's own and one's partner's interpersonal behaviors and model-confirming social perceptions could affect stability and change in baseline levels of ambivalence. Generally speaking, attachment orientations should change when people perceive that either their *own* behavior or their *partner's* behavior is starkly incongruent with their current working models (see Path N). On the other hand, attachment orientations should be reinforced when perceptions are highly congruent with existing working models. According to Bowlby (1973), attachment orientations ought to be fairly self-sustaining because they slant perceptions and behavior in directions that assimilate, confirm, and "justify" current working models. As the findings reviewed earlier indicate, ambivalence is systematically related to individuals' interpersonal behavior, the interpersonal behavior of their romantic partners, and their relationship-relevant social perceptions (Paths D, E, F, and G) in ways that bolster the view that attachment figures cannot be counted on for sufficient emotional support in times of need. Model-incongruent perceptions, of course, must be triggered by situations or events that are external to current working models, such as an attachment figure's unexpected attachment behavior, a radically new experience, or a life-altering experience (see Path N). There is likely to be constant tension between model-incongruent information (which may be common in everyday life) and model-congruent information (which ought to be preferentially perceived, assimilated, and behaviorally evoked in many cases).

Attachment orientations should be most susceptible to change during major life transitions. Many transitions involve either physical or psychological separations from attachment figures, dramatic changes in how attachment figures are related to, or the formation of new attachment bonds. Other theorists have proposed similar ideas. Epstein (1980), for example, has argued that emotional experiences that sharply confirm or disconfirm cherished interpersonal expectancies are necessary for internal models to be modified. Similarly, Caspi and Bem (1990) have proposed that major life transitions, which typically force people to enter new roles and deal with novel interpersonal issues, may be required to instigate a complete reevaluation and reorganization of internal models.

Guided by this reasoning, we next examined stability versus change in ambivalence among participants in our transition-to-parenthood project (Simpson et al., 2003). Systematic pre- to postpartum changes in ambivalence were related to women's perceptions of their husbands' amount of prenatal support. Specifically, women who perceived that their husbands provided less prenatal support had become significantly more ambivalent at the postnatal period, whereas those who perceived greater prenatal support had become less ambivalent. In addition, women who perceived that their husbands behaved in an angrier, more rejecting manner during the prenatal period also experienced significant increases in ambivalence from the pre- to postnatal periods. These findings suggest that attachment-relevant perceptions that are consistent with ambivalent models may strengthen them, whereas model-inconsistent perceptions might weaken or erode these models.

Individuals who are more ambivalent during the prenatal period should perceive greater spousal anger and less support than less ambivalent individuals, and these negative perceptions should at least stabilize and perhaps enhance their degree of ambivalence across the transition periods. Mediation analyses confirmed that these perceptions forecasted increases in ambivalence at 6 months postpartum. Ambivalent models, in other words, may have "reinforced" themselves through elevated and perhaps excessive perceptions of spousal anger.

Women's perceptions of their husbands' supportiveness or anger also could have shaped their beliefs about themselves, which might also have undermined or reinforced their ambivalence. It has long been recognized that self-perceptions can be influenced by how significant others perceive and act toward oneself (Mead, 1934). The effects of this process have been amply documented in recent research on close relationships. Murray, Holmes, and Griffin (1996), for example, have shown that romantic partners tend to shift their self-views in positive or negative directions, depending on their romantic *partners'* views of them. Similarly, Drigotas and colleagues (1999) have documented that people view themselves as closer to their ideal self if their *partners'* views of them are closer to their ideal self. Accordingly, women's perceptions of their husbands' levels of support and anger in our transition project might have strengthened or undermined their ambivalence by making them feel either more or less worthy of love, support, and affection.

Experiences with adult romantic partners might also affect working models by reinstating emotions or cognitions associated with experiences that occurred with attachment figures during childhood. As mentioned earlier, working models are composed in part of episodic memories of experiences with attachment figures, which can be memories from early childhood or from more contemporary periods. When adult attachment figures behave in ways that resemble the emotions or behavior of uncaring attachment figures from the past, these memories may be activated and may increase levels of insecurity. Conversely, when adult attachment figures act in ways that resemble good caregiving received in the past, feelings of greater security should be fostered. Andersen and her colleagues have documented how such "transference" processes influence social perceptions and behavior in interactions with people who resemble significant others from an individual's past (see Chen & Andersen, 1999, for a review).

In summary, the third study from our transition project provides preliminary support for Path H in our model. For pragmatic reasons, Figure 14.1 does not depict the process of change in attachment orientations across time. If this temporal dimension was included in the model, paths E, F, G, H, and D would form loops that might grow in strength over time, producing increasingly negative outcomes for highly ambivalent individuals until events intervene to derail these recursive processes or an asymptote is reached. Intervening events could include new external situations (e.g., becoming involved with a new partner who convincingly disconfirms one's existing working models) or factors more directly under the control of highly ambivalent individuals (e.g., deciding to seek therapy). If highly ambivalent people become aware of their relationship-destabilizing tendencies and learn to monitor and regulate the perceptions and behaviors that produce them, they might be able to short-circuit these processes on their own.

CONCLUSIONS

For more than two decades, interpersonal processes have been considered critical to understanding the onset and maintenance of depressive symptoms (Joiner, Coyne, & Blaylock, 1999). Until recently, however, most research on the interpersonal foundations of depression has been couched in a social learning perspective. Attachment theory has many important insights to offer about the interpersonal origins of depression. It provides, for example, a powerful, integrative framework for understanding how and why certain early childhood experiences (or at least the perception of early experiences) might increase vulnerability to depression and depressive symptoms in adulthood. It also offers a rich theoretical perspective on how working models could trigger dysfunctional perceptions and behaviors in highly stressful situations, which then might instigate, sustain, or exacerbate depressive symptoms.

The primary goal of this chapter was to introduce an integrative conceptual model that highlights some (but certainly not all) of the pathways that might link early attachment experiences and attachment ambivalence in adulthood to adult depressive symptoms. We have reviewed several lines of evidence that are consistent with some (but not all) pathways in the model. We have also introduced two new constructs—dysfunctional relationship attitudes and feelings of relationship deprivation—that may prove useful in guiding future research on the interpersonal origins of depressive symptoms. In addition, we have addressed a largely neglected issue in the attachment literature by providing some provisional evidence that memories (or perceptions) of early attachment experiences and current attachment ambivalence have *independent* effects on depressive symptoms in adulthood. That is, the impact of early relationship experiences (perceptions of parental risk) is *not* mediated through attachment ambivalence in adulthood; rather, it appears to have a direct effect on adult depressive symptoms that is moderated (amplified) by attachment ambivalence. These new findings suggest that the working models through which early experiences are filtered may affect susceptibility to depressive symptoms.

Our model remains tentative and preliminary. Certain potential paths that could lead to depressive symptoms, for instance, are not shown in our model, principally because they are more difficult to generate from attachment theory. There are no paths, for example, from the partner's model-confirming behavior to dysfunctional relationship attitudes or relationship deprivation, even though both paths could exist. The model also does not make a distinction between the events or interpersonal processes that might instigate depressive symptoms and those that might sustain or aggravate such symptoms. Despite the fact that attachment theory makes no distinctions between the origins that may underlie the initiation, maintenance, and exacerbation of depressive symptoms, the processes that generate these different types of symptoms could be slightly different. Finally, the origins of depressive symptoms for highly avoidant people are likely to be different from those depicted in our model. We suspect that major failures or disappointments in life domains other than close relationships (e.g., regarding work, finances, health, or independence) may play a larger role in precipitating and maintaining depressive symptoms among highly avoidant people.

In conclusion, our model and program of research suggests that the working models of highly ambivalent individuals may lead them to engage in self-fulfilling perceptual and behavioral processes that, if left unchecked, may create what they dread the most—interpersonal difficulties with attachment figures that increase the likelihood of eventual relationship loss. Identifying how highly ambivalent people can break or extricate themselves from these vicious self-fulfilling cycles should be a central mission of future research.

ACKNOWLEDGMENTS

Jeffry A. Simpson and W. Steven Rholes contributed equally to this chapter. This work was supported by National Institutes of Health Grant No. MH49599–05. We would like to thank Ramona Paetzold for her insightful comments on an earlier version of this chapter.

NOTES

1. A significant correlation was not found between parental behavior and romantic attachment ambivalence. Unlike previous measures of early attachment experiences, Grich's (2001) index of parental risk did not assess respondents' interpretations of the care they received from their parents; rather, trained raters assessed respondents' *probable* experiences during childhood based on their memories, their defensive predispositions, and other components of the AAI scoring procedure. AAI category scores (secure, dismissive, and preoccupied) were not differentially associated with the number of depressive symptoms. However, these null results could be attributable to low statistical power in the sample or the small percentage of people classified as preoccupied.

2. Women also provide support to their husbands during the transition to parenthood, which should influence their husbands' adjustment to this period. We are currently investigating this issue. Because our initial research focused on the effects of ambivalence in wives, some readers might infer that wives bear greater responsibility than their husbands for marital problems that might occur during the transition to parenthood. This inference is not justified. Husbands are likely to be equally responsible for any marital difficulties. In addition, we have confined our model and literature review to ambivalence because of space limitations and, more critically, because our findings indicate that ambivalence predicts depressive symptoms more strongly than avoidance does, especially during the opening months of the transition to parenthood. According to attachment theory (Bowlby, 1988), ambivalence and avoidance should be related to depressive symptoms via different pathways.

3. The support scale used in this project assessed emotional rather than instrumental support.

4. Consistent with Path G, husbands' perceived (self-reported) provision of support and their wives' perceptions of received support were significantly correlated.

5. As part of this process, wives may selectively define supportiveness to emphasize behaviors that are not in their husbands' repertoire. Alternatively, they may discount or overlook the supportive behaviors their husbands actually display.

6. Those few ambivalent women who perceived high levels of spousal support were very satisfied with their marriages, both prenatally and at 6 months postpartum.

7. It is important to make a clear distinction between attitudes or beliefs about partners (i.e., that they cannot be counted on for support or can never understand one's feelings) that are likely to be dysfunctional for interpersonal inter-

actions with the new concept we are proposing. Dysfunctional relationship attitudes tap beliefs that happiness is highly *contingent* on obtaining certain types of gratification from one's partner or relationship and believing that one will never be totally happy unless they are attained.

REFERENCES

Ainsworth, M. D. S., Blehar, M. C., Waters, E., & Wall, S. (1978). *Patterns of attachment: A psychological study of the Strange Situation.* Hillsdale, NJ: Erlbaum.

Anton, W. D., & Reed, J. R. (1991). *The College Adjustment Scales: Professional manual.* Odessa, FL: Psychological Assessment Resources.

Arieti, S., & Bemporad, J. R. (1980). The psychological organization of depression. *American Journal of Psychiatry, 137,* 1360–1365.

Beck, A. T., Rush, A. J., Shaw, B. F., & Emery, G. (1979). *Cognitive therapy of depression.* New York: Guilford Press.

Belsky, J., Lang, M. E., & Rovine, M. (1985). Stability and change in marriage across the transition to parenthood: A second study. *Journal of Marriage and the Family, 47,* 855–865.

Belsky, J., & Pensky, E. (1988). Marital change across the transition to parenthood. *Marriage and Family Review, 13,* 133–156.

Belsky, J., Spanier, G. B., & Rovine, M. (1983). Stability and change in marriage across the transition to parenthood. *Journal of Marriage and the Family, 45,* 553–556.

Bowlby, J. (1969). *Attachment and loss: Vol. 1. Attachment.* New York: Basic Books.

Bowlby, J. (1973). *Attachment and loss: Vol. 2. Separation: Anxiety and anger.* New York: Basic Books.

Bowlby, J. (1980). *Attachment and loss: Vol. 3. Loss: Sadness and depression.* New York: Basic Books.

Bowlby, J. (1988). *A secure base: Clinical applications of attachment theory.* New York: Basic Books.

Brennan, K. A., Clark, C. L., & Shaver, P. R. (1998). Self-report measurement of adult attachment: An integrative overview. In J. A. Simpson & W. S. Rholes (Eds.), *Attachment theory and close relationships* (pp. 46–76). New York: Guilford Press.

Brennan, K. A., & Shaver, P. R. (1998). Attachment styles and personality disorders: Their connections to each other and to parental divorce, parental death, and perceptions of parental caregiving. *Journal of Personality, 66,* 835–878.

Burge, D., Hammen, C., Davila, J., Daley, S. E., Paley, B., Lindberg, N., et al. (1997). The relationship between attachment cognitions and psychological adjustment in late adolescent women. *Development and Psychopathology, 9,* 151–167.

Campbell, L., Simpson, J. A., Boldry, J., & Kashy, D. A. (2003). *Perceptions of conflict and support in romantic relationships: The role of attachment anxiety.* Unpublished manuscript, University of Western Ontario, London, Ontario, Canada.

Caspi, A., & Bem, D. J. (1990). Personality continuity and change across the life course. In L. A. Pervin (Ed.), *Handbook of personality: Theory and research* (pp. 549–575). New York: Guilford Press.

Cassidy, J., & Berlin, L. (1994). The insecure/ambivalent pattern of attachment: Theory and research. *Child Development, 65,* 971–991.

Chen, S., & Andersen, S. M. (1999). Relationships from the past in the present: Significant-other representations and transference in interpersonal life. In M. Zanna (Ed.), *Advances in experimental social psychology* (Vol. 31, pp. 123–190). San Diego, CA: Academic Press.

Cole-Detke, H., & Kobak, R. (1996). Attachment processes in eating disorder and depression. *Journal of Consulting and Clinical Psychology, 64,* 282–290.

Collins, N. L., & Allard, L. M. (2001). Cognitive representations of attachment: The content and function of working models. In G. J. O. Fletcher & M. S. Clark (Eds.), *Blackwell handbook of social psychology: Vol. 2. Interpersonal processes* (pp. 60–85). Malden, MA: Blackwell.

Collins, N. L., & Feeney, B. C. (2000). *Working models of attachment: Implications for the perception of partner behavior.* Paper presented at the International Conference on Personal Relationships, Brisbane, Australia.

Cooper, M. L., Shaver, P. R., & Collins, N. L. (1998). Attachment styles, emotion regulation, and adjustment in adolescence. *Journal of Personality and Social Psychology, 74,* 1380–1397.

Cowan, C., Cowan, P., Core, L., & Core, J. (1978). Becoming a family: The impact of a first child's birth on the couple's relationship. In L. Newman & W. Miller (Eds.), *The first-child and family formation* (pp. 296–326). Chapel Hill, NC: Carolina Population Center.

Cowan, C. P., & Cowan, P. A. (2000). *When partners become parents: The big life change in couples.* Mahwah, NJ: Erlbaum.

Cowan, C. P., Cowan, P. A., Heming, G., Coysh, W. S., Curtis-Boles, H., & Boles, A. J. (1985). Transition to parenthood: His, hers, and theirs. *Journal of Family Issues, 6,* 451–481.

Crockenberg, S. C., & Leerkes, E. M. (2003). Parental acceptance, postpartum depression, and maternal sensitivity: Mediating and moderating processes. *Journal of Family Psychology, 17,* 80–93.

Crocker, J., & Wolfe, C. T. (2001). Contingencies of self-worth. *Psychological Review, 108,* 593–623.

Derogatis, L. R., & Melisaratos, N. (1983). The Brief Symptom Inventory: An introductory report. *Psychological Medicine, 13,* 595–605.

Downey, G., Freitas, A. L., Michaelis, B., & Khouri, H. (1998). The self-fulfilling prophecy in close relationships: Rejection sensitivity and rejection by romantic partners. *Journal of Personality and Social Psychology, 75,* 545–560.

Dozier, M., Stovall, K. C., & Albus, K. E. (1999). Attachment and psychopathology in adulthood. In J. Cassidy & P. R. Shaver (Eds.), *Handbook of attachment: Theory, research, and clinical applications* (pp. 497–519). New York: Guilford Press.

Drigotas, S. M., Rusbult, C. E., Wieselquist, J., & Whitton, S. W. (1999). Close partner as sculptor of the ideal self: Behavioral affirmation and the Michelangelo phenomenon. *Journal of Personality and Social Psychology, 77,* 293–323.

Epstein, S. (1980). The stability of behavior: II. Implications for psychological research. *American Psychologist, 35,* 790–806.

Feeney, J. A. (1999). Adult romantic attachment and couple relationships. In J. A.

Cassidy & P. R. Shaver (Eds.), *Handbook of attachment: Theory, research, and clinical applications* (pp. 355–377). New York: Guilford Press.

Fonagy, P., Leigh, T., Steele, M., Steele, H., Kennedy, R., Mattoon, G., et al. (1996). The relation of attachment to status, psychiatric classification, and response to psychotherapy. *Journal of Consulting and Clinical Psychology, 64,* 22–31.

Grich, J. (2001). *Earned secure attachment in young adulthood: Adjustment and relationship satisfaction.* Unpublished doctoral dissertation, Texas A&M University, College Station.

Griffin, D. W., & Bartholomew, K. (1994). Models of the self and other: Fundamental dimensions underlying measures of adult attachment. *Journal of Personality and Social Psychology, 67,* 430–445.

Hammen, C. (1995). The social context of risk for depression. In K. D. Craig & K. S. Dobson (Eds.), *Anxiety and depression in adults and children* (pp. 82–96). Thousand Oaks, CA: Sage.

Hammen, C. (2000). Interpersonal factors in an emerging developmental model of depression. In S. L. Johnson, A. M. Hayes, T. M. Field, N. Schneiderman, & P. M. McCabe (Eds.), *Stress, coping, and depression* (pp. 71–88). Mahwah, NJ: Erlbaum.

Hammen, C. L., Burge, D., Daley, S. E., Davila, J., Paley, B., & Rudolph, K. D. (1995). Interpersonal attachment cognitions and prediction of symptomatic responses to interpersonal stress. *Journal of Abnormal Psychology, 104,* 436–443.

Hazan, C., & Shaver, P. R. (1987). Romantic love conceptualized as an attachment process. *Journal of Personality and Social Psychology, 52,* 511–524.

Heinicke, C. M. (1995). Determinants of the transition to parenthood. In M. H. Bornstein (Ed.), *Handbook of parenting, Vol. 3: Status and social conditions of parenting* (pp. 277–303). Mahwah, NJ: Erlbaum.

Ingram, R. E. (2003). Origins of cognitive vulnerability to depression. *Cognitive Therapy and Research, 27,* 77–88.

Joiner, T., Coyne, J. C., & Blaylock, J. (1999). On the interpersonal nature of depression: Overview and synthesis. In T. Joiner & J. C. Coyne (Eds.), *Interactional nature of depression* (pp. 3–21). Washington, DC: American Psychological Association Press.

Kobak, R. R., & Duemmler, S. (1994). Attachment and conversation: Toward a discourse analysis of adolescent and adult security. In K. Bartholomew & D. Perlman (Eds.), *Advances in personal relationships: Vol. 5. Attachment processes in adulthood* (pp. 121–149). London: Kingsley.

Levy, K. N., Blatt, S. J., & Shaver, P. R. (1998). Attachment styles and parental rejection. *Journal of Personality and Social Psychology, 74,* 407–419.

Levy-Shiff, R. (1994). Individual and contextual correlates of marital change across the transition to parenthood. *Developmental Psychology, 30,* 591–601.

Main, M., & Goldwyn, R. (1994). *Adult attachment scoring and classification systems.* Unpublished manual, University College, London, United Kingdom.

Main, M., Kaplan, N., & Cassidy, J. (1985). Security in infancy, childhood, and adulthood: A move to the level of representation. *Monographs of the Society for Research in Child Development, 50* (1 & 2, Serial No. 209), 66–104.

Mead, G. H. (1934). *Mind, self, and society.* Chicago: University of Chicago Press.

Mickelson, K. D., Kessler, R. C., & Shaver, P. R. (1997). Adult attachment in a nationally representative sample. *Journal of Personality and Social Psychology, 73,* 1092–1106.

Mikulincer, M., Florian, V., & Weller, A. (1993). Attachment styles, coping strategies, and posttraumatic psychological distress: The impact of the Gulf War in Israel. *Journal of Personality and Social Psychology, 64,* 817–826.

Murray, S. L., & Holmes, J. G. (1997). A leap of faith? Positive illusions in romantic relationships. *Personality and Social Psychology Bulletin, 23,* 586–604.

Murray, S.L., Holmes, J.G., & Griffin, D.W. (1996). The self-fulfilling nature of positive illusions in romantic relationships: Love is not blind, but prescient. *Journal of Personality and Social Psychology, 71,* 1155–1180.

Patrick, M., Hobson, R. P., Castle, D., Howard, R., & Maughan, B. (1994). Personality disorder and the mental representation of early social experience. *Development and Psychopathology, 6,* 375–388.

Pearson, J. L., Cohn, D. A., Cowan, P. A., & Cowan, C. P. (1994). Earned- and continuous-security in adult attachment: Relation to depressive symptomatology and parenting style. *Development and Psychopathology, 6,* 359–373.

Rholes, W. S., & Simpson, J. A. (2004). Ambivalent attachment and depressive symptoms: The role of romantic and parent-child relationships. *Journal of Cognitive Psychotherapy, 18,* 67–78.

Rholes, W. S., Simpson, J. A., Campbell, L., & Grich, J. (2001). Adult attachment and the transition to parenthood. *Journal of Personality and Social Psychology, 81,* 421–435.

Rholes, W. S., Simpson, J. A., & Oriña, M. M. (1999). Attachment and anger in an anxiety-provoking situation. *Journal of Personality and Social Psychology, 76,* 940–957.

Roberts, J. E., Gotlib, I. H., & Kassel, J. D. (1996). Adult attachment security and symptoms of depression: The mediating roles of dysfunctional attitudes and low self-esteem. *Journal of Personality and Social Psychology, 70,* 310–320.

Rosenstein, D. S., & Horowitz, H. A. (1996). Adolescent attachment and psychopathology. *Journal of Consulting and Clinical Psychology, 64,* 244–253.

Scott, R. L., & Cordova, J. V. (2002). The influence of adult attachment styles on the association between marital adjustment and depressive symptoms. *Journal of Family Psychology, 16,* 199–208.

Shaver, P. R., Belsky, J., & Brennan, K. A. (2000). The Adult Attachment Interview and self-reports of romantic attachment: Associations across domains and methods. *Personal Relationships, 7,* 25–43.

Shaver, P. R., & Mikulincer, M. (2002). Attachment-related psychodynamics. *Attachment and Human Development, 4,* 133–161.

Simpson, J. A., Ickes, W., & Grich, J. (1999). When accuracy hurts: Reactions of anxious–ambivalent dating partners to a relationship-threatening situation. *Journal of Personality and Social Psychology, 76,* 754–769.

Simpson, J. A., & Rholes, W. S. (1994). Stress and secure base relationships in adulthood. In K. Bartholomew & D. Perlman (Eds.), *Advances in personal relationships: Vol. 5. Attachment processes in adulthood* (pp. 181–204). London: Kingsley.

Simpson, J. A., Rholes, W. S., Campbell, L., Tran, S., & Wilson, C. L. (2003). Adult attachment, the transition to parenthood, and depressive symptoms. *Journal of Personality and Social Psychology, 84,* 1172–1187.

Simpson, J. A., Rholes, W. S., Campbell, L., & Wilson, C. L. (2003). Changes in attachment orientations across the transition to parenthood. *Journal of Experimental Social Psychology, 39,* 317–331.

Simpson, J. A., Rholes, W. S., & Nelligan, J. S. (1992). Support seeking and support giving within couples in an anxiety-provoking situation: The role of attachment styles. *Journal of Personality and Social Psychology, 62,* 434–446.

Simpson, J. A., Rholes, W. S., & Phillips, D. (1996). Conflict in close relationships: An attachment perspective. *Journal of Personality and Social Psychology, 71,* 899–914.

Sroufe, L. A., & Waters, E. (1977). Attachment as an organizational construct. *Child Development, 48,* 1184–1199.

Sund, A. M., & Wichstrom, L. (2002). Insecure attachment as a risk factor for future depressive symptoms in early adolescence. *Journal of the American Academy of Child and Adolescent Psychiatry, 41,* 1478–1485.

Swann, W. B., Jr. (1990). To be adored or to be known? The interplay of self-enhancement and self-verification. In E. T. Higgins & R. M. Sorrentino (Eds.), *Handbook of motivation and cognition: Foundations of social behavior* (Vol. 2, pp. 408–448). New York: Guilford Press.

Tidwell, M. O., Reis, H. T., & Shaver, P. R. (1996). Attachment, attractiveness, and social interaction: A diary study. *Journal of Personality and Social Psychology, 71,* 729–745.

Tucker, P., & Aron, A. (1993). Passionate love and marital satisfaction at key transition points in the family life cycle. *Journal of Social and Clinical Psychology, 12,* 135–147.

van IJzendoorn, M. H. (1995). Adult attachment representations, parental responsiveness, and infant attachment: A meta-analysis on the predictive validity of the Adult Attachment Interview. *Psychological Bulletin, 117,* 387–403.

van IJzendoorn, M. H., & Bakermans-Kranenburg, M. (1996). Attachment representations in mothers, fathers, adolescents and clinical groups: A meta-analytic search for normative data. *Journal of Consulting and Clinical Psychology, 64,* 8–21.

Waters, E., Merrick, S. K., Treboux, D., Crowell, J., & Albersheim, L. (2000). Attachment security in infancy and early adulthood: A 20-year longitudinal study. *Child Development, 71,* 684–689.

Waters, E., Weinfield, N. S., & Hamilton, C. E. (2000). The stability of attachment security from infancy to adolescence and early adulthood: General discussion. *Child Development, 71,* 703–706.

Weissman, A. N., & Beck, A. T. (1978). *Development and validation of the Dysfunctional Attitude Scale: A preliminary investigation.* Paper presented at the annual meeting of the American Educational Research Association, Toronto.

CHAPTER 15

Attachment Styles
and Intrapersonal Adjustment

A Longitudinal Study
from Adolescence into Young Adulthood

M. Lynne Cooper
Austin W. Albino
Holly K. Orcutt
Natalie Williams

During adolescence, the hierarchy of attachment figures (Bowlby, 1969/ 1982) is gradually reshuffled as young people increasingly direct their attachment behaviors and concerns toward peers rather than parents (Furman & Buhrmester, 1992; Hazan & Zeifman, 1994). Although parents are generally not completely displaced as attachment figures, during adolescence they slowly become what Weiss (1982) called "attachment figures in reserve." By the end of this period, some time in early adulthood, most people settle on a single romantic partner who will serve as a primary attachment figure. While making this transition, many adolescents alter their conceptions of and feelings about themselves and experiment with a range of exploratory behaviors (e.g., sex and substance use) that may be developmentally functional but nonetheless carry substantial risk of harm (Baumrind, 1987).

Despite the normativeness of such experiences, little is known about how individual differences in attachment patterns shape the unfolding of these experiences throughout adolescence and into young adulthood. Do individual differences in attachment styles during adolescence forecast intrapersonal adjustment in young adulthood? Do adolescents with different attachment types follow different pathways, or differently timed pathways, through this developmental period? Unfortunately, virtually no longitudinal or prospective data exist to inform these important questions. This study, therefore, used longitudinal data from a representative, community sample of black and white adolescents to examine individual differences in attachment styles, assessed during adolescence, as predictors of intrapersonal adjustment approximately 4½ years later.

ATTACHMENT THEORY AND ATTACHMENT STYLES

Bowlby (1969, 1973) theorized that attachment behaviors in infancy and childhood are regulated by an innate behavioral system that functions to promote safety and survival by maintaining a child's proximity to a nurturing caretaker. A child's ability to rely on his or her attachment figure as a safe haven in times of need and as a secure base from which to explore the environment are key components of well-functioning attachment bonds and essential to healthy emotional development. According to Bowlby, early caregiving experiences are internalized as working models of oneself as worthy or unworthy of love and of others as responsive or unresponsive. Once developed, these models become core features of personality that are carried forward and guide attachment-related thought, feeling, and action.

At least three distinct patterns of attachment-related cognitions, emotions, and behaviors, known as attachment styles, have been identified among adolescents and adults (see Mikulincer & Shaver, 2003, for a review). Securely attached individuals are self-confident, socially skilled, open to and interested in close relationships with romantic partners, and likely to form relatively stable and satisfying long-term relationships. Anxious or anxious–ambivalent people lack self-confidence, are worried about rejection and abandonment, and are prone to bouts of jealousy and anger with relationship partners who are perceived as untrustworthy. Despite their unease, anxiously attached individuals are nevertheless eager to be involved in romantic relationships and often enter into relationships with ill-advised partners. In contrast, avoidant individuals are uncomfortable with closeness, self-disclosure, and dependence on others and are relatively inhibited and socially unskilled. Although genetic and temperamental differences may contribute to these patterns (e.g., Seifer, Scheller, Sameroff, Resnick, & Riordan, 1996), attachment theory underscores the contributions made by interactions with key attachment figures during infancy and childhood. Theoretically, caregivers who were sensitive and responsive induced feelings of support and security; those who were inconsistent in their responding induced anxiety, vigilance, and anger; and those who were cool, rejecting, and unsupportive induced premature self-reliance and suppression of vulnerabilities.

INDIVIDUAL DIFFERENCES IN ATTACHMENT STYLES
AND INTRAPERSONAL ADJUSTMENT

The implications of attachment theory for interpersonal functioning have by now been documented in hundreds of studies (see Feeney, 1999, for a review). Also central to Bowlby's original theory (1969, 1973), but much less well researched, are attachment theory's implications for *intra*personal adjustment. In particular, Bowlby believed that early caregiver exchanges provide a critical context within which the child organizes emotional experience and learns to regulate feelings of security. According to Bowlby, the desire to maintain feelings of security is a universal goal, although the specific strategies people use to achieve this goal vary with their attachment histories. When, for example, the attachment figure is available and responsive to the child's distress signals, the child learns that he or she can effectively regulate distressing emotions and experiences. Under less optimal circumstances, however, the child learns that the experience of distress is associated with negative outcomes and that distressing emotions cannot be effectively regulated. Based on these early experiences, Bowlby argued that expectancies regarding the experience of negative emotions and preferred styles of coping with these emotions are also internalized as part of an individual's working model.

Specifically, he proposed that secure individuals should be able to acknowledge and then cope effectively with negative emotions. In contrast, avoidant individuals try not to acknowledge negative emotions, may act emotionally without full knowledge of the reasons, and are uncomfortable seeking support. Finally, anxious individuals are highly emotionally expressive but often cannot regulate their emotions or emotionally driven behavior effectively in line with personal goals or social norms.

Numerous studies provide evidence consistent with Bowlby's original notions about attachment style differences in the experience and expression of emotion. For example, insecure attachment has been associated with greater loneliness, anger, resentment, anxiety, depression, paranoia, self-consciousness, and somatic symptoms, as well as with lower self-esteem and less self-confidence (see Mikulincer & Shaver, 2003, for a review). Also consistent with these notions, a number of recent studies suggest that people with different attachment styles cope with or regulate negative emotions in theoretically expected ways. In one study (Simpson, Rholes, & Nelligan, 1992), for example, women who were more securely attached were found to use their partners as a source of comfort and reassurance in an anxiety-provoking situation, whereas women who were more avoidant withdrew from their partners both emotionally and physically. Similarly, Mikulincer, Florian, and Wells (1993) found that securely attached adults used more support-seeking strategies in the aftermath of the Gulf War, anxious adults used more emotion-focused coping, and avoidant adults used more distancing strategies. Mikulincer and Orbach (1995) found that avoidant individuals have poorer memories of emotional experiences and take longer to recall those experiences, an effect that Fraley, Garner, and Shaver (2000) showed was due to avoidant individuals' poorer memory encoding at the time of the experience rather than to differential forgetting. Together these data suggest that avoidant people pursue a defensive strategy in the presence of distressing information, attempting to insulate themselves by minimizing its self-relevance and failing to encode it, whereas anxious individuals are more likely to ruminate on negative information and overestimate its importance.

In perhaps the most comprehensive study of these ideas and their implications for intrapersonal adjustment conducted to date, Cooper, Shaver, and Collins (1998) found consistent and theoretically meaningful patterns of attachment style differences in emotional experience, self-views, and risky or problem behaviors in a large and representative sample of adolescents 13 to 19 years old. In line with the notion that secure attachment leads to the development of adaptive ways of coping with negative emotions and a sense of self-efficacy, secure adolescents reported generally superior functioning across multiple developmentally relevant domains. They viewed themselves in the most positive terms; they reported the lowest levels of psychological distress; and they engaged in what can be interpreted as developmentally appropriate exploratory behaviors. For example, although the majority of secure youths drank alcohol and had sex, they were significantly less likely to have had drinking problems or casual sex partners than their insecure counterparts. In contrast, anxious–ambivalent adolescents appeared to be the most poorly adjusted group overall. They reported the most negative self-concepts and the most distress, as well as the highest levels of problematic or risky behaviors. Although avoidant adolescents experienced as many anxious, paranoid, psychotic, obsessive–compulsive, and somatic symptoms as their anxious–ambivalent counterparts and were actually less socially skilled, they were otherwise better adjusted. They were less hostile and depressed, more academically able, and less involved in delinquent, substance-use, and sexual behaviors. In fact, avoidant adolescents did not differ from their secure counterparts on the majority of the risk or problem behaviors and were significantly *less* likely than secure adolescents ever to have had sex or used substances. Finally, mediation analyses suggested that the effects of attachment styles on risky behaviors were at least partly attributable to underlying differences in social competence and, more important for the present study, the experience of negative emotions.

Although the results of this study were broadly consistent with Bowlby's notions about attachment style effects on the experience, expression, and regulation of emotions and emotionally driven behaviors, we were unable to convincingly address the core assumption that attachment styles *predispose* individuals to these experiences because our study (like the overwhelming majority of studies in this area) was cross-sectional. Indeed, although a small number of longitudinal studies examining attachment outcomes in adolescence and young adulthood have been published in the past 10 years, they shed only limited light on the issues at hand for several reasons.

First, the majority of longitudinal studies (e.g., Collins, Cooper, Albino, & Allard, 2002; Duemmler & Kobak, 2001; Hammond & Fletcher, 1991; Herzberg et al., 1999; Kirkpatrick & Davis, 1994; Kirkpatrick & Hazan, 1994) have focused on relationship or interpersonal outcomes and processes to the exclusion of a broader range of adaptive outcomes. In fact, we are aware of only five studies (viz., Burge, Hammen, Davila, Daley, Paley, Herzberg, & Lindberg, 1997; Burge, Hammen, Davila, Daley, Paley, Lindberg, et al., 1997; Hammen et al., 1995; Simpson, Rholes, Campbell, Tran, & Wilson, 2003; Vasquez, Durik, & Hyde, 2002) that have examined links between prior attachment and later intrapersonal functioning or changes in intrapersonal functioning using adolescent or young adult samples. However, two of these studies (Simpson et al., 2003; Vasquez et al., 2002) were conducted with samples of pregnant women and their partners, thus minimizing their relevance to issues of growth and change among unselected adolescent and young adult samples. Unfortunately, the remaining three longitudinal studies (Burge, Hammen, Davila, Daley, Paley, Herzberg, & Lindberg, 1997; Burge, Hammen, Davila, Daley, Paley, Lindberg, et al., 1997; Hammen et al., 1995) used the same sample of approximately 130 recent high school graduates, all of whom were women. In addition to sample limitations, these studies also focused on a limited range of intrapersonal adaptive outcomes. Although all five studies examined depressive symptoms, only one study (Hammen et al., 1995) examined a second psychological symptom (anxiety). In addition, only two studies (Burge, Hammen, Davila, Daley, Paley, Herzberg, & Lindberg, 1997; Vasquez et al., 2002) examined dimensions of perceived self-competence or self-views; and only two studies—both using the same sample of women—examined any type of externalizing behavior. Thus, taken as a whole, these studies form a very limited data base from which to draw conclusions about attachment effects on intrapersonal adaptation during adolescence and young adulthood, particularly among young men.

GOALS OF THE PRESENT STUDY

Using data from a longitudinal follow-up of the same sample who participated in our earlier study (Cooper et al., 1998), the present study affords a more comprehensive examination of the prospective effects of attachment styles on changes in intrapersonal adaptation from adolescence into young adulthood. Building on our earlier findings, as well as on those from the aforementioned longitudinal studies, we examine three broad issues regarding the longitudinal and prospective effects of attachment styles on psychological distress, self-views, and risky or problem behaviors. Although we generally expected differences between the attachment groups present at baseline to be maintained across time, expectations regarding differential change are less clear-cut given the limited evidentiary base. Nevertheless, we outline here several general expectations regarding the distinct nature of change among the three attachment types across multiple domains of functioning.

First, we examine whether the three attachment types show differential patterns of change across time in multiple domains of adjustment, including psychological distress, self-concept, and risky or problem behaviors. In general, we expect that anxiously attached youths, relative to their nonanxious counterparts, will experience the greatest difficulties adjusting to the demands of what can be a turbulent developmental period (Arnett, 1999). These adjustment difficulties will be evidenced in steeper increases in psychological distress and in a range of risk-taking or problematic behaviors, as well as by steeper decreases (or less steep increases) in positive self-views. Based on the results of our earlier study (Cooper et al., 1998), we know that anxious youths in our sample were the most distressed and had the fewest resources for coping at baseline. Because of this, we expect these youths to follow a more adverse course over time, as their liabilities and limitations continue to place them at a disadvantage in coping with the unavoidable demands posed by this developmental period.

In contrast, although avoidant youths will likely continue to be plagued by elevated levels of distress and poor self-concepts, their ability to divert attention away from emotionally upsetting issues (Fraley, Garner, & Shaver, 2000) may serve to ameliorate the adverse impact of some of the difficulties they will face during this developmental period. We also speculate that avoidant youths' lack of social competence may "protect" them from increasing involvement in risky or problematic behaviors, most of which are heavily socially regulated during adolescence (for supporting evidence, see Moore & Arthur, 1989; White, Bates, & Johnson, 1990). Thus, because increasing involvement in risk behaviors is normative from adolescence into young adulthood (Moffitt, 1993; Steinberg & Morris, 2001) and is thought to serve at least some adaptive functions (Baumrind, 1987), avoidant youths may well continue to lag behind secure youths in their levels of risk involvement, at least in the more benign forms of these behaviors (e.g., alcohol use). At the same time, avoidant adolescents may show steeper increases than their secure counterparts in those risk behaviors that are more deviant and potentially harmful (e.g., illicit drug use, violence, property crimes, etc.).

Finally, we expect that securely attached young people will follow the most adaptive course throughout adolescence into young adulthood. Specifically, we expect that secure youths, given their superior adjustment at the outset, will continue to show lower levels of distress and more positive self-views over time. To the extent that experimentation with some risky behaviors signals developmentally appropriate exploratory behavior, we also expect that secure adolescents will show moderate and generally increasing levels of involvement in a range of risky or problem behaviors, as is normative during this life stage (Steinberg & Morris, 2001).

Second, we examine the onset of risky or problem behaviors among individuals who reported no prior experience with these behaviors at Time 1. Relative to the change analyses discussed previously, these analyses provide a stronger test of the causal effects of attachment style on risk behavior by ruling out the possibility that prior involvement in risk behaviors caused both initial attachment style and later risk behaviors. Similar to the reasoning outlined previously, we generally expect that anxiously attached youths will exhibit the highest rates of onset of risky or problem behaviors due to their high levels of distress, poor self-concepts, and strong social orientations. In contrast, we expect that avoidant youths will continue to lag behind their securely attached peers in making what are for most people developmentally appropriate transitions into responsible adult sexual behavior and alcohol use. At the same time, avoidant adolescents who do engage in these behaviors may have greater difficulty in regulating them and thus be more likely to report problematic or deviant levels of involvement.

Finally, we examine the robustness of these findings across gender, race, and age groups. Doing so enhances the external validity of the study by identifying specific limits, if any, on the generalizability of our findings (Shadish, Cook, & Campbell, 2002). This is particularly important with regard to gender because the bulk of existing longitudinal research has been conducted among female-only samples.

BACKGROUND AND METHODS OF THE PRESENT STUDY

Sample

Data for the present study were obtained from a longitudinal study of adolescents that examined psychosocial factors that affect health risk behavior (Cooper & Orcutt, 1997; Cooper et al., 1998). Participants were interviewed first in 1989–1990 and in 1994–1995, approximately 4½ years later. At Time 1 (T1), random-digit-dialing techniques were used to identify a sample of 2,544 adolescents, ages 13–19, residing within the city limits of Buffalo, New York. Interviews were completed with 2,052 of the adolescents, yielding an 81% completion rate. Telephone exchanges in areas populated primarily by African Americans were intentionally over-sampled, thus yielding a final sample that included nearly equally numbers of black and white respondents (44% vs. 48%). Completion rates did not differ by race or age, though a slightly higher percentage of females than males were interviewed (83% vs. 79%). Parental education level was also slightly higher among respondents than among nonrespondents (13.1 years vs. 12.8 years), although occupation ranks (using U.S. Census Bureau categories) did not differ.

At Time 2 (T2), 88% of the T1 sample (n = 1,815) was reinterviewed (or 71% of the initially eligible sample). Although the T2 sample did not differ from the initially eligible sample in racial composition or socioeconomic status, more females than males were retained across both waves of data (77% of initially eligible females vs. 66% of initially eligible males). In addition, despite the lack of age differences in initial participation rates at T1, younger participants were more likely to be reinterviewed at T2 (m = 16.7 years at T1 for reinterviewed respondents vs. 17.2 years for respondents who were not reinterviewed).

Respondents were included in the present study if they were reinterviewed at Time 2 and had answered the attachment questions at Time 1 in a consistent manner (n = 1,410). Somewhat more females than males (54% vs. 47%) were included in this sample, largely due to higher completion rates at Time 2 among female respondents. Approximately half of the retained sample members were white; 42% were black, and 8% were members of other racial groups (mostly Hispanic and Asian American). Respondents were 16.8 (± 2.0) years old, on average, at T1, and 21.5 (± 2.1) years, on average, at T2. The youngest respondents were 13 at Time 1 (n = 131), whereas the oldest were 25 at Time 2 (n = 32). Finally, the majority of respondents were classified as having a secure attachment style at T1 (56%); 21% were classified as avoidant, and 23% as anxiously attached. As noted in our prior study (Cooper et al., 1998), this distribution is similar to the proportions observed in other studies.

Interview Protocol and Procedures

T1 data were collected from the fall of 1989 through the end of 1990. Face-to-face interviews were conducted by 30 professionally trained interviewers using a structured interview schedule. Interviewers and participants were always matched on sex and were matched on race whenever possible (approximately 75% of interviews). Average interview length was 2 hours, and respondents were paid $25 for their participation. Prior to the interview, written informed consent was obtained from respondents, as well as from parents of underage respondents. The interview contained both interviewer-administered and self-administered portions, with private self-administration of more sensitive questions (e.g., delinquency and sexual behavior). Respondents were provided with simply worded definitions of sexual behavior to ensure common understanding of key terms.

T2 data were collected from the fall of 1994 through 1995 by a staff of 24 professionally trained interviewers following a protocol identical to that used at T1, with two exceptions. First, both the interviewer- and self-administered portions of the interview were computerized. Computer administration allowed for more reliable implementation of complex skip patterns, for elimination of out-of-range and missing responses, and for automated data entry (Rosenfeld, Booth-Kewley, & Edwards, 1993). Nevertheless, because computer administration relative to paper-and-pencil administration appears to reduce underreporting of sensitive behaviors (Rosenfeld et al., 1993), at least some of the increase observed in risk behaviors across time may be due to the shift from pencil-and-paper to computer presentation. Second, whereas all interviews were conducted face-to-face at T1, 68 respondents who had moved out of the greater Buffalo area during the intervening period were interviewed by telephone at T2. Notably, although comparisons of phone and face-to-face interview respondents on the T2 outcome measures revealed a number of significant differences, these differences were largely explainable in terms of demographic differences between individuals who moved and those who stayed in the local community.

Measures

Attachment Style

Descriptive information (including change over time) on key study variables can be found in Table 15.1. Attachment style was measured in two ways using a slightly modified version of Hazan and Shaver's (1987, 1990) questionnaire. This questionnaire was selected for use because it was the only self-report measure available when the study was designed. Each respondent was first asked whether he or she had ever been involved in a serious romantic relationship. If the answer was yes, the respondent was asked to answer the attachment questions with respect to experiences during those relationships. If the answer was no, the respondent was asked to imagine what his or her experiences *would* be like in such relationships. Respondents read each of three attachment style descriptions and rated how self-characteristic each style was on a 7-point Likert-type scale (which produced three quantitative ratings). They were then asked to choose which one of the three styles was most self-descriptive (a categorical measure). The three answer alternatives were worded as follows:

TABLE 15.1. Descriptive Statistics for Study Variables

Variable	Valid n	T1 M	T1 SD	T2 M	T2 SD	Observed range	Δ (T2 − T1)	α T1	α T2
				Psychological symptomatology					
Distress									
Hostility	1,408	1.20	0.89	1.05	0.85	0.00–4.00	−.15**	.79	.82
Anxiety	1,410	0.81	0.68	0.83	0.68	0.00–4.00	.02	.77	.79
Depression	1,408	0.75	0.71	0.89	0.77	0.00–4.00	.14**	.81	.83
Self-concept									
Social competence	1,410	4.52	0.81	4.62	0.81	T1 = 1.38–6.00 T2 = 1.00–6.00	.10**	.78	.82
Athletic	1,410	4.52	1.38	4.47	1.39	1.00–6.00	−.07†	.88	.87
Intellectual	1,410	4.25	0.95	4.28	0.87	T1 = 1.75–6.00 T2 = 1.00–6.00	.03	.55	.66
Body image	1,408	4.24	1.33	3.86	1.44	1.00–6.00	−.38**	.82	.77
Physical attractiveness	1,405	4.24	0.99	4.22	1.00	1.00–6.00	.02	.75	.84
				Risky or problem behaviors					
Sexual behavior									
Number of partners	1,388	1.76	1.86	3.97	2.32	T1: 0.00–7.00 T2: 0.00–8.00	2.21**		
Risky practices	1,385	0.53	0.81	1.71	1.49	T1: 0.00–3.00 T2: 0.00–8.00	1.18**		
Pregnancy/STDs	1,388	0.43	0.55	0.55	0.58	0.00–2.00	.12**		
Substance use									
Heavy/problem drinking	1,399	1.00	1.50	1.41	1.59	T1: 0.00–6.67 T2: 0.00–7.33	.41**		
Illicit drug use	1,410	0.49	0.70	1.54	1.60	T1: 0.00–4.00 T2: 0.00–8.00	1.05**		
Tobacco use	1,410	0.31	0.66	0.62	0.79	0.00–2.00	.31**		
Delinquency									
Truancy	1,409	1.83	1.44	2.80	1.45	0.00–5.00	.97**		
Violent behavior	1,409	1.46	1.29	1.89	1.33	0.00–4.00	.43**		
Property crime	1,409	0.56	0.80	1.00	1.03	0.00–4.00	.44**		
Educational underachievement									
Poor grades	1,243	3.32	1.38	3.25	1.26	1.00–8.00	−.07		
Low educational aspirations	1,388	1.39	1.50	1.41	1.65	T1: 0.00–8.00 T2: 0.00–9.00	−.02		
Years lost	1,243	0.36	0.67	0.51	0.89	0.00–6.00	.15*		

Note. Alphas are provided only for multi-item scales that conform to the assumptions of the factor model.
†$p < .10$; *$p < .01$; **$p < .001$.

1. *Avoidant.* "I am somewhat uncomfortable being close to others; I find it difficult to trust them completely, difficult to allow myself to depend on them. I am nervous when anyone gets too close, and often, love partners want me to be more intimate than I feel comfortable being."

2. *Anxious–Ambivalent.* "I find that others are reluctant to get as close as I would like. I often worry that my partner doesn't really love me or won't want to stay with me. I want to get very close to my partner, and this sometimes scares people away."

3. *Secure.* "I find it relatively easy to get close to others and am comfortable depending on them. I don't often worry about being abandoned or about someone getting too close to me."

In the present study, a procedure used by Mikulincer and colleagues (e.g., Mikulincer & Nachshon, 1991) was used to distinguish consistent from inconsistent responders. Consistent responders were defined as those whose categorical choice matched their highest Likert rating, whereas inconsistent responders chose an attachment style on the categorical measure that did not correspond to their highest Likert rating. According to this method, 404 respondents provided inconsistent responses and were thus eliminated from further analyses. (See Cooper et al., 1998, for a comparison of consistent and inconsistent responders.)

Psychological Distress

Three subscales from the Brief Symptom Index (BSI; Derogatis & Melisaratos, 1983) were administered at both time points: depression, general anxiety, and hostility. The depression subscale assesses a range of depressive symptoms, including lack of motivation, feeling hopeless about the future, and thoughts of suicide. The anxiety subscale taps both cognitive (e.g., feelings of apprehension and fear) and somatic (e.g., feeling tense) components of anxiety. Finally, the BSI hostility subscale assesses thoughts, feelings, and actions associated with the experience of anger, such as getting into arguments and having temper outbursts that cannot be controlled. For all items, respondents rated on a 5-point scale (1 = *not at all*, 5 = *extremely*) the extent to which they had been bothered or distressed by each symptom in the preceding month.

Self-Concept

Positive self-concept, or perceived self-competence, was assessed across five specific domains: (1) general social competence with one's peers (primarily opposite-sex peers) and with adults; (2) perceived athletic skill and ability; (3) perceived intellectual competence; (4) subjective physical attractiveness; and (5) body image. Each scale consisted of four to eight items, answered on a 6-point scale ranging from *disagree strongly* to *agree strongly*. Items were taken from three well-established self-concept measures (Marsh & O'Neill's SDQ-III, 1984; Petersen, Schulenberg, Abramowitz, Offer, & Jarcho's Self-Image Scale for Young Adolescents, 1984; Shrauger's Personal Evaluation Inventory [reviewed in Blascovich & Tomaka, 1991]) and adapted to a common format.

Risky Behaviors

Four clusters of risky or problem behaviors (sexual behavior, substance use, delinquency, educational underachievement) were examined in the present study. Three measures were included in each cluster, and all measures, with two exceptions (described later), were identical at both points in time. (For additional detail on the measures, see Cooper, Wood, Orcutt, & Albino, 2003; Cooper et al., 1998; Huselid & Cooper, 1994.)

Sexual behavior was measured by (1) the number of lifetime sexual partners, (2) a count of the number of risky sexual practices in which the respondent had ever engaged, and (3) a count of two adverse outcomes associated with sexual risk taking (having ever had an STD or an unplanned pregnancy). At T1, three risky practices were assessed (e.g., sex with a stranger), whereas a total of eight such practices (including the three from T1) were assessed at T2.

Substance use was assessed in three different areas. Heavy or problem drinking during the previous 6 months was assessed by a composite of three items: frequency of drinking five or more drinks on a single occasion; the frequency of drinking to intoxication; and the number of drinking problems reported, including having problems with friends, partners, or parents or difficulties at school, work, or with the law due to drinking. Tobacco use was assessed by a three-level variable in which 0 = *do not currently smoke,* 1 = *smoke fewer than 10 cigarettes a day,* and 2 = *smoke 10 or more cigarettes a day.* Finally, illicit drug use was assessed by a count of the number of different illicit drugs ever used. At Time 1, the use of four drugs was assessed, whereas nine (including the four from T1) were assessed at T2.

Delinquent behaviors were assessed by three composites: (1) a count of the number of truant acts (skipping school, suspension or expulsion, running away from home, and staying out all night) in which the adolescent had ever engaged; (2) a count of the number of property-related crimes (breaking and entering, car theft, shoplifting, and fire setting); and (3) a similar count of the number of violent behaviors (fistfights or shoving matches, gang fights, causing injury to another person, and use of weapons).

Educational underachievement was assessed by: (1) average grades received in school, with 1 = *mostly A's* and 8 = *mostly D's and F's*; (2) total number of years held back in school, adjusted among dropouts to include the number of years that they dropped out *before* completing the 12th grade (e.g., a person who was held back 2 years in school *and* dropped out in the 10th grade would receive a score of 4); and (3) educational aspirations, coded as the highest year in school the respondent expected to complete (reverse scored to maintain consistency across indicators).

OVERVIEW OF RESEARCH QUESTIONS AND ANALYSES

The present study examines whether attachment styles assessed during adolescence forecast adjustment in young adulthood in three broad domains of functioning: (1) psychological distress; (2) self-concepts; and (3) risky or problem behaviors. We do this in two ways. First, we examine whether the three attachment types show differential patterns of change over time in psychological distress, self-concept, and risky or problem behaviors. Second, we examine the onset of specific risk or problem behaviors among individuals who reported no prior experience with these behaviors at Time 1. These prospective or onset analyses provide a stronger test of attachment style effects because the possibility that prior risk behaviors caused both attachment style and later risk behaviors is effectively ruled out. Finally, we examine the robustness of both sets of findings across gender, race, and age subgroups.

Does Attachment Type at Time 1 Forecast Different Patterns of Change across Time?

Repeated-measures analysis of covariance (ANCOVA) was used to examine differential patterns of change across time. In each analysis, the outcome (e.g., depression) assessed at both waves served as the repeated (within-persons) factor, and attachment style at Time 1 served as the independent (between-persons) factor. Gender, race, and age were treated as covariates. In addition, to help rule out the possibility that observed differences in change by attachment style were instead due to differential change across demographic subgroups, we ran a series of preliminary repeated-measures analyses in which gender × change, race × change, and age × change interactions were tested. Based on results of these analyses, significant demographic covariate × change interactions were identified and included in the final models.

These analyses (referred to subsequently as change analyses) were conducted in the full sample for most outcomes. However, change analyses for risk and problem behaviors with discrete onset (e.g., alcohol use) were conducted among the subset of adolescents reporting prior involvement in each respective behavior at Time 1. This allowed us to examine attachment effects on the maintenance, escalation, or desistance of involvement in specific risk behaviors separate from its effects on the initial onset and development of these behaviors. Unfortunately, lifetime measures of psychological disorders (e.g., clinically significant depression or anxiety) and of tobacco use were not included at Time 1. Thus we were unable to conduct parallel analyses for these outcomes. Finally, adolescents who did not attend school between Time 1 and Time 2 ($n = 160$) were dropped from change analyses of grades and educational loss because no change could have occurred on these variables among this subset of individuals.

Because our primary focus in the present study is on the longitudinal effects of attachment styles, we first present the results of the attachment × change interaction tests, followed by the results of the between-persons tests. The interaction tests are of particular interest in the present study because they provide an explicit test of the stability of attachment style differences across time. A significant interaction indicates that the three groups changed differentially across time, whereas a nonsignificant interaction suggests that between-group differences in place at Time 1 were maintained across time.

Attachment × Change Interactions

The results of the interaction tests (not shown) revealed a significant pattern of differential change for 5 of the 20 outcome variables examined (depression, social competence, general appearance, lifetime partners, negative sex-related events). The covariate adjusted means and change scores for these five outcomes are presented in Table 15.2.

As shown in the top portion of Table 15.2, and contrary to expectation, securely attached youths showed the least positive trajectories of change over time in depression, social competence, and perceptions of physical attractiveness. They reported significantly greater increases in depression, as well as the smallest increase in social competence and the largest decline in perceived attractiveness. Avoidant youths, in contrast, showed the most positive trajectories on all three outcomes, whereas anxious youths followed an intermediate pathway. Despite the relative gains of insecurely attached youths over time, however, secure adolescents maintained their advantaged position, reporting significantly better adjustment on all three outcomes at Time 2.

Examination of the pattern of means in the bottom portion of Table 15.2 revealed a very different scenario, however. Securely attached youths

TABLE 15.2. Predicted Means for Significant Attachment × Time Interactions

	Depression (n = 1,408)			Social competence (n = 1,410)			Physical attractiveness (n = 1,405)		
	T1	T2	Δ	T1	T2	Δ	T1	T2	Δ
Avoidant	$.88_a$	$.95_a$	$.07_a$	4.20_a	4.43_a	$.23_a$***	3.98_a	4.15_a	$.17_a$**
Anxious	1.02_b	1.11_b	$.09_a$	4.36_b	4.51_a	$.15_a$**	4.00_a	3.99_b	$-.01_b$
Secure	$.59_c$	$.79_c$	$.20_b$***	4.71_c	4.75_b	$.04_b$	4.42_b	4.34_c	$-.08_b$**

	No. of lifetime partners (n = 876)			No. of pregnancies/ STDs (n = 876)		
	T1	T2	Δ	T1	T2	Δ
Avoidant	2.73_a	5.08_a	2.35_a***	$.26_a$	$.62_a$	$.32_a$***
Anxious	2.85_a	4.98_a	2.13_a***	$.32_a$	$.78_b$	$.43_b$***
Secure	2.71_a	4.58_b	1.87_b***	$.29_a$	$.67_a$	$.36_a$***

Note. Values within each column that do not share a common subscript differ from one another at the $p <$ .05 level.

*$p < .05$; **$p < .01$; ***$p < .001$.

experienced the most positive (i.e., least risky) trajectories of change on both sexual behavior outcomes; they had significantly fewer new sex partners between Time 1 and Time 2 than either insecure group and significantly fewer unplanned pregnancies and STDs than anxious youths. In contrast, anxious youths followed the riskiest trajectory, whereas avoidant youths followed an intermediate pathway, reporting the largest increase in sex partners but the smallest increase in pregnancies and STDs. As a result of these differential change patterns, although none of the groups differed from one another on either outcome at Time 1, secure youths reported the lowest overall levels on both behaviors by Time 2.

Invariance of Attachment × Change Interactions across Demographic Groups

To determine whether the basic patterns of change observed for the three attachment types were invariant across major demographic subgroups, attachment × change × gender, attachment × change × race (black vs. nonblack), and attachment × change × age group interactions were also tested. For these analyses, age was divided into three groups, roughly corresponding to early ($\leq$14 years old), middle (15 to 17 years old), and late ($\geq$ 18 years old) adolescence. Across a total of 60 demographic × attachment × change interactions tested, only two were marginally significant, thus indicating that results of the attachment × change interaction analyses were robust across gender, race, and age subgroups.

Stable, between-Person Differences among Attachment Style Groups

As previously discussed, the presence of a significant attachment × change interaction indicates that the three attachment groups changed differentially over time, whereas a nonsignificant interaction suggests that between-group differences present at Time 1 were maintained across time. Thus, for those outcomes not qualified by a significant attachment × change interaction, the between-persons averaged (across wave) effects can be seen as providing the most reliable estimates of stable differences among the three attachment groups. Results of these analyses are summarized in Table 15.3, omitting results for outcomes where the between-persons attachment effect either was not significant (violence, illicit drug use) or was qualified by time (depression, social competence, general appearance, lifetime partners, pregnancy/STDs).

As shown in the top portion of Table 15.3, significant attachment style differences in average levels (collapsed across waves) were found on all psychological-distress and self-concept measures. Examination of the covariate adjusted means (also shown in Table 15.3) revealed that secure adolescents reported both the lowest levels of psychological distress and the most positive self-concepts. In contrast, anxious youths reported the highest levels of hostility and the lowest levels of intellectual competence. On the three remaining indices (anxiety, athletic competence, body image), the two insecure groups reported significantly worse adjustment than secures, but they did not differ from each other.

As shown in the bottom portion of Table 15.3, the three attachment style groups differed significantly or marginally significantly on six of the averaged risk or problem behaviors. In addition, although the overall omnibus test was not significant for either alcohol use or property violations, post hoc pairwise comparisons revealed significant subgroup differences. Examination of the patterns of covariate adjusted means revealed that anxious youths reported the highest overall levels of problem behavior among the three groups. Indeed, anxious adolescents reported significantly higher levels of involvement than their nonanxious counterparts on 5 of the outcomes examined and, along with avoidant youths, reported significantly higher involvement than secure youths on two of the remaining outcomes. Avoidant youths, in contrast, did not differ from secure youths on the majority of outcomes (with the primary exception being risky sexual practices) and in fact reported significantly less problematic alcohol involvement than either secure or anxious adolescents, who did not differ from each other.

TABLE 15.3. Predicted Means for Significant, Unqualified (by Time) between-Persons Attachment Style Effects

	Attachment η^2	Attachment classification								
		Avoidant			Anxious			Secure		
		n	M	SD	n	M	SD	n	M	SD
		Psychological symptomatology								
Distress										
Hostility	.022**	300	1.15_a	0.70	327	1.30_b	0.76	781	1.04_c	0.71
Anxiety	.037***	300	0.91_a	0.61	328	0.97_a	0.64	782	0.72_b	0.49
Self-concept										
Athletic	.020***	300	4.18_a	1.32	328	4.27_a	1.31	782	4.71_b	1.20
Intellectual	.040***	300	4.21_a	0.76	328	4.08_b	0.81	782	4.35_c	0.74
Body image	.013***	299	3.94_a	1.29	328	3.82_a	1.24	781	4.18_b	1.12
		Risky or problem behaviors								
Sexual behavior										
Risky practices[1]	.006***	149	2.21_a	0.94	220	2.18_a	1.04	506	1.89_b	0.97
Substance use										
Heavy/problem drinking[2]	.004	187	2.57_a	1.24	228	2.87_{ab}	1.33	542	2.88_b	1.28
Tobacco use	.009**	277	0.41_a	0.64	316	0.60_b	0.69	747	0.48_a	0.63
Delinquency										
Truancy[3]	.007*	210	3.85_a	1.15	277	4.11_b	1.09	613	3.82_a	1.07
Property offense[4]	.005	118	2.06_{ab}	.67	144	2.19_a	.80	327	2.03_b	.70
Educational underachievement										
Poor grades	.011***	272	3.21_a	1.14	283	3.47_b	1.12	688	3.24_a	1.09
Low educational aspirations	.017***	295	1.32_a	1.27	321	1.69_b	1.41	772	1.31_a	1.31
Years lost[5]	.007†	138	1.11_{ab}	0.75	186	1.16_b	0.93	387	0.94_a	0.83

Note. Means within a row that do not share a common subscript differ from one another at $p < .05$.

[1] Analyses conducted among subset who had ever had sex at Time 1 ($n = 878$).

[2] Analyses conducted among subset who had ever consumed alcohol at Time 1 ($n = 957$).

[3] Analyses conducted among subset who had ever engaged in a truant act at Time 1 ($n = 1100$).

[4] Analyses conducted among subset who had ever committed a property crime at Time 1 ($n = 589$).

[5] Analyses conducted among subset who had ever failed a grade or dropped out of high school at Time 1 ($n = 711$).

†$p < .10$; *$p < .01$; ***$p < .001$.

Does Attachment Type at Time 1 Predict Onset of Risky or Problem Behaviors among Initially Problem-Free Youths?

In this series of analyses, the prospective effects of attachment styles on the onset and escalation of involvement in risk or problem behaviors was examined among adolescents reporting no prior involvement in these behaviors at Time 1.

Onset Analyses

To address the question of differential onset among the three attachment groups, a series of logistic regression models was estimated in which onset (yes vs. no) of risk or problem behaviors was treated as the dependent variable and regressed on a pair of dummy-coded attachment style variables, controlling for gender, race, and age at Time 1. To test all possible pairwise contrasts among the three attachment groups, each model was run twice with different pairings of the dummy-coded attachment variables, and nonredundant results for the attachment contrasts were recorded. Onset analyses were estimated among the following partially overlapping subgroups, each defined with respect to their lack of self-reported involvement in specific risk or problem behaviors at Time 1: (1) 519 Time 1 virgins; (2) 451 Time 1 alcohol abstainers; (3) 867 youths reporting no prior illicit drug use; (4) 415 youths reporting no prior violent behaviors; (5) 820 youths reporting no prior property-related offenses; (6) 309 youths reporting no prior history of truancy, and (7) 962 youths who had neither failed a grade nor dropped out of school. As in the prior analyses, adolescents who did not attend school at any point between Time 1 and Time 2 were excluded from the onset analyses of educational loss.

As shown in the second column of Table 15.4, attachment style differences at Time 1 prospectively predicted onset of both drug and alcohol use (at $p < .10$). Examination of the covariate adjusted means revealed that initially abstinent avoidant youths were the least likely of the three groups to begin to drink alcohol (71%) or use drugs (49%). Securely attached youths were the most likely to begin to drink (81%), whereas secure and anxious youths reported equally high rates of onset of illicit drug use (60% and 63%, respectively). In addition, although the χ^2 test for the overall attachment style effect was not significant for onset of sexual behavior, avoidant youths were nevertheless significantly less likely to become sexually active over time than their anxious counterparts (78% vs. 87%). No remaining differences in rates of onset of risky or problematic behaviors were found among the three attachment groups.

TABLE 15.4. Prospective Analyses of Attachment Style Effects on Time 2 Risky Behaviors among Initially Problem-Free Adolescents

Dependent variable	n	χ^2	η^2	Covariate adjusted means		
				Avoidant	Anxious	Secure
Sexual behavior						
Ever had intercourse	519	3.57	—	0.78_a	0.87_b	0.80_{ab}
No. of lifetime partners	420	—	0.025**	2.63_a	3.36_b	3.21_b
No. of risky sex practices	420	—	0.007	1.21_a	1.55_b	1.36_{ab}
No. of pregnancies/STDs	420	—	$0.012^\dagger$	0.26_a	0.39_b	0.29_a
Substance use						
Ever drank alcohol	451	$5.23^\dagger$	—	0.71_a	0.74_{ab}	0.81_b
Heavy/problem alcohol use	349	—	0.020*	0.67_a	1.24_b	1.06_b
Ever used illicit drugs	867	8.98*	—	0.49_a	0.63_b	0.60_b
No. of illicit drugs used	504	—	0.002	1.49	1.59	1.60
Delinquent behaviors						
Ever engaged in ≥ 1 truant acts	309	1.37	—	0.63	0.72	0.66
Ever engaged in ≥ 1 violent acts	415	1.11	—	0.37	0.44	0.40
Ever engaged in ≥ 1 property offenses	820	0.39	—	0.33	0.35	0.35
Educational underachievement						
Ever lost ≥ 1 year of education	962	1.09	—	0.08	0.08	0.07

Note. Results for "ever had intercourse," "drank alcohol," "used drugs," "engaged in specific delinquent behaviors," and "lost ≥ 1 year of education" were taken from logistic regression analyses; the remaining results were taken from a one-way analysis of covariance. Means within a row that do not share a common subscript differ from one another at $p < .05$.
$^\dagger p < .10$; $^* p < .05$; $^{**} p < .001$.

Level of Involvement among the Onset Groups

Whereas the preceding analyses examined onset of any involvement in risk or problem behaviors among initially abstinent adolescents, the present set of analyses examines differences in level of involvement, or degree of escalation, among initially abstinent youth who first became involved in these behaviors between Time 1 and Time 2. To address this issue, a series of ANCOVAs was estimated in which continuous measures of Time 2 risk and problem behaviors were treated as the dependent variables and attachment type at Time 1 was treated as the independent variable. As before, gender, race, and Time 1 age were controlled. These ANCOVAs were estimated among the following subsets of adolescents: (1) 420 Time 1 virgins who had had sex by Time 2; (2) 349 Time 1 abstainers who had ever drunk alcohol by Time 2; and (3) 504 adolescents who had never used illicit drugs at Time 1 but had done so by Time 2. Because only a relatively small number of adolescents met parallel criteria for the three delinquent behaviors and for the educational loss variable, and because there was little variability among those who did in level of involvement at Time 2, we did not run analyses for these outcomes. Results of the remaining analyses are also summarized in Table 15.4.

As shown in Table 15.4, attachment style prospectively predicted level of involvement among initially abstinent (from sex or alcohol) adolescents for number of lifetime partners, number of pregnancies or STDs, and heavy or problem drinking. Attachment styles also discriminated among attachment groups on a fourth outcome (risky sex practices), even though the omnibus test of differences was neither significant nor marginally significant. Examining the covariate-adjusted means showed that initially abstinent avoidant youths who had become sexually active or begun to drink by Time 2 reported the lowest overall levels of involvement in both behaviors. In contrast, initially abstinent anxious youths generally reported the highest levels of involvement in Time 2 risk behaviors, though they differed significantly from secure adolescents only on unplanned pregnancies and STDs.

Invariance of Attachment Style Effects on Onset of Risk Behaviors across Demographic Groups

To determine whether the basic patterns of onset observed for the three attachment types were invariant across major demographic subgroups, attachment × gender, attachment × race (black vs. nonblack), and attachment × age group interactions were also tested. As before, age was trichotomized for these analyses. Across a total of 36 demographic × attachment interactions tested, four were significant. Two involved onset of initial involvement in alcohol and drug use, and two involved degree of involvement in alcohol and drug use among those who initiated use.

An examination of the adjusted means broken down by demographic subgroups showed that attachment style predicted onset of alcohol use among males but not females and that it predicted degree of drug involvement among white but not black youths. Mirroring patterns observed in the overall sample, avoidant male adolescents were significantly less likely than their nonavoidant counterparts to have ever drunk alcohol, and avoidant white youths who began to use drugs reported significantly less use than their nonavoidant counterparts.

Both of the remaining interactions involved age. Examination of adjusted means for onset of drug use broken down by age group revealed that roughly 80% of all individuals who were 18 or older at Time 1 had ever used drugs by Time 2, regardless of their attachment type. However, rates of onset among the two younger cohorts suggested different time trajectories in which onset was accelerated among anxious youths and delayed among avoidant youths relative to their secure counterparts. Finally, examination of the pattern of adjusted means for the 6-month heavy-drinking composite showed that insecurely attached youths who first began to drink at an earlier age drank relatively more than those who first began to drink at a later age. In contrast, secure youths who first began to drink at an earlier age drank less than those who first began to drink at a later age.

SUMMARY AND DISCUSSION

The present study examined attachment styles assessed in adolescence and their ability to forecast intrapersonal adjustment in young adulthood. Consistent with expectation, individual differences in attachment styles predicted unique patterns of adjustment across multiple developmentally relevant domains nearly 5 years later. These differences were found in both longitudinal change and true prospective analyses and were largely invariant across gender, race, and age subgroups. Key findings are discussed more fully in the following.

First, each attachment style group exhibited a unique pattern or profile of adjustment. Securely attached youths exhibited the healthiest profile overall, reporting relatively low levels of distress, positive self-concepts, and moderate levels of involvement in risk or problem behaviors. To the extent that risk behaviors provide opportunities to explore alternative identities and to acquire important life skills, moderate involvement can be seen as developmentally appropriate exploratory behavior (cf. Shedler & Block, 1990). Anxious adolescents, in contrast, were the most poorly adjusted group, reporting the highest overall levels of involvement in risky or problematic behaviors, as well as the highest levels of psychological distress and the poorest self-concepts. Finally, avoidant adolescents presented the most complex profile. Although they reported levels of distress and negative self-concepts that were nearly equal to those observed among their anxious counterparts, they were much less involved in risk or problem behaviors. Indeed, avoidant youths exhibited levels of involvement in most risk behaviors that were comparable to, or in the case of substance use, even less than, those of their securely attached counterparts. In the only clear exception to this pattern, avoidant youths reported significantly more lifetime sex partners, more risky sex practices, and more (though not significantly more) educational loss than their secure counterparts.

This pattern of differences was evident in strictly between-persons comparisons (averaged across waves), as well as in longitudinal change analyses and in true prospective analyses. Indeed, anxious and avoidant youths, who were more distressed and perceived themselves less positively at baseline than their secure counterparts, remained less well adjusted across time. Likewise, insecure and especially anxious youths who were more heavily involved in risk or problem behaviors at Time 1 continued their relatively high levels of involvement across time in the vast majority of cases. In fact, in no case did a significant secure versus insecure difference that was present at Time 1 completely dissipate by Time 2. Although data indicating continuity of differences over time are typically considered equivocal regarding cause and effect, they are nevertheless important in ruling out transient point-in-time influences as plausible alternative explanations for attachment style differences. Thus the fact that differences were maintained over a nearly 5-year period enhances confidence in the substantive meaningfulness of the observed relationships between attachment styles and intrapersonal adjustment.

Although the majority of differences in place at Time 1 were simply maintained across time, evidence of differential change was also found for 5 of 20 outcomes. In general, differential change by the three groups served to decrease, but not eliminate, overall differences between secure and insecure youths on depression, social competence, and perceived attractiveness at Time 2 and to exacerbate differences in number of lifetime partners and adverse sex-related outcomes. Indeed, no significant attachment style differences existed at Time 1 among the sexually active subset on number of partners or adverse sex-related outcomes, though such differences were found by Time 2 due to the relatively greater increases among insecure youths on both variables.

In true prospective analyses, attachment style differences predicted the onset of sexual behavior, alcohol use, and illicit drug use among initially abstinent youths. Mirroring the general patterns described earlier, avoidant youths were the least likely of the three attachment groups to initiate these behaviors, whereas anxious youths were the most likely. Moreover, among those who did initiate these behaviors between Time 1 and Time 2, avoidant youths reported the fewest lifetime partners, the fewest risky sex practices, the fewest pregnancies and STDs (though not significantly fewer than secure youths), and the lowest rates of heavy drinking, whereas anxious youths reported the highest level of involvement across all four of these behaviors. Given that prior involvement in sex and substance use behaviors could not have caused individuals' attachment styles in this subgroup, these data provide strong support for individual differences in attachment as causal factors shaping initial involvement in substance use and sexual behaviors.

Implications

The results of the present study hold a number of potentially important implications for future research and theory on attachment styles and processes. First, these data indicate that, when a broad range of outcomes is examined, the three attachment groups exhibit distinctive profiles. Although the secure–insecure distinction accounted for most of the variance in psychological symptoms and self-concept, consistent differences between the two insecure groups emerged for the more overt behavioral indicators of adjustment. These findings highlight the benefits of examining a broad range of adaptive outcomes in future research. Had we focused simply on distress symptoms, self-concept, or risk behaviors in isolation, we would have missed the uniqueness of these profiles altogether and have drawn (at best) incomplete conclusions about the nature of attachment style differences in intrapersonal adjustment.

The particular profiles of differences that emerged in the present study also serve to highlight a potentially important link to the larger personality literature, and in particular to Block and Block's (1980) personality dimensions of ego resilience and ego control. Although attachment types have historically been interpreted in terms of two underlying dimensions—models of self versus other (Bartholomew & Horowitz, 1991) or anxiety versus avoidance (Brennan, Clark, & Shaver, 1998)—the pattern of differences observed in the present study also appears explicable in terms of the Blocks' ego-resilience and control dimensions. Ego resilience is closely related to emotional stability (Klohnen, 1996) and refers specifically to the tendency to respond flexibly rather than rigidly to changing situational demands, especially stressful ones. Ego control refers to the tendency to contain versus express emotional and motivational impulses. Block and Block assumed that high resiliency was related to moderate levels of ego control and that both extremely low and extremely high ego control were related to low resiliency. Thus the dimension of ego resilience is thought to bifurcate on the low end into two relatively discrete classes—undercontrol and overcontrol (cf. Asendorpf & van Aken, 1999).

Applied to attachment types, this model suggests that securely attached youths are highly resilient and moderately controlled, whereas anxious youths are low in resilience and low in control and avoidant youths are low in resilience and high in control. Consistent with this speculation, a number of studies using ego resilience and ego control as the core dimensions have identified three personality types that bear striking resemblance to the attachment groups described here (e.g., Asendorpf & van Aken, 1999; Hart, Hofmann, Edelstein, & Keller, 1997; Robins, John, Caspi, Moffitt, & Stouthamer-Loeber, 1996). For example, Robins and colleagues (1996) distinguished three groups on the basis of caregiver responses on Block and Block's (1980) California Child Q-Set. Similar to our secure group, their well-adjusted or resilient group reported the lowest overall levels of distress, the most positive self-concepts, and relatively low levels of acting-out behaviors. Of the two poorly adjusted groups, their undercontrolled group, like our anxious group, was generally viewed as the most problematic and troubled group: They reported the most distress, the poorest self-concepts, and the highest levels of acting-out or risk behaviors. Finally, their overcontrolled group closely resembled our avoidant group. They experienced high levels of distress symptoms and poor self-concepts but levels of acting-out behaviors that were, for the most part, indistinguishable from those found among the best-adjusted group. Similar subtypes have also been identified in Eisenberg's work (e.g., Eisenberg & Fabes, 1992) based on a joint consideration of two highly similar dimensions, negative emotionality and emotional constraint. The resemblance of these independently derived subtypes to the three attachment types examined in the present study suggests the potential utility of efforts to link attachment theory and research to these underlying dimensions and, in particular, to more carefully consider the role of ego control, which is not well represented by either of the existing dimensional models of attachment.

Finally, our findings suggest that attachment styles may be more consequential for some areas or domains of intrapersonal adjustment than others, as well as for certain stages of the etiology and development of these behaviors and conditions. Specifically, attachment processes appeared to be related to the maintenance of differences among the three groups over time but generally not to increases or decreases in adjustment difficulties once these differences were established. Individual differences in attachment styles also appeared influential in the onset and development of sexual behavior and substance use during this developmental period, though not to the development of delinquent behaviors or school failure. Although these findings must be considered preliminary pending replication, they nevertheless underscore the need to distinguish individuals on the basis of prior experience or lifetime history and to examine these etiological processes separately in future research.

Caveats and Conclusions

Before concluding, several limitations of the present study should be acknowledged. First, this study relied solely on self-report data. Although every effort was made to increase the validity and reliability of responding, self-report data (even under optimal circumstances) are subject to a host of both random and systematic errors of reporting (e.g., forgetting, telescoping, etc.; for a review, see Schwartz, 1999). Realistically, however, many of the outcomes examined in this study are difficult if not impossible to assess otherwise. Others—even close others—do not have direct access to an individual's internal experience of distress or of self. Others also are unlikely to have accurate information on involvement in risky or problem behaviors, most of which are illegal or sanctioned. Official records are both incomplete and biased by race, class, and gender. Thus, self-report data, despite their limitations, remain the single best source of information for addressing many of the issues examined in the present study.

A second issue, separate from the limitations of self-report methodology per se, concerns the limitations of our measure of attachment style. Hazan and Shaver's (1987) simple, three-category measure of attachment style was the only self-report measure available at the time of our baseline interview. Although this measure has been validated and widely used in prior research, it has some important weaknesses (see Crowell, Fraley, & Shaver, 1999, for a review). More sensitive and reliable measures of attachment style have now been developed (e.g., Brennan et al., 1998) and should be used in future replications of these findings. A related limitation concerns our inability to distinguish among subtypes of avoidant individuals (Bartholomew & Horowitz, 1991), which may have contributed to the complex pattern of effects (particularly regarding sexual behavior) observed for avoidant adolescents in our sample.

Finally, although the longitudinal, prospective design of our study allows us to rule out some alternative causal processes, these data are correlational, and we cannot draw unambiguous causal inferences about the impact of attachment style differences on intrapersonal adjustment over time. In particular, it remains possible that some unmeasured third variable better accounts for the observed effects.

These issues notwithstanding, the present study provides the strongest evidence to date of the importance of individual differences in attachment for intrapersonal adjustment during this crucial developmental period. We found theoretically meaningful patterns of differences among the three attachment groups that were maintained across time, as well as increases in differences among the groups over time. Such findings are unusual in longitudinal studies, in which trait and type differences instead tend to wash out over time (see, e.g., Caspi, 1998). Even more important, we found evidence of true prospective effects in which attachment type assessed during adolescence predicted the onset and development of both substance use and sexual behaviors nearly 5 years later. Taken as a whole, these data add substantially to a growing body of evidence for the usefulness of attachment theory as a framework for understanding human functioning across the lifespan.

ACKNOWLEDGMENTS

This research was supported by Grant No. AA08047 from the National Institute on Alcohol Abuse and Alcoholism to M. Lynne Cooper. We thank Jeremy Skinner for his thoughtful comments on an earlier draft of this chapter.

REFERENCES

Arnett, J. J. (1999). Adolescent storm and stress, reconsidered. *American Psychologist, 54,* 317–326.

Asendorpf, J. B., & van Aken, M. A. (1999). Resilient, overcontrolled, and undercontrolled personality prototypes in childhood: Replicability, predictive power, and the trait-type issue. *Journal of Personality and Social Psychology, 77,* 815–832.

Bartholomew, K., & Horowitz, L. M. (1991). Attachment styles among young adults: A test of a four-category model. *Journal of Personality and Social Psychology, 61,* 226–244.

Baumrind, D. (1987). A developmental perspective on adolescent risk taking in contemporary America. *New Directions for Child Development, 37,* 93–125.

Blascovich, J. J., & Tomaka, J. (1991). Measures of self-esteem. In J. P. Robinson, P. R. Shaver, & L. S. Wrightsman (Eds.), *Measures of personality and social psychological attitudes* (pp. 115–160). San Diego, CA: Academic Press.

Block, J. H., & Block, J. (1980). *The California Child Q-set.* Palo Alto, CA: Consulting Psychologists Press.

Bowlby, J. (1969). Disruption of the affectional bonds and its effects on behavior. *Canada's Mental Health Supplement, 59.*

Bowlby, J. (1973). *Attachment and loss: Vol. 2. Separation: Anxiety and anger.* New York: Basic Books.

Bowlby, J. (1982). *Attachment and loss: Vol. 1. Attachment* (Rev. ed.). New York: Basic Books. (Original work published 1969)

Brennan, K. A., Clark, C. L., & Shaver, P. R. (1998). Self-report measurement of adult attachment: An integrative overview. In J. A. Simpson & W. S. Rholes (Eds.), *Attachment theory and close relationships* (pp. 46–76). New York: Guilford Press.

Burge, D., Hammen, C., Davila, J., Daley, S. E., Paley, B., Herzberg, D. S., & Lindberg, N. (1997). Attachment cognitions and college and work functioning two years later in late adolescent women. *Journal of Youth and Adolescence, 26,* 285–301.

Burge, D., Hammen, C., Davila, J., Daley, S. E., Paley, B., Lindberg, N., et al. (1997). The relationship between attachment cognitions and psychological adjustment in late adolescent women. *Development and Psychopathology, 9,* 151–167.

Caspi, A. (1998). Personality development across the life course. In W. Damon (Series Ed.) & N. Eisenberg (Vol. Ed.), *Handbook of child psychology, Vol. 3: Social, emotional, and personality development* (pp. 311–388). New York: Wiley.

Collins, N. L., Cooper, M. L., Albino, A., & Allard, L. (2002). Psychosocial vulnerability from adolescence to adulthood: A prospective study of attachment style differences in relationship functioning and partner choice. *Journal of Personality, 70,* 965–1008.

Cooper, M. L., & Orcutt, H. K. (1997). Drinking and sexual experience on first dates among adolescents. *Journal of Abnormal Psychology, 106,* 191–202.

Cooper, M. L., Shaver, P. R., & Collins, N. L. (1998). Attachment styles, emotion regulation, and adjustment in adolescence. *Journal of Personality and Social Psychology, 74,* 1380–1397.

Cooper, M. L., Wood, P. K., Orcutt, H. K., & Albino, A. (2003). Personality and the predisposition to engage in risky or problem behaviors during adolescence. *Journal of Personality and Social Psychology, 84,* 390–410.

Crowell, J. A., Fraley, R. C., & Shaver, P. R. (1999). Measurement of individual differences in adolescent and adult attachment. In J. Cassidy & P. R. Shaver (Eds.), *Handbook of attachment: Theory, research, and clinical applications* (pp. 434–465). New York: Guilford Press.

Derogatis, L. R., & Melisaratos, N. (1983). The Brief Symptom Inventory: An introductory report. *Psychological Medicine, 13,* 595–605.

Duemmler, S. L., & Kobak, R. (2001). The development of commitment and attachment in dating relationships: Attachment security as relationship construct. *Journal of Adolescence, 24,* 401–415.

Eisenberg, N., & Fabes, R. A. (1992). Emotion, regulation, and the development of social competence. In M. S. Clark (Ed.), *Emotion and social behavior: Review of personality and social psychology* (Vol. 14, pp. 119–150). Newbury Park, CA: Sage.

Feeney, J. A. (1999). Adult romantic attachment and couple relationships. In J. Cassidy & P. R. Shaver (Eds.), *Handbook of attachment: Theory, research, and clinical applications* (pp. 355–377). New York: Guilford Press.

Fraley, R. C., Garner, J. P., & Shaver, P. R. (2000). Adult attachment and the defensive regulation of attention and memory: Examining the role of preemptive and postemptive defensive processes. *Journal of Personality and Social Psychology, 78,* 816–826.

Furman, W., & Buhrmester, D. (1992). Age and sex differences in perceptions of networks of personal relationships. *Child Development, 63,* 103–115.

Hammen, C. L., Burge, D., Daley, S. E., Davila, J., Paley, B., & Rudolph, K. D. (1995) Interpersonal attachment cognitions and prediction of symptomatic responses to interpersonal stress. *Journal of Abnormal Psychology, 104,* 436–443.

Hammond, J. R., & Fletcher, G. J. O. (1991). Attachment styles and relationship satisfaction in the development of close relationships. *New Zealand Journal of Psychology, 20,* 56–62.

Hart, D., Hofmann, V., Edelstein, W., & Keller, M. (1997). The relation of childhood personality types to adolescent behavior and development: A longitudinal study of Icelandic children. *Developmental Psychology, 33,* 195–205.

Hazan, C., & Shaver, P. R. (1987). Romantic love conceptualized as an attachment process. *Journal of Personality and Social Psychology, 52,* 511–524.

Hazan, C., & Shaver, P. R. (1990). Love and work: An attachment-theoretical perspective. *Journal of Personality and Social Psychology, 59,* 270–280.

Hazan, C., & Zeifman, D. (1994). Sex and the psychological tether. In K. Bartholomew & D. Perlman (Eds.), *Advances in personal relationships: Vol. 5. Attachment processes in adulthood* (pp. 151–177). London: Kingsley.

Herzberg, D. S., Hammen, C., Burge, D., Daley, S. E., Davila, J., & Lindberg, N. (1999). Attachment cognitions predict perceived and enacted social support during late adolescence. *Journal of Adolescent Research, 14,* 387–404.

Huselid, R. F., & Cooper, M. L. (1994). Gender roles as mediators of sex differences in expressions of pathology. *Journal of Abnormal Psychology, 103,* 595–603.

Kirkpatrick, L. A., & Davis, K. E. (1994). Attachment style, gender, and relationship stability: A longitudinal analysis. *Journal of Personality and Social Psychology, 66,* 502–512.

Kirkpatrick, L. A., & Hazan, C. (1994). Attachment styles and close relationships: A four-year prospective study. *Personal Relationships, 1,* 123–142.

Klohnen, E. C. (1996). Conceptual analysis and measurement of the construct of ego-resilience. *Journal of Personality and Social Psychology, 70,* 1067–1079.

Marsh, H. W., & O'Neill, R. (1984). Self-Description Questionnaire III: The construct validity of multidimensional self-concept ratings by late adolescents. *Journal of Educational Measurement, 21,* 153–174.

Mikulincer, M., Florian, V., & Weller, A. (1993). Attachment styles, coping strategies, and posttraumatic psychological distress: The impact of the Gulf War in Israel. *Journal of Personality and Social Psychology, 64,* 817–826.

Mikulincer, M., & Nachshon, O. (1991). Attachment styles and patterns of self-disclosure. *Journal of Personality and Social Psychology, 61,* 321–331.

Mikulincer, M., & Orbach, I. (1995). Attachment styles and repressive defensiveness: The accessibility and architecture of affective memories. *Journal of Personality and Social Psychology, 68,* 917–925.

Mikulincer, M., & Shaver, P. R. (2003). The attachment behavioral system in adulthood: Activation, psychodynamics, and interpersonal processes. In M. P. Zanna (Ed.), *Advances in experimental social psychology* (Vol. 35, pp. 53–152). New York: Academic Press.

Moffitt, T. (1993). Adolescence-limited and life course persistent antisocial behaviour: A developmental taxonomy. *Psychological Review, 100,* 674–701.

Moore, D. R., & Arthur, J. L. (1989). Juvenile delinquency. In T.H. Ollendick & M. Hersen (Eds.), *Handbook of child psychopathology* (2nd ed., pp. 197–217). New York: Plenum Press.

Petersen, A. C., Schulenberg, J. F., Abramowitz, R. H., Offer, D. E., & Jarcho, H. D. (1984). A self-image questionnaire for young adolescents (SIQYA): Reliability and validity studies. *Journal of Youth and Adolescence, 13,* 93–111.

Robins, R. W., John, O. P., Caspi, A., Moffitt, T. E., & Stouthamer-Loeber, M. (1996). Resilient, overcontrolled, and undercontrolled boys: Three replicable personality types. *Journal of Personality and Social Psychology, 70,* 157–171.

Rosenfeld, P., Booth-Kewley, S., & Edwards, J. E. (1993). Computer-administered surveys in organizational settings: Alternatives, advantages, and applications. *American Behavioral Scientist, 36,* 485–511.

Schwartz, N. (1999). Self reports: How the questions shape the answers. *American Psychologist, 54,* 93–105.

Seifer, R., Schiller, M., Sameroff, A., Resnick, S., & Riordan, K. (1996). Attachment, maternal sensitivity, and infant temperament during the first year of life. *Developmental Psychology, 32,* 12–25.

Shadish, W. R., Cook, T. D., & Campbell, D. T. (2002). *Experimental and quasi-experimental designs for generalized causal inference.* Boston: Houghton Mifflin.

Shedler, J., & Block, J. (1990). Adolescent drug use and psychological health: A longitudinal inquiry. *American Psychologist, 45,* 612–630.

Simpson, J. A., Rholes, W. S., Campbell, L., Tran, S., & Wilson, C. L. (2003). Adult attachment, the transition to parenthood, and depressive symptoms. *Journal of Personality and Social Psychology, 84,* 1172–1187.

Simpson, J. A., Rholes, W. S., & Nelligan, J. S. (1992). Support seeking and support giving within couples in an anxiety-provoking situation: The role of attachment styles. *Journal of Personality and Social Psychology, 62,* 434–446.

Steinberg, L., & Morris, A. S. (2001). Adolescent development. *Annual Review of Psychology, 52,* 83–110.

Vasquez, K., Durik, A. M., & Hyde, J. S. (2002). Family and work: Implications of adult attachment styles. *Personality and Social Psychology Bulletin, 28,* 874–886.

Weiss, R. S. (1982). Attachment in adults. In C. M. Parkes & J. Stevenson-Hinde (Eds.), *The place of attachment in human behavior* (pp. 171–194). New York: Basic Books.

White, H. R., Bates, M. E., & Johnson, V. (1990). Social reinforcement and alcohol consumption. In M. Cox (Ed.), *Why people drink* (pp. 233–261). New York: Gardner Press.

Index

Page numbers followed by an *f* indicate figure, *t* indicate table.